Insights Into Drug Resistance in *Staphylococcus aureus*

Edited by Amjad Aqib

Published in London, United Kingdom

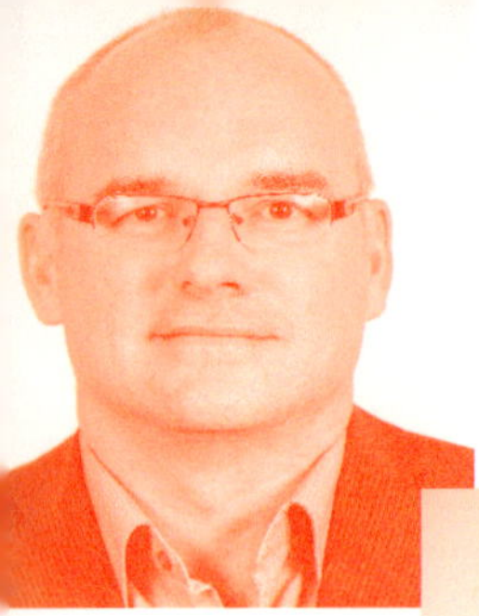
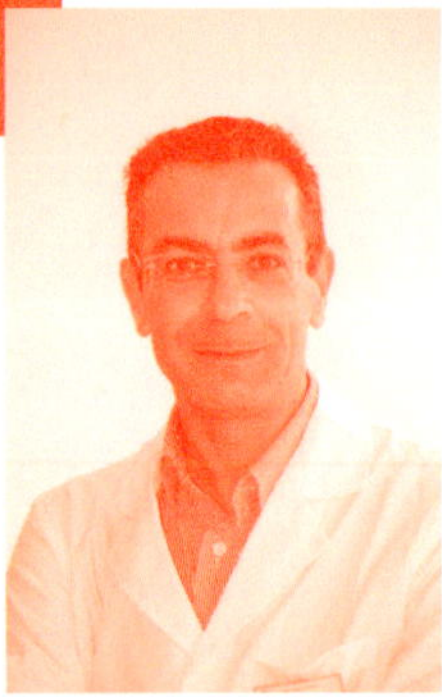
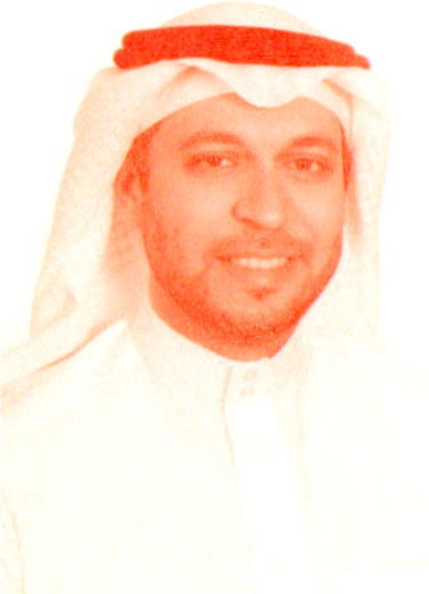
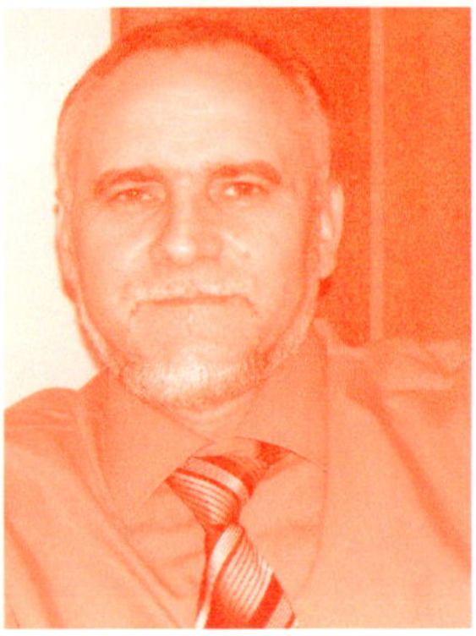
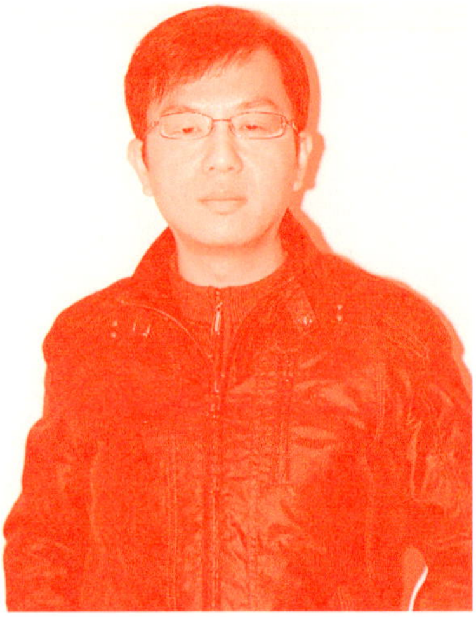
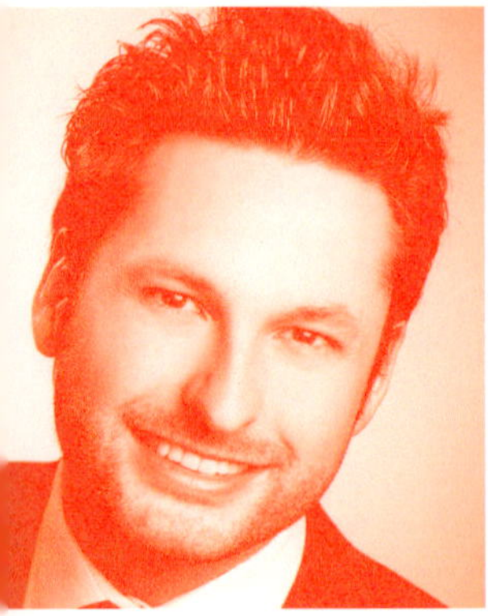
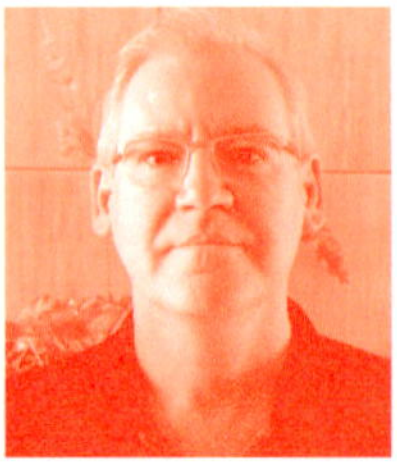

IntechOpen

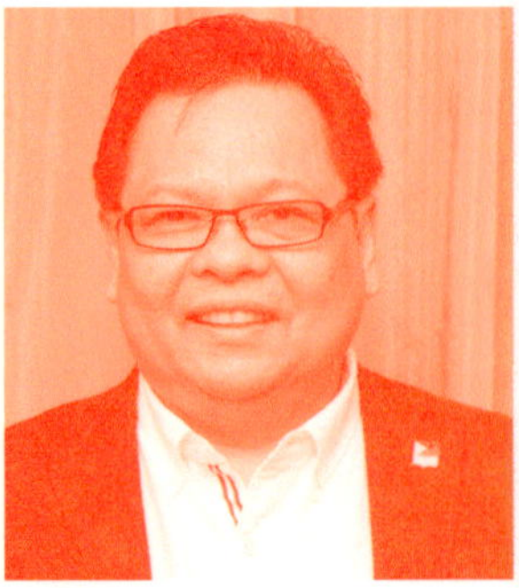
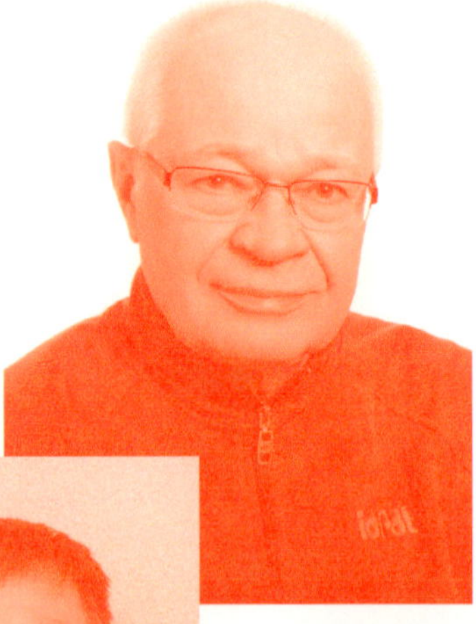
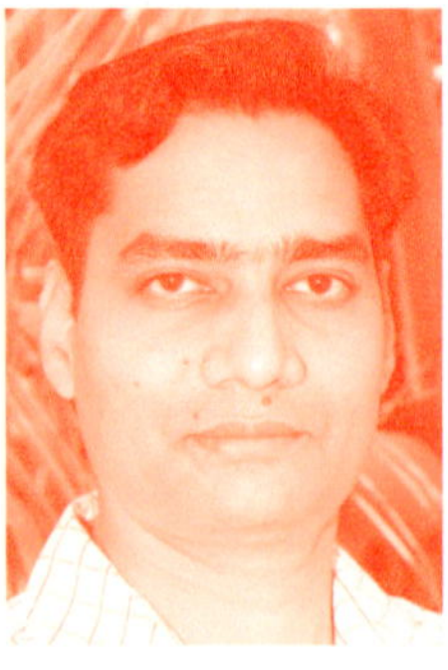
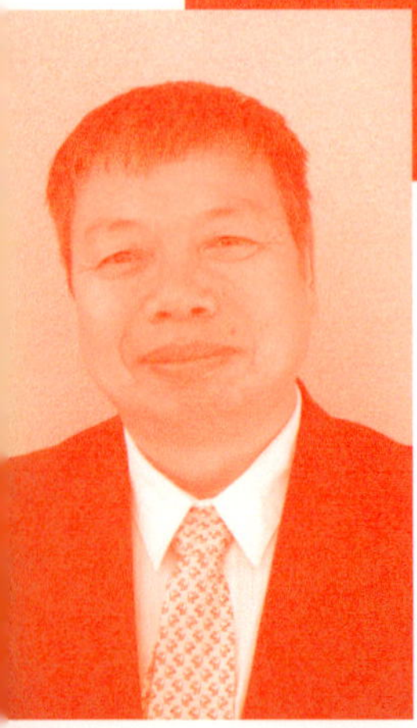
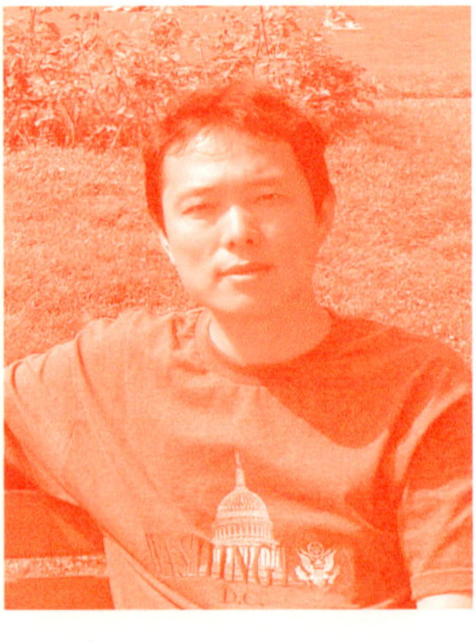
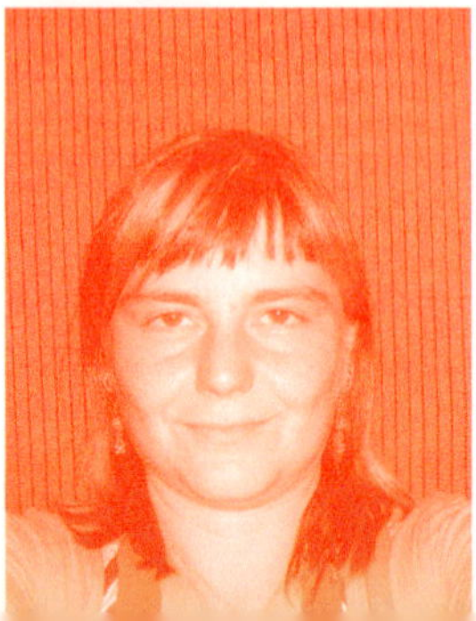

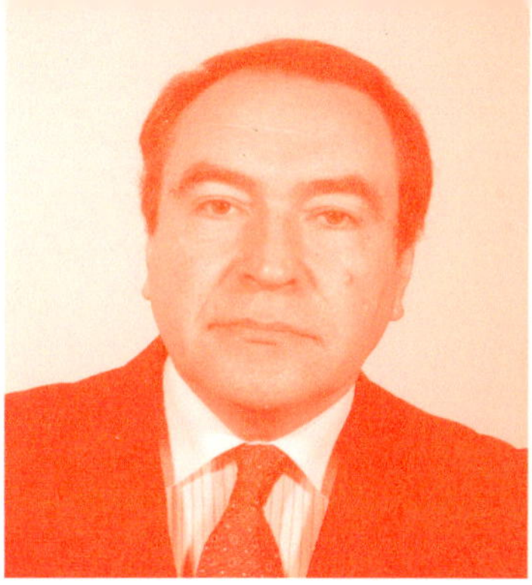
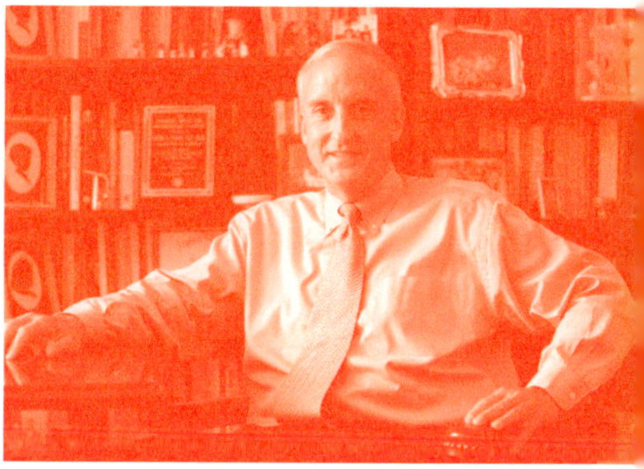
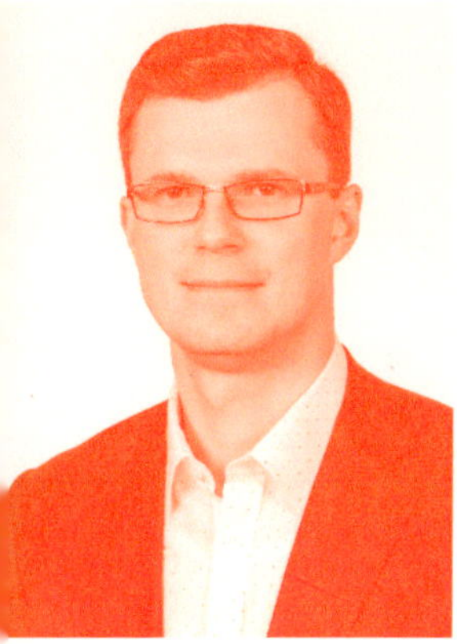
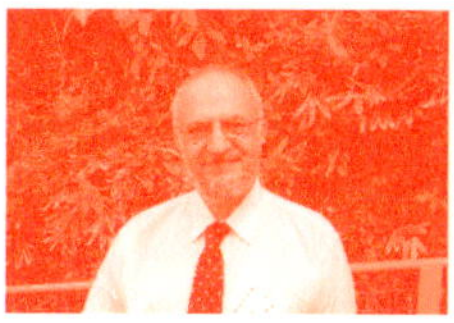
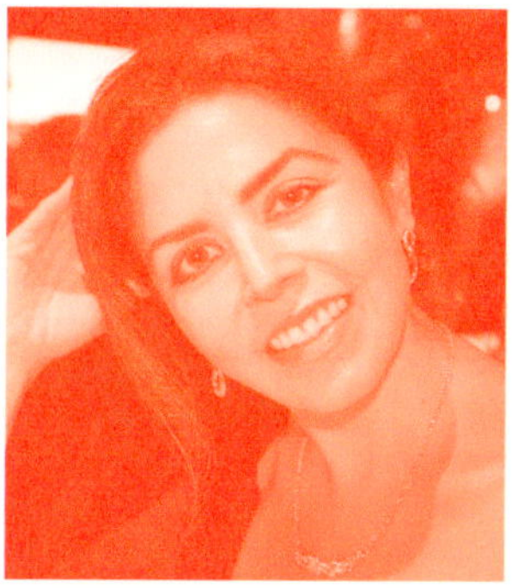

Supporting open minds since 2005

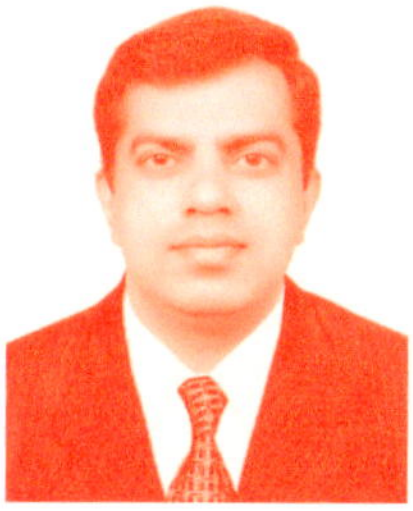
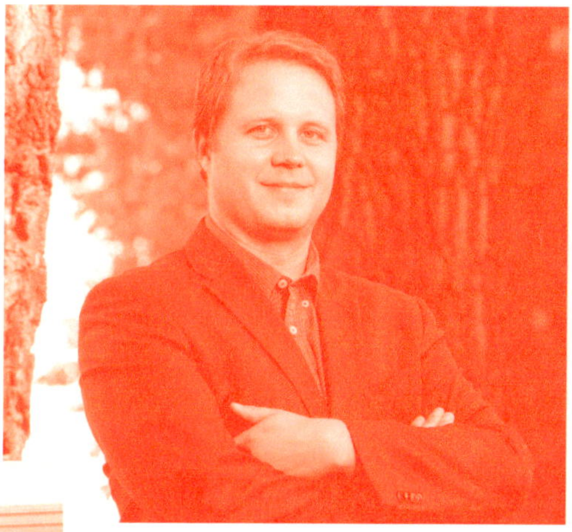
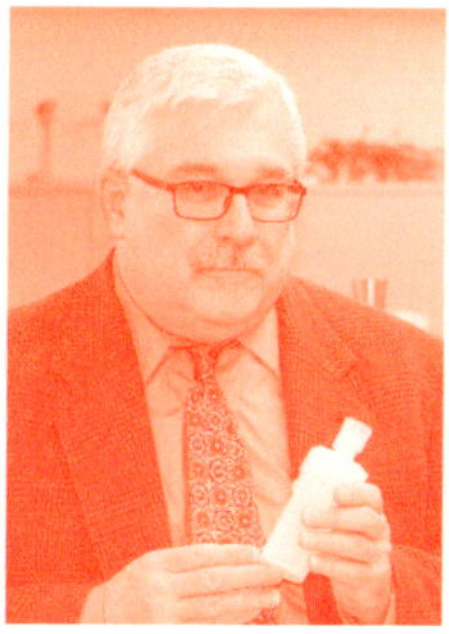
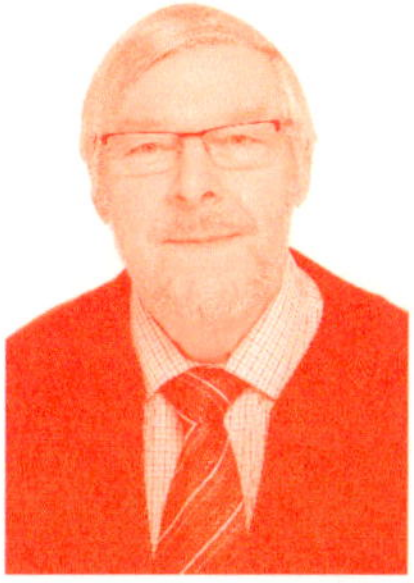
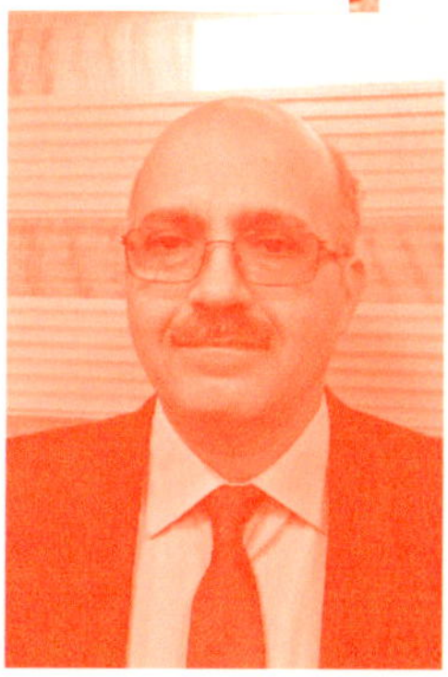
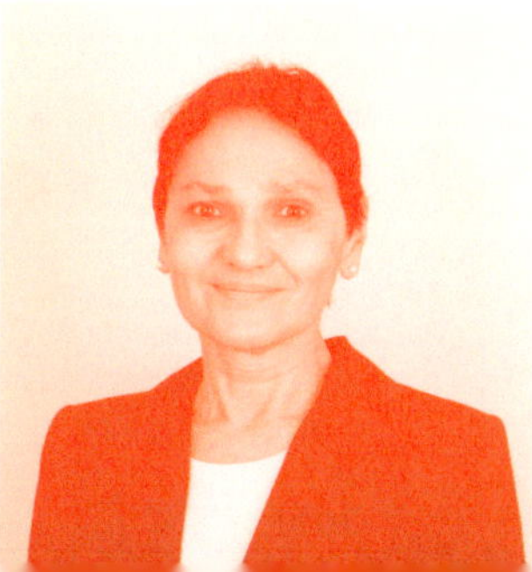
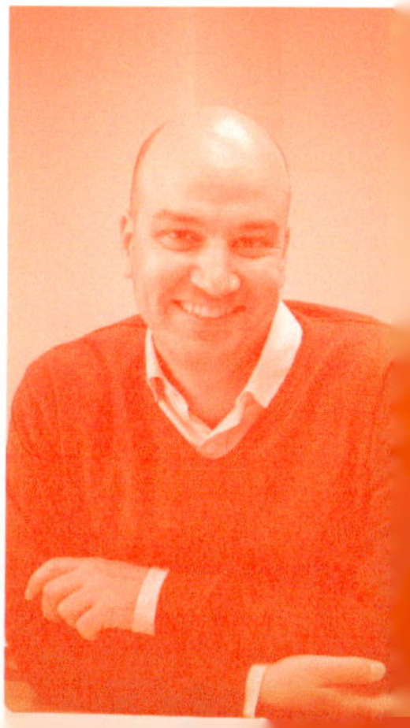

Insights Into Drug Resistance in *Staphylococcus aureus*
http://dx.doi.org/10.5772/intechopen.87320
Edited by Amjad Aqib

Part of IntechOpen Book Series: Infectious Diseases, Volume 10
Book Series Editor: Shailendra K. Saxena

Contributors
Nada Khazal Kadhim Hindi, Mohammed Malih Radhi, Fatima Malik AL-Rubea, Rusull Hamza Kh. AL-Jubori, Muhammad Farhab, Amjad Islam Aqib, Muhammad Shahid Khan, Muhammad Tahir Aleem, Shakseema Shaukat, Ayesha Qadry, Muhammad Zeeshan Ul Haq, Muhammad Jawad, Muhammad Farooq, Ifra Siddique, Zia Ullah, Atamjit Singh, Kirandeep Kaur, Komalpreet Kaur, Shilpa Heer, Preet Mohinder Singh Bedi, Neena Bedi, Saroj Arora, Pallvi Mohana, Avneet Kaur, Antresh Kumar, Manisha Kaushal, Muhammad Ijaz, Iqra Muzamil, Aamir Naseer, Iftikhar Hussain, Rais Ahmad, Yasir Razzaq Khan, Tean Zaheer, Iqra Sarwar, Muhammad Shoaib, Simone Ulrich Ulrich Picoli, Nicole Mariele Santos Röhnelt, Tiago Sfredo Schenkel, Ramendra Pati Pandey, Vethakkani Samuel Raj, Anjali Priyadarshini, Riya Mukherjee, Vasco Azevedo, Brenda Silva Rosa da Luz, Yves Le-Loir, Eric Guédon, Rudra Mishra, Bhama Mishra, Kodiveri Muthukaliannan Gothandam, Nalini Easwaran, Arun Kumar, Roma A. Chougale, Furqan Awan, Muhammad Muddassir Ali, Muhammad Hassan Mushtaq

First published in London, United Kingdom, 2021 by IntechOpen
IntechOpen is the global imprint of INTECHOPEN LIMITED, registered in England and Wales, registration number: 11086078, 5 Princes Gate Court, London, SW7 2QJ, United Kingdom
Printed in Croatia

British Library Cataloguing-in-Publication Data
A catalogue record for this book is available from the British Library

Additional hard and PDF copies can be obtained from orders@intechopen.com

Insights Into Drug Resistance in *Staphylococcus aureus*
Edited by Amjad Aqib
p. cm.
Print ISBN 978-1-83962-742-2
Online ISBN 978-1-83962-743-9
eBook (PDF) ISBN 978-1-83962-744-6
ISSN 2631-6188

For EU product safety concerns:
IN TECH d.o.o., Prolaz Marije Krucifikse Kozulić 3, 51000 Rijeka, Croatia, info@intechopen.com or visit our website at intechopen.com.

IntechOpen Book Series

Infectious Diseases

Volume 10

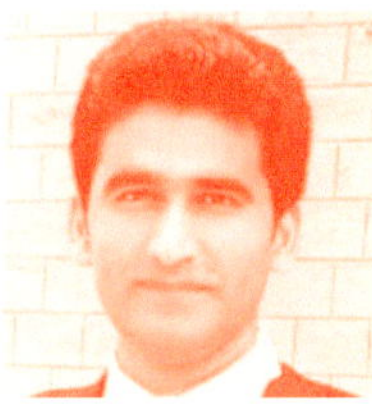

Dr. Amjad Islam Aqib obtained a DVM and MSc (Hons) from University of Agriculture Faisalabad (UAF), Pakistan, and a Ph.D. from the University of Veterinary and Animal Sciences Lahore, Pakistan. Dr. Aqib joined the Department of Clinical Medicine and Surgery at UAF for one year as an assistant professor where he developed a research laboratory designated for pathogenic bacteria. Since 2018, he has been Assistant Professor/ Officer in-charge, Department of Medicine, Manager Research Operations and Development-ORIC, and President One Health Club at Cholistan University of Veterinary and Animal Sciences, Bahawalpur, Pakistan. He has nearly 100 publications to his credit. His research interests include epidemiological patterns and molecular analysis of antimicrobial resistance and modulation and vaccine development against animal pathogens of public health concern.

Editor of Volume 10:
Amjad Aqib
Department of Medicine, Cholistan University of Veterinary and Animal Sciences, Bahawalpur, Pakistan

Book Series Editor:
Shailendra K. Saxena
King George's Medical University

Scope of the Series

The series will give a most comprehensive overview of recent trends in various infectious diseases (as per the most recent Baltimore classification), as well as general concepts of infections, immunopathology, diagnosis, treatment, epidemiology and etiology to current clinical recommendations in management of infectious diseases, highlighting the ongoing issues, recent advances, with future directions in diagnostic approaches and therapeutic strategies. This book series will focus on various aspects and properties of infectious diseases whose deep understanding is very important for safeguarding human race from more loss of resources and economies due to pathogens.

Contents

Preface

Staphylococcus aureus is the most ubiquitous microorganism in humans, animals, and the environment, existing as commensal as well as pathogenic bacterium. The pathogen is a major etiology of bovine mastitis that compromises economy and public health. Its greater prevalence in dairy farms results in culling of animals from the production system due to its contagious nature. Several preventive and therapeutic approaches have been applied to stop *S. aureus* from infecting animals. Inability to control this pathogen from spreading from animals to humans and back to animals may result in extensive resistance.

Due to the rise in antibiotic resistance, new strains and types of *S. aureus* are developing. These include methicillin-resistant *S. aureus* (MRSA) and its different types, which include hospital-acquired MRSA (HA-MRSA), livestock-acquired MRSA (LA-MRSA), and community-acquired MRSA (CA-MRSA). Moreover, newer strains have recently developed against the antibiotic vancomycin: vancomycin-resistant *S. aureus* (VRSA) and vancomycin-intermediate *S. aureus* (VISA). Further isolates are expected to emerge against other antibiotics, including penicillin, cephalosporins, tetracycline, aminoglycosides, mupirocin, and macrolide. It is evident that resistance in *S. aureus* may spread both vertically (from parent to offspring) as well as horizontally (transformation, transduction, and conjugation) by modifying drug target, limited uptake, inactivation of drug, and active efflux.

Several anti-methicillin-resistant *S. aureus* drugs are now becoming ineffective. Food and food products are harboring resistant strains of *S. aureus*, which is a threat to the environment. In humans, skin infections are a typical representation of strains that take longer than normal to treat. In addition to antibiotics, several other methods are being used to combat *S. aureus*, such as vaccines and bacteriophages. The use of lytic bacteriophages and their byproducts is a promising alternative for bacterial control, since they infect and lyse the pathogen without the inconvenience of side effects as well as contribute to lower consumption of antimicrobials, reflected in the reduction of rates of antibiotic resistance.

This book highlights mechanisms of resistance in *S. aureus* against different antibiotics. The first section discusses the status of resistance and reasons for its increase. The second section discusses the pathogenesis of *S. aureus* in animals and humans, as well as possible solutions. The book summarizes insights into drug resistance in *S. aureus* and its impacts on animals and humans. It opens up new horizons for further research to better cope with *S. aureus* infection.

Amjad Aqib
Department of Medicine,
Cholistan University of Veterinary and Animal Sciences,
Bahawalpur, Pakistan

Section 1

Resistant Strains and Mechanisms

Chapter 1

Antibiotic Resistant *Staphylococcus aureus*

Arun Kumar Parthasarathy and Roma A. Chougale

Abstract

Staphylococcus is an adaptable pathogen and leads to rapid development of antibiotic resistance. The major targets for antibiotics are (i) the cell wall, (ii) the ribosome and (iii) nucleic acids. Resistance can either develop intrinsically or extrinsically via horizontal gene transfer, drug site modification, and efflux pumps etc. This review focuses on development of resistance to currently used antibiotics in Staphylococcal infection, novel therapeutic approaches resistance pattern of antibiotics and also the future prospectus for new antibiotics usage.

Keywords: Staphylococcus aureus, MRSA, antibiotic resistant

1. Introduction

Staphylococcus is normal resident bacterium that lives in nasal cavity, throat, skin and mucous membrane of humans as well as a variety of animals and birds [1]. Approximately 20% of healthy populations are persistent nasal carriers and 30% are intermittent carriers of *S. aureus*. Individuals who are colonized with *S. aureus* are at a great risk of infection and also serve as an important source of transferring *S. aureus* in the community and hospital settings [2].

Based on the Coagulase production, Staphylococci are classified into Coagulase negative staphylococci (CONS) and Coagulase positive staphylococci (COPS). Of these, CONS causing infections are mostly seen in immune-compromised patients [3]. COPS (eg. *S. aureus*) is a pathogen of great concern, because of its intrinsic virulence property, its ability to cause a variety of life-threatening infections (superficial skin infections to deep seated infections), and its capacity to adapt to different environmental conditions [4].

S. aureus is a major problem in animals. It causes mastitis or intramammary infections and is a cause of major financial losses in the dairy industry. In Poultry industry, *S. aureus* causes a variety of disease manifestations such as comb necrosis, bacterial chondronecrosis and also leads to leg weakness, lameness and septicemia [5].

In the modern world, antibiotics are used in treatment and prophylaxis of human and animal infection. They are also used in poultry industry to prevent bacterial infection and reduce the financial loss [6]. In some developing and under-developed countries, antibiotics are used as growth promoters in animal feed, especially in poultry industry to increase the yield of meat production. Due to irrational use of antibiotics, *S. aureus* has emerged to become increasingly antibiotic resistant. This leads to treatment failure and leaves us with limited choice of antibiotics to be used in future [7]. Resistant bacteria can be transmitted from animals to humans among poultry workers and other agricultural workers, who are in close contact with these animals. It is documented that, after using the antibiotic, 'Avoparcin' as growth promoter in animal feed, there is emergence of glycopeptide- resistant Enterococcus. These resistant determinants are transferred to other gram positive bacteria such as MRSA via horizontal gene transfer method. These leads to development of resistance to Vancomycin, a drug of choice for the treatment of MRSA. Simarily, 'Tylosin' or Enrofloxacin (a derivative of fluoroquinolones) is used as a supplement in animal feeds. This has resulted in the development of Erythromycin and Ciprofloxacin- resistant Staphylococci [8].

2. Mechanisms of antibiotic resistant

2.1 Methicillin resistant *Staphylococus aureus* (MRSA)

Alexander Flemming introduced the antibiotic, Penicillin in 1940s for the treatment of bacterial infection. At that time, *S. aureus* infections were well controlled. However, with the widespread use of this antibiotic in the 1950s, Penicillin-resistant *S. aureus* appeared. It produces pencillinase enzyme, which can hydrolyze the beta-lactum ring of Penicillin. In 1959, substitution of the natural aminoadipoyl chain from Penicillin with bulkier moieties, developed a semi-synthetic Penicillin, named Methicillin. However, it was not widely used because of its toxicity. It was replaced by similar, more stable Penicillins like Oxacillin, Flucloxacillin and Dicloxacilllin. These antibiotics show good antibacterial activity and are resistant to beta-lactamase substrate. In 1961 the British scientist, Jevons isolated the penicillin stable resistant *S. aureus*. However, the name Methicillin resistant *S. aureus* (MRSA) continues to be used [9].

Bifunctional Transglycolylase-transpeptidase (Penicillin binding protein 'a' or PBPa) is the inhibitory target of beta-lactam antibiotics in *S. aureus*. The transglycolylase domain is responsible for transferring the disaccharide pentapeptide (L-alanine, D-glutamine, Lysine and 2 D-alanines) from membrane bound lipid to growing chains of polysaccharide. Domain of Transpeptidase (TP) cross-links the glycine bridge and links the D-alanine of 4th position to adjacent chain of peptidoglycan layer to make the cell-wall strong. The active site of Transpeptidase (TP) serine is blocked (i.e., PBP2a) by causing structural analogous changes of D-Ala4 to D-Ala5. This leads to breakdown of beta lactam ring and a penicilloyl-O-serine intermediate is formed [10].

PBP2a is encoded by mec A gene. This mecA gene is a mobile genetic element integrated into the chromosomal element (SCCmec) of Methicillin sensitive *S. aureus*. The mecA gene is transfered to other *S. aureus* via horizontal gene transfer mechanisms. Resistance confered by mec A gene is broad spectrum and shows resistance to all beta-lactum antibiotics except Ceftaroline and Ceftobiprole [11].

SCCmec contains two essential components such as mec gene complex and ccr gene complex. The mec gene complex contains mecA and is associated with regulatory and insertion sequences. It has been classified into 6 different classes (A, B, C1, C2, D and E) along with ccr complex (Cassette chromosome recombinase) genes. It encodes for the enzyme, 'recombinase' that helps in integration and excision of SCCmec into the chromosome. There are 3 different types of recombinase enzymes, namely ccrA, ccrB, and ccrC. Recombinase enzymes are further classified into eight different types based on the existing recombinase and allotypes in the different characteristics.

SCCmecs are classified into 8 types and subtypes according to 'International Working Group on the Staphylococcal Cassette Chromosome elements' [12].

2.2 Vancomycin resistant *S. aureus*

Vancomycin is a glycopeptide antibiotic which has been used as the first line drug in the treatment of MRSA infections. It was introduced for human use in late 1958 [13] and resistance to Vancomycin was reported in *Enterococci* by 1980s. Thereafter slowly *S. aureus* showed reduced susceptibility to Teicoplanin (structurally similar to Vancomycin) in European countries [14]. The first VRSA (Vancomycin Resistant *S. aureus*) was identified in 2002, in Michigan, USA. In the same year, total 52 isolates carrying Van gene were identified in USA, India, Iran, Pakistan, Brazil and Portugal [15]. *S. aureus* having reduced susceptibility to Vancomycin is classified into 3 groups based on the MIC value by CLSI as follows [16]:

1. Vancomycin Susceptible *S. aureus* (VSSA) with MIC ≤2 μg/ml

2. Vancomycin Resistant *S. aureus* (VRSA) with MIC ≥16 μg/ml

3. Vancomycin Intermediate *S. aureus* (VISA) with MIC 4-8 μg/ml

2.2.1 VISA

The first vancomycin intermediate *S. aureus* was reported in 1997 from Japan with MIC value of 8 μg/ml [17]. VISA strains are generally preceded from heterogeneous Vancomycin resistant *S. aureus* (hVISA). hVISA is the precursor of VISA and is composed of cell subpopulations with various degrees of Vancomycin resistance. Vancomycin-intermediate *S. aureus* (VISA) are those isolates with a MIC between 4 and 8 mg/l, whereas heterogeneous VISA (hVISA) strains appear to be sensitive to Vancomycin with susceptible range of 1–2 mg/l, but containing subpopulation of Vancomycin-intermediate daughter cells (MIC ≥4 μg/ml). Vancomycin-resistant *S. aureus* (VRSA) are defined as those having MICs of at least 16 mg/l [16]. This means that, in the same culture plate, some strains are sensitive and some strains show Intermediate resistance to Vancomycin which may lead to treatment failure [18]. The underlying mechanism is still not completely known. However, scientists have put some efforts to identify the genetic determininants of VISA via different molecular identification methods such as comparative genomics, proteomics, transcriptomics etc. This lead to identification of genes responsible for VISA such as WalKR, GraSR, and VraSR [19]. The following are the fundamental characteristics of VISA phenotypes [14]:

1. Increased cell wall thickness

2. Reduced cross- linking of peptidoglycan

3. Decreased autolytic activity of bacteria

4. Changes in surface protein profile

5. Dysfunction of *agr* system (The accessory gene regulator *(agr)* of *S. aureus* is a global regulator which secretes virulence factors and surface proteins) and changes the growth profile of bacteria.

GraRs gene regulates the transcription of cell wall biosynthesis and specifically up-regulates the genes responsible for capsule biosynthesis operon. It also up-regulates the *dlt* operon and the *mprF/fmtC* genes, which are linked to teichoic acid alanylation and alters the cell wall charge. Moreover, the GraRS mutation can modify the expression of *rot* (repressor of toxins) and *agr* (accessory gene regulator). This leads to downstream effect of global regulators [20].

2.2.2 VRSA

Vancomycin resistance is mediated by Van cluster which are found in bacteria such as S. *aureus, E.fecalis, E.faceium, Clostridium difficile*, Acintomycetes (Amycolotopsis orientalis, *Actinoplanes teichomyceticus, and* Streptomyces toyocaensis) as well as anaerobic bacteria from the human bowel flora such as *Ruminococcus* species and *Paenibacillus popilliae* [21].

Based on the Van gene, homologues Vancomycin resistance is classified into several gene (Van) clusters which encode for the enzymes which synthesize D-Alanyl-D-lactate and D-alanyl-D-serine. Eleven van gene clusters have been discovered till now, namely, *VanA, VanB, VanD, Van F, VanI, VanM, VanC, VanE, VanG, VanL, and VanN* [22].

1. *vanA*, *vanB*, *vanD*, *van F*, *vanI*, and *vanM* encode for synthesis of d-Alanyl-Lac ligase and are responsible for high-level Vancomycin resistance with MIC range > *256 mg/ml*

2. *vanC, vane, vanG, vanL, and vanN* clusters encode for synthesis of D-ala-ser-ligases and are responsible for low level Vancomycin resistance with MIC range 8-6 mg/ml [23].

VRSA resistance mechanism is mediated by van A operon, which is carried on the mobile genetic element (Transposon) Tn1546. VanA cluster is encoded by 5 proteins such as VanS, VanR, VanH, VanA and VanX, having the following functions;

1. *vanS and vanR* together form two-component system and upregulate the vanA gene clusters in the presence of Vancomycin

2. *VanH, VanA, and VanX* are responsible in modifying D-ala-ala precursors of cell wall to D-ala-D-lac, which confer resistance to Vancomycin

3. *vanH* produces dehydrogenase enzyme which reduces pyruvate to D-lac.

4. *vanX* produces D,D dipeptidase that hydrolyses the native precursors and prevents the synthesis and cros- linking of cell wall peptidoglycan [24].

Enterococcus spp. is the major reservoir of Vancomycin resistance and it is transferred to other bacterial species by the horizontal gene transfer method of bacterial conjugation. The Inc18 incompatibility conjugative plasmid naturally occurs in Enterococcus but not in Staphylococci spp. The Inc18 contains pSK41-like multi-resistant conjugative plasmids. These plasmids are transferred from *E. faecalis* to *S. aureus* [25].

2.2.3 Treatment challenges

Deletion of Van cluster components has lead to recovery of Vancomycin sensitivity. This is a promising target for new drug development [26]. For example, hydroxyethylamines, posphinate and phosphonate transition-state analogues have

DOI: http://dx.doi.org/10.5772/intechopen.100057

been used for the inhibiton of VanA [27, 28]. Phosphinate based covalent inhibitors, and sulfur-containing compounds have been demonstrated in VanX inhibitors [29]. These inhibitors can be used in combination with Vancomycin to increase uptake of the antibiotic inside the bacterial cell [21].

2.3 Mechanisms of tetracycline resistance

Three different tetracycline resistance mechanisms have been described:

1. Ribosomal protection, which is the most common resistance mechanism,

2. Active efflux of the antibiotic and

3. Enzymatic inactivation of the drug.

All these mechanisms are based on the acquisition of one or several tetracycline resistant determinants, which are widely distributed among bacterial genera [30]. Additionally, mutations in the rRNA, multidrug transporter systems or permeability barriers may be involved in developing resistance to several antibiotics including Tetracyclines [31].

Efflux of the drug occurs through some export proteins from the major facilitator super family (MFS). These export proteins are membrane-associated proteins which are coded for by *tet* efflux genes and export Tetracycline from the cell. Export of Tetracycline reduces the intracellular drug concentration and thus protects the ribosomes within the cell.

Ribosome protection proteins that protect the ribosomes from the action of Tetracyclines [32] are cytoplasmic proteins. They are similar to elongation factors EF-Tu and EF-G that bind to the ribosome and cause changes in ribosomal conformation. This prevents Tetracycline from binding to the ribosome, without altering or stopping protein synthesis. This occurs by a ribosome-dependent GTPase activity, which confers resistance mainly to Doxycycline, Minocycline and a wider spectrum of resistance to tetracyclines than is seen with bacteria that carry tetracycline efflux proteins.

2.3.1 Tetracycline resistance genes

There are at least 38 different characterized tetracycline resistance (*tet*) genes and three Oxytetracycline resistance genes (*otr*) to date [33]. These genes include 23 genes which code for efflux proteins, 11 genes for ribosomal protection proteins, three genes for an inactivating enzyme and one gene with unknown resistance mechanism. Most environmental *tet* genes encode for transport proteins, which pump the antibiotic out of the bacterial cell and keep the intracellular concentrations low to make the ribosomes function normally [34]. The most common genes found in *S. aureus* are *tet(K), tet(L), tet(M), tet(O).*

tet (K) gene is a mobile genetic element originally detected in *S. aureus* plasmids of pT181 family [35]. It is a 4.45-kb plasmid protein consisting of 459 amino acids and belongs to the incompatibility group inc3 [36]. PT181-like plasmids have also been detected either integrated in the large plasmids or in the bacterial chromosome. They are always flanked by directly repeated insertion sequences of the type IS257 [37].

tet (L) gene carrying plasmid pSTE1 was identified in *Staphylococcus hyicus* in 1992. In 1996, tet(L) was also found to be carried on the naturally occurring plasmid pSTS7 of *Staphylococcus epidermidis* [38]. It is the second most prevalent tetracycline resistant gene in Streptococci and Enterococci [39]. It consists of 458 amino acids.

tet (M) gene is the most widely distributed tetracycline resistant gene in gram-positive bacteria [40]. It was first identified in *Streptococcus spp*. Subsequently, it has been isolated in a large number of gram-positive and gram-negative bacteria, including Mycoplasmas and Ureoplasmas [40]. The *tet(M)* gene is frequently associated with conjugative transposons of the Tn916-Tn1545 family [41, 42]. which also carry additional antibiotic resistance genes. According to the study of Schmitz et al. [34], *tet(M)* is the most prevalent single tetracycline resistance determinant in MRSA (Methicillin Resistant *Staphylococcus aureus*). The majority of *tet(M)*-positive *S. aureus* isolates also carry *tet(K).* Hence, MRSA isolates are typically of *tet(M) or tet(K,M)* genotype [43].

tet (O) genes also have been detected very rarely in Staphylococci.

2.4 Mechanisms of macrolide resistance

Macrolides inhibit protein synthesis by stimulating dissociation of the peptidyl-tRNA molecule from the ribosomes during elongation. This results in polypeptide chain termination and a reversible stoppage of protein synthesis. The first described mechanism of Macrolide resistance was due to post-transcriptional modification of the 23S rRNA by the adenine-N6 methyltransferase. These enzymes add one or two methyl groups to a single adenine (A2058 in *Escherichia coli*) in the 23S rRNA moiety. Over the last 30 years, a number of adenineN6-methyltransferases from different species, genera, and isolates have been described. In general, genes encoding these methylases have been designated *erm* (erythromycin ribosome methylation), although there are exceptions, especially in the antibiotic-producing organisms. As the number of *erm* genes described has increased, the nomenclature for these genes has varied and has been inconsistent. In some cases, unrelated genes have been given the same letter designation, while in other cases, highly related genes (90% identity) have been given different names [33].

2.4.1 Macrolide resistance genes

Although structurally unrelated to each other, Macrolides, Lincosamide, and Streptogramin, are often investigated simultaneously for microbial resistance, as some Macrolide resistance genes (*erm*) encode for resistance to two or all three of these compounds. In total, more than 60 different genes conferring resistance to one or more of the MLS antibiotics have been identified, including genes associated with rRNA methylation, efflux and inactivation.

The ***erm (A) gene*** is associated with the transposon, Tn554. It is integrated into SCCmec II elements, and is a non-conjugative or conjugative transposon. It is mostly seen in Methicillin resistant staphylococci [43].

The ***erm (B) gene*** is seen in transposons Tn917/Tn551. It is 2.3 and 4.4 kb in size and does not carry additional resistant genes [44].

The ***erm (C) gene*** is commonly located on small plasmids. It is widely spread in Methicillin susceptible strains [45].

The **msr (A)** gene is efflux- pump mediated, codes for 488 amino acids, ABC transporters system and is encoded by plasmid borne *msr (A)* genes [46]. It is an ATP-binding transport protein which mediates the active efflux of 14-membered ABC transporters system and confers resistance to Macrolides and B-compounds of the Streptogramins.

2.5 Aminoglycosides resistant *S. aureus*

Aminoglycosides are broad spectrum antibiotics that inhibit protein synthesis of the bacteria. They were first isolated from the Actinomycetes spp. namely

Streptomyces griseus and introduced for clinical use in 1944. They were used as the first-line drugs worldwide but were replaced by Cephlaosporins, Carbapenems and Flouoroquinolones due to lesser toxicity and broader coverage than Aminoglycosides [47]. Members of these groups include Neomycin, Amikacin, Gentamicin, Netilmicin, Tobramycin, Kanamycin etc. The novel Aminoglycosides recently developed, namely Arbekacin and Plazomicin were meant to overcome the Aminoglycoside resistance mechanisms [48]. Clinical studies reported a higher incidence of nephrotoxicity in patients on Aminoglycosides. Hence, screening the patients for serum urea and creatinine after injection of Aminoglycosides is impor tant to monitor the severity of the toxic effects. Aminoglycosides have got a substantial activity against *S. aureus* infections including MRSA, VISA, and VRSA [47].

Entry of Aminoglycosides inside the bacteria mostly comprises of three distinct stages [49]:

1. **Increase in permeability of bacterial cell membrane:** Binding of polycationic Aminoglycoside antibiotics to the bacterial membrane which has negative charged components such as phospholoipids and teichoic acids occurs by electrostatic attraction. This leads to disruption of the outer membrane of the bacterial cells.

2. **Energy dependent:** Entry of Aminoglycoside antibiotics into cytoplasm is mediated by slow, energy dependent and electron transport mechanisms.

3. **Mistranslation of protein synthesis and inhibition of protein synthesis**: This occurs once the Aminoglycoside molecules enter into the cytoplasm. Mistranslation leads to cytoplasmic damage and facilitates rapid uptake of more Aminoglycosides inside the bacterial cell.

Aminoglycoside resistance mostly occurs by

1. Enzymatic modification

2. Target site modification

3. Efflux pump proteins on bacterial cell.

1. **Enzymatic methylation of the rRNA**: Methylation at N7 of guanine residues of the 16 s rRNA produces high level resistance, but this has not been reported among clinically important bacteria.

The major mechanism of aminoglycoside resistance among both gram negative and gram positive clinical isolates is the enzymatic modification of amino or hydroxyl group of these antibiotics. Three families of enzymes are responsible in performing co-factor dependent drug modification:

i. Aminoglycoside phosphotransferases (APHs)

ii. Aminoglycoside acetyltransferases (AACs)

iii. Aminoglycoside nucleotidyltranferases (ANTs)

These are further subdivided into many types (designated by Roman numerals). AAC (6′)-I enzymes are aminoglycoside acetyltransferases, modifying the antibiotic at position 6′ [50, 51].

Aminoglycoside resistance in clinical strains of *S. aureus* is due to the acquisition of cytoplasmic Aminoglycoside Modifying Enzyme (AME) by plasmids. For example, Gentamicin and Neomycin resistance is confered by bifunctional Acetyl Transferase –Phosphotransferase (aac-aphD) encoded by Tn4001.

Neomycin resistance occurs by aphA encoded adenyl transferase which is encoded by PUB 110 or Tn 5405. It is seen in SSC II mec [52].

2. **Modifications of the target** include mutational changes in the ribosomal proteins or 16S rRNA. The mutational changes are mostly seen in Streptomycin

3. **Efflux pump proteins on bacterial cell** is an intrinsic aminoglycoside resistance mechanism in various pathogens. In the opportunistic pathogen, *P. aeruginosa*, intrinsic low-level resistance to Aminoglycosides, Tetracycline and Erythromycin is mediated by the expression of the multiple efflux (Mex) XY-OprM system. In *S. aureus*, efflux pump proteins causing resistance to aminoglycosides have not been identified [46].

2.6 Linezolid

2.6.1 Mechanism of action

It is an Oxazolidinone, useful in treatment of resistant gram positive coccal and bacillary infection. It is primarily bacteriostatic but can exert bactericidal action against some *Streptococci, Pneumococci and B. fragilis* [53, 54].

It acts mainly by inhibiting bacterial protein synthesis, acting at an early step. It binds to the central loop of domain V in the 23S fraction (P site) of the 50S ribosome and interferes with the formation of tertiary N-formylmethionine- tRNA- 70S initiation complex. Hence it stops protein synthesis before it starts.

2.6.2 Mechanism of resistance

Since Linezolid is a synthetic drug, natural resistance to this drug does not occur; hence mutations are mostly acquired.

1. Mutations in the 23srRNA subunit domain V region of ribosomes lead to alteration of peptidyltransferase center (PTC), where conserved regions of ribosome interact directly with Linezolid. Gram positive bacteria passes 4 to 6 allelic copies of 23S rRNA; hence, development of Linezolid resistance requires more than one allele to be mutated.

2. Mutations in the genes of ribosomal proteins L3 (rplC gene), L4 (rplD gene), and L22 (rplV) gene arefound in some gram positive bacteria.

3. Acquired resistance by Natural cfr (Chloramphenicol –Florfenicol Resistance) gene from Chloramphenicol resistant bacteria, which is a plasmid mediated gene, encodes a protein to catalyze the post transcriptional methylation of the C-8 atom (A2503) in the 23S rRNA. Methylation by the cfr leads to development of multidrug resistance to Linezolid, Lincosamide and Streptomycin [52].

Genes encoding for Ribosomal proteins have been analyzed by PCR and Amplicon sequencing.

Whole molecular background is elucidated by PCR- Amplicon sequencing and whole genome sequencing [56].

2.7 Mupirocin (MUP)

2.7.1 Mechanism of action

Mupirocin is a mixture of several pseudomonic acids. It binds to its target site of the enzyme isoleucyl-tRNA synthetase and inhibits protein synthesis. However it does not bind to the mammalian enzyme counterparts, making it non-toxic for human beings. The synthesis of bacterial isoleucine tRNA gets depleted which leads to cessation of protein and RNA synthesis in the bacteria. At the concentrations near Minimum Inhibitory Concentration (MIC) Mupirocin is bacteriostatic and at higher concentrations it becomes bactericidal. It is mainly used against the gram positive bacteria [57].

2.7.2 Mechanism of resistance

Mupirocin-resistant (mupR) *S. aureus* was first reported in the United Kingdom in 1987.

Mupirocin resistance is classified into two types.

1. **Low Level MUP resistance**- MIC value of 8-64 mcg/ml is mainly due to chromosomal point mutations in the native ileS1 gene leading to a Val-to-Phe change in the MUP- binding site.

2. **High Level MUP resistance**- At a MIC of 128- 256 μg/ml. there is plasmid mediated resistance, which occurs by two mechanisms:

    1. Acquiring an alternate isoleucine - tRNA synthetase i.e. by acquisition of a plasmid mediated mupA or isleS2 gene.

    2. Acquisition of mupB gene [58, 59].

2.8 Fusidic acid

2.8.1 Mechanism of action

It was isolated from a strain of *Fusidium coccineum*, which is a steroid like antibiotic. It is mainly bacteriostatic in nature but may become bactericidal at higher concentrations. It acts by binding with Elongation factor G i.e. Translocase which is necessary for translocation on the bacterial ribosome after peptide bond formation during protein synthesis. However eukaryotes have another enzyme which is not affected by the drug. This specific mode of action explains the absence of intrinsic cross- resistance between Fusidic acid and other antibiotics. It has a limited spectrum of activity, mainly against Gram positive bacteria i.e. *Staphylococcus aureus, S.epidermidis, Clostridium spp. and Corynebacterium*. However, *Streptococci* are moderately susceptible. But most Gram Negative Bacteria are resistant to it [60].

2.8.2 Mechanism of resistance

Two major Fusidic acid resistance mechanisms are discovered in *S. aureus*:

1. Alteration of the drug target site which is due to the mutations in fusA gene (encoding elongation factor G, EF-G), rplF or fusE (encoding ribosome protein L6)

2. Point mutation in fusA gene occurs in domain III of EF-G.

Other resistant mechanisms include:

i. Fusidic acid resistant small colony variant (SCV) isolates, referred to as fusA-SCV class mostly occur due to mutations in domain V of EF-G

ii. Acquired Fusidic acid resistance of *Staphylococcus* spp. includes *fusB*, *fusC*, and *fusD.* The genes *fusB (found in plasmid pUB 101 in S. aureus)* and *fusC* were found in *S. aureus* and coagulase-negative Staphylococci

iii. *fusD* is an intrinsic factor causing Fusidic acid resistance in *Staphylococcus saprophyticus* [61].

3. Alternative to antibiotic therapy

3.1 Spread of antibiotic resistant

3.1.1 Antimicrobial peptides

Antimicrobial peptides or host defense peptides are biologically active molecules produced by variety of organisms [62]. AMPs have board spectrum of antimicrobial activity against pathogenic microorganisms and are the first line defense against the foreign attacks [63]. AMPs also serve as immune-modulators in higher animals [64]. AMP'S are expressed by specific genes and their expression is by either constitutive or specific external factors [64]. AMPS are classified into several types based on the source, activity Amino acid sequences and structural characteristics. AMPS are usually 1. Cationic and Hydrophophic in nature with helical polypeptides of short amino acid sequences mostly lysine and arginine amino acids. 2. Some are Cationic and Amphiphilic (Both hydrophobic and Hydrophilic).

3.1.2 Membrane target mechanism

Amphiphilic peptides are alpha helix and their amphiphilicity interacts with bacterial cell membrane. These alpha helices peptides are folded and adsorbed with both hydrophilic and hydrophobic sides of lipid bilayer membranes. Positive charged AMPS interact with negative charged cell membranes by electrostatic interactions and undergo conformational changes of the cell membrane.

3.1.3 Non membrane target mechanism

AMPS bind to hydrophobic and negative charged cell membrane of lipid bilayer at their N-terminal ends containing basic amino acids and their C-terminal ends are amidated with neutral hydrophobicity. The number of positive net charge are related to the antibacterial activity and their hemolytic activity is related to the hydrophobicity of the peptides. Multiple models to explain the action of these peptides, include the toroidal pore model, the barrel-stave model, and the carpet model etc. [65].

3.1.4 Advantages of AMPs

1. AMPs have rapid germ killing abilities with low bactericidal concentration

2. No toxic effects

3. Hard to induce bacterial resistance

4. AMPs have broad spectrum antimicrobial activity

5. AMPs have good thermal stability and good water stability

6. AMPs are small molecules with low synthetic cost

7. AMPs show inhibitory ability to cancer cells [66].

3.1.5 Disadvantage of AMPs

AMPs have mostly L-amino acids; are sensitive to protease degradation and rapid renal clearance.

AMPs are not specific to microorganisms and display systemic toxicity

Oral administration of AMPS can lead to proteoloytic degradation by gastric enzymes such as trypsin and pepsin.

Systemic administration results in short half life time in vivo and cytotoxicity in blood

Chemical modification of AMPS and the use of drug delivery vehicles such as Nanoparticles, lipid system can improve the properties of AMPS for their clinical use [26].

3.2 Nanoparticles

Nanoparticles are smaller in size (less than 10 nm in diameter) that exhibit high surface area to volume ratio [27]. Nano particles have significant application in the medical fields. Nano-drugs or Nanoparticles can act individually or synergistically with antibiotic components against the multi-drug resistant pathogens. Nanoparticles are used as drug delivery vehicle that improve the therapeutic efficacy and enhance their physicochemical characteristics [28]. Metal and metal oxide Nanoparticles such as gold, silver, titanium, copper, zinc etc. are the most studied Nanoparticles against the multi-drug resistant pathogens [28].

3.2.1 Interaction and penetration of nanoparticle to bacteria

Electric charges present on the nanoparticles are the most important property in terms of antimicrobial effect. Interactions of nano-particles with bacteria membrane depend on the different factors such as electrostatic interactions, hydrophobic interactions, receptor ligand interaction and Van der Val forces [29].

The phosphates present in the teichoic acids of gram positive bacterial cell wall are responsible for bacterial negative charge and acts as binding site of divalent cation ions. Gram Negative bacteria consists of plasma or cytoplasmic membrane followed by peptidoglycan layer and hydrophobic lipid bilayer consisting of lipopolysaccharides (Phosphates and Carboxylates) which are responsible for negative charge of gram negative bacterial cell wall. The interaction of NPs with membrane structure leads to blebbing, tubule formation and other membrane defects [67].

Nanoparticles can bind to cell wall by electrostatic interactions and disrupt cytoplasmic membrane leading to leakage of cytoplasmic content of the bacterial cell. Nano particles also bind to intracellular components such as DNA and other enzymes responsible for normal cellular machinery causing disruption in cellular machinery by creating oxidizing stress, electrolytic imbalance and enzyme inhibition followed by cell death. For example, free copper ions (CU2+) from CU Nanoparticles generates reactive oxygen species that disrupts the amino acid synthesis and DNA [67].

3.2.2 Nanoparticles as a drug delivery vehicle

Nano-particles based drug delivery system provides increased drug retention time in blood. Reduced non-specific distribution at targeted site of infections, Opsonin proteins in blood rapidly attach to Nanoparticles, promoting macrophages to bind and remove NPs from blood circulation [68].

3.2.3 Bacterial resistance to NPS

Bacterial cells acquire resistant towards NPs by multiple mutations. NPs resistance to bacteria is a clinical concern but it is rare. Some studies suggest that bacteria develop resistance to Ag, Au, and Cu NPs after continuous exposure. For example: CU++ NPs sowed reduced susceptibility to TiO2 NPS after continuous exposure to *Schewanella oneidensis* [69].

Increased use of Ag NPS in clinical application raises the NP bacterial drug resistance to *K.pneumoniae and Enterobacter cloacae.* Hemeg et al. showed, Al_2O_3 NPs increased the expression of conjugation-promoting genes and are responsible for horizontal gene transfer of resistant genes [70].

3.3 Probiotics

Probiotics are living Microorganisms that confers a health benefit to the host when administered in adequate amount. For example, *Lactobacilli and bifidobacteria*. Probiotics bacteria have many beneficial properties:

1. Controlling the activity of pathogenic bacteria

2. Improving intestinal barrier function

3. Reducing adherence to pathogenic bacteria cells,

4. Co-aggregation

5. Production of organic acids which antagonize the pathogenic bacteria.

6. Many Probiotics produce antimicrobial compounds such as short chain fatty acids, Nitric oxide, bacteriocins [71].

3.3.1 Spread of antibiotic resistant

Gastrointestinal bacteria act as a major reservoir for resistance genes that can be acquired from ingested bacteria and it is responsible for transfer of resistant gene from one bacteria cell to another by plasmid mediated conjugation. Intrinsic resistance of probiotic bacteria is a major concern. Vancomycin, Tetracycline and Chloramphenicol antibiotic resistance have been reported in lactobacillus spp. intrinsically [71].

3.4 Vaccines

See **Table 1** [72].

Target antigen	**Clinical trails**	**Out come**
CP 5and CP8	Phase III	Failed
CP-5 CRM197, CP8-CRM and CIfA (SA3 ag)	Phase I	Significant antibody response
CP5-CRM 197, CP8-CRM197, MntC and CIfA (SA4 ag)	Phase I	robust immune response, safe, and well-tolerated and phase 2b is ongoing
Alpha toxin and Panton-Valentine leukocidin	Phase I	good toxin neutralizing sero-positive response
EsxA and Esx B	Preclinical	protection with improving survival of murine model
Surface Protein A (SpA)	Preclinical	protection in mouse model
D-alanine auxotrophic *S. aureus*	Preclinical	protection from the formation of abscesses and improved survival in immunized mice
AdsA	Preclinical	protection in the immunized mouse model
Coa (Hc-CoaR6)	Preclinical	strong T-cell response and protection in mice against lethal dose of *S. aureus*
Staphylococcal enterotoxin B	Preclinical	efficient protection in BALB/c mice

Table 1.
List of vaccines in clinical trials and outcomes (adapted from Ansari et al., [72]).

4. Conclusion

Staphylococcus is an adaptable pathogen and has ability to develop rapid antibiotic resistance. After 1980s development of newer classes of antibiotics is very limited. Rapid development of resistance will reduce the availability of antibiotic in clinical practice and this will cause serious health problem in future. Development of newer molecules in expensive clinical trials, the huge investment in target based discovery with the structural biology did not yield the hope for newer break throughs. Microorganisms are very crucial in developing resistance to novel therapeutic agent rapidly. This will development of more strategies to combat the antibiotic resistance. Antibiotic stewardship policy is mandatory to control the development and spread of antibiotic resistance in community and hospital settings.

Author details

Arun Kumar Parthasarathy and Roma A. Chougale*
Department of Microbiology, D.Y. Patil Medical College,
Kolhapur, Maharashtra, India

*Address all correspondence to: neetiroma@gmail.com

References

[1] Smith "Livestock-Associated *Staphylococcus aureus*: The United States Experience". PLoS Pathog 2015. 11(2): e1004564. https://doi.org/10.1371/journal.ppat.1004564

[2] Abiye Tigabu, Moges Tiruneh, Feleke Mekonnen, "Nasal Carriage Rate, Antimicrobial Susceptibility Pattern, and Associated Factors of *Staphylococcus aureus* with Special Emphasis on MRSA among Urban and Rural Elementary School Children in Gondar, Northwest Ethiopia: A Comparative Cross-Sectional Study", *Advances in Preventive Medicine*, vol. 2018, ArticleID 9364757, 11 pages, 2018. https://doi.org/10.1155/2018/9364757.

[3] Chambers HF, Deleo FR. Waves of resistance: *Staphylococcus aureus* in the antibiotic era. Nat Rev Microbiol. 2009 Sep;7(9):629-41. doi: 10.1038/nrmicro 2200. PMID: 19680247; PMCID: PMC2871281.

[4] Karsten Becker, Christine Heilmann, Georg Peters "Coagulase-Negative Staphylococci" Clinical Microbiology Reviews Oct 2014, 27 (4) 870-926; DOI: 10.1128/CMR.00109-13

[5] Fluit AC. Livestock-associated Staphylococcus aureus. Clin Microbiol Infect. 2012 Aug;18(8):735-744. doi: 10.1111/j.1469-0691.2012.03846.x. Epub 2012 Apr 18. PMID: 22512702.

[6] Landers TF, Cohen B, Wittum TE, Larson EL. A review of antibiotic use in food animals: perspective, policy, and potential. Public Health Rep. 2012;127(1):4-22. doi:10.1177/0033354 91212700103

[7] Butaye P, Devriese LA, Haesebrouck F. Antimicrobial growth promoters used in animal feed: effects of less well known antibiotics on gram-positive bacteria. Clin Microbiol Rev. 2003 Apr;16(2):175-88. doi: 10.1128/cmr.16.2.175-188.2003. PMID: 12692092; PMCID: PMC153145.

[8] Mehndiratta PL, Bhalla P. Use of antibiotics in animal agriculture & emergence of methicillin-resistant Staphylococcus aureus (MRSA) clones: need to assess the impact on public health. Indian J Med Res. 2014;140(3):339-344.

[9] Kelly M. Craft, Johny M. Nguyen, Lawrence J. Berg and Steven D. Townsend Methicillin-resistant *Staphylococcus aureus* (MRSA): antibiotic-resistance and the biofilm phenotype. The Royal Society of Chemistry 2019. 10.1039/ c9md00044e

[10] Timothy J. Foster, Antibiotic resistance in *Staphylococcus aureus*. Current status and future prospects, *FEMS Microbiology Reviews*, Volume 41, Issue 3, May 2017, Pages 430-449, https://doi.org/10.1093/femsre/fux007

[11] Franklin D. LowyAntimicrobial resistance: the example of *Staphylococcus aureus* J Clin Invest. 2003 May 1; 111(9): 1265-1273. doi: 10.1172/JCI18535

[12] unlei Guo, Guanghui Song, Meiling Sun, Juan Wang and Yi Wang Prevalence and Therapies of Antibiotic-Resistance in *Staphylococcus aureus*. Front. Cell. Infect. Microbiol., 17 March 2020 | https://doi.org/10.3389/fcimb.2020. 00107

[13] Sorrell TC, Packham DR, Shanker S. et al. Vancomycin therapy for methicillin-resistant *Staphylococcus aureus*. Ann Intern Medd. 1982;97(3): 344-350.

[14] McGuinness WA, Malachowa N, DeLeo FR. Vancomycin Resistance in *Staphylococcus aureus*. Yale J Biol Med. 2017;90(2):269-281. Published 2017 Jun 23.

[15] Murray BE. Vancomycin-resistant enterococcal infections. N Engl J Med. 2000;342(10):710-721.

[16] CLSI Guidelines 2020. https://clsi.org/

[17] Hiramatsu K, Hanaki H, Ino T. et al. Methicillin-resistant *Staphylococcus aureus* clinical strain with reduced vancomycin susceptibility. J Antimicrob Chemother. 1997;40(1):135-136

[18] Keiichi Hiramatsu, Vancomycin-resistant Staphylococcus aureus: a new model of antibiotic resistance,The Lancet Infectious Diseases. 2001; 1(3): 147-155

[19] Q. Hu, H. Peng, X. Rao Molecular events for promotion of vancomycin resistance in vancomycin intermediate *Staphylococcus aureus* Front Microbiol, 7 (2016), p. 1601

[20] Meehl M, Herbert S, Götz F. et al. Interaction of the GraRS two-component system with the VraFG ABC transporter to support vancomycin-intermediate resistance in *Staphylococcus aureus*. Antimicrob Agents Chemother. 2007;51(8):2679-2689.

[21] Yanguang Cong, Sijin Yang, Xiancai Rao, Vancomycin resistant Staphylococcus aureus infections: A review of case updating and clinical features, Journal of Advanced Research. 2020; 21: 169-176

[22] P. Courvalin Vancomycin resistance in Gram-positive cocci. Clin Infect Dis, 42 (Suppl 1) (2006), pp. S25-S34

[23] B.L. Hollenbeck, L.B. Rice Intrinsic and acquired resistance mechanisms in *Enterococcus* Virulence, 3 (5) (2012), pp. 421-433

[24] M. Arthur, P. Courvalin Genetics and mechanisms of glycopeptide resistance in *enterococci* Antimicrob Agents Chemother, 37 (8) (1993), pp. 1563-1571

[25] Zhu W, Clark N, Patel JB. pSK41-like plasmid is necessary for Inc18-like vanA plasmid transfer from Enterococcus faecalis to Staphylococcus aureus in vitro. Antimicrob Agents Chemother. 2013 Jan;57(1):212-219

[26] Mathew Drayton, Jayachandran N. Kizhakkedathu and Suzana K.Straus "Towards Robust Deliver of Antimicrobial Peptides to Combat Bacterial Resistance" Molecules 2020, 25 3048; doi: 10.3390/molecules25133048.

[27] Hulkoti NI, Taranath TC. Biosynthesis of nanoparticles using microbes—a review. Colloids Surf B Biointerfaces. 2014;121:474-483. doi: 10.1016/j.colsurfb.2014.05.027.

[28] Niño-Martínez N, Salas Orozco MF, Martínez-Castañón GA, Torres Méndez F, Ruiz F. Molecular Mechanisms of Bacterial Resistance to Metal and Metal Oxide Nanoparticles. Int J Mol Sci. 2019;20(11):2808. Published 2019 Jun 8. doi:10.3390/ijms20112808

[29] Wang L, Hu C and Shao L, Int. J. Nanomedicine, 2017, 12, 1227-1249. [PubMed: 28243086]

[30] Schnappinger D and Hillen W. Tetracyclines: antibiotic action, uptake, and resistance mechanisms. Arch. Microbiol 1996; 165:359-369

[31] Michalova E, Novotna P, and Schelegelova J. Tetracycline in veterinary medicine and bacterial resistance to them.Vet. Med.Czech 2004; 49:79-100

[32] Taylor DE and Chau A. Tetracycline resistance mediated by ribosomal protection. Antimicrob.Agents Chemother 1996; 40:1-5.

[33] Roberts MC, Sutcliffe J, Courvalin P, Jensen LB, Rood J, Seppala H. Nomenclature for macrolide and macrolide-lincosamide-streptogramin B

resistance determinants. Antimicrob. Agents.Chemother1999; 43: 2823-2830.

[34] Schmitz FJ, Krey A, Sadurski R, Verhoef J, Milatovic D, Fluit AC. and for the European SENTRY participants. Resistance to tetracycline and distribution of tetracycline resistance genes in European Staphylococcus aureus isolates. Antimicrob. Agents Chemother 2001;47: 239-240

[35] Khan SA, and Novick RP. Complete nucleotide sequence of pT181, a tetracycline resistance plasmid from Staphylococcus aureus. Plasmid 1983;30:163-166.

[36] Projan SJ and Novick R. Comparative analysis of five related staphylococcal plasmids.Plasmid.1988; 19:203-221

[37] Morse SA, Johnson SJ, Biddle JW, and Roberts MC. Highlevel tetracycline resistance in Neisseria gonorrhoeaedue to the acquisition of the tetMdeterminant. Antimicrob.Agents Chemother. 1986; 30:664-670

[38] Schwarz S, Gregory PD, Werckenthin C, Curnock S, Dyke KG. A novel plasmid from Staphylococcus epidermidis specifying resistance to kanamycin, neomycinand tetracycline.J. Med. Microbiol 1996; 45:57-63.

[39] Poyart-Salmeron C, Trieu-Cuot P, Carlier C, MacGowan A, McLauchlin J, Courvalin P. Genetic basis of tetracycline resistance in clinical isolates of Listeriamonocytogenes. Antimicrob. Agents Chemother 1992;36:463-466

[40] Roberts MC. Tetracycline resistant determinants: mechanisms of action, regulation of expression, genetic mobility and diatribution. FEMS Microbial.Rev 1996; 19: 1-24.

[41] Clewell DB, Flannagan SE, and Jaworski DD. Unconstrained bacterial promiscuity: the Tn916-Tn1545 family of conjugative transposons. Trends Microbiol 1995; 3: 229-236.

[42] Bismuth R, Zillah R, Sakamoto H, Guesdon JL, Courvalin P. Gene heterogeneity for tetracycline resistance in Staphylococcus spp. Antimicrob. Agents Chemother1990; 34: 1611-1614.

[43] Wendlandt Sarah, Andrea T, Febler, Monecke Stefan, Ehricht Ralf, Schwarz Stefan. The diversity of antimicrobial resistance genes among staphylococci of animal origin.Inter. J. Med. Microbiol 2013; 303: 338-349.

[44] Lina G, Quaglia A, Reverdy ME, Leclercq R, Vandenesch F, Etienne J. Distribution of genes encoding resistance to macrolides, lincosamides,and streptogramins among staphylococci. Antimicrob Agents Chemother 1999; 43: 1062-1066.

[45] Ross JI, Eady EA, Cove JH, Cunliffe WJ, Baumberg S, Wootton JC. Inducible erythromycin resistance in staphylococci is encoded by a member of the ATP-binding transport super-gene family. Mol. Microbiol 1990; 4: 1207-1214

[46] Kevin M. Krause, Alisa W. Serio, Timothy R.Kane and Lynn E. Connolly. Aminoglycosides: An overview. Cold Spring Harb Perspect Med 2016;6:a027029

[47] *Armstrong ES, Miller GH* Combating evolution with intelligent design: the neoglycoside ACHN-490. Curr Opin Microbiol. *2010 Oct; 13(5):565-573.*

[48] Davis BD Mechanism of bactericidal action of aminoglycosides. Microbiol Rev. 1987 Sep; 51(3):341-350.

[49] *Shaw KJ, Rather PN, Hare RS, Miller GH* Molecular genetics of aminoglycoside resistance genes and familial relationships of the aminoglycoside-modifying enzymes. Microbiol Rev. *1993 Mar; 57(1):138-163.*

[50] *Ramirez MS, Tolmasky ME.* Aminoglycoside modifying enzymes. Drug Resist Updat. *2010 Dec; 13(6):151-171.*

[51] Rahimi F. Characterization of Resistance to Aminoglycosides in Methicillin-Resistant *Staphylococcus aureus* Strains Isolated From a Tertiary Care Hospital in Tehran, Iran. *Jundishapur J Microbiol*. 2016;9(1): e29237. Published 2016 Jan 2. doi:10.5812/jjm.29237

[52] Essentials of Medical Pharmacology by KD Tripathi 8th edition Jaypee Publications

[53] Linezolid update- stable in vitro activity following more than a decade of clinical use and summary of associated resistant mechanisms, by Rodreigo E Mendes, et al. Drug resist update t. 2014

[54] Linezolid resistant enterococci in Polish hospitals; species, clonality and determinants of linezolid resistance by I. Gawryszewska, D. zabicka, E. Sadowy. European journal of clinical microbiology and infectious diseases.

[55] Molecular Investigations of linezolid investigations in enterococci octravariants from a hospital In Shanghai by Pei li et al. infect drug resist. 2020

[56] A Review of mechanism of action, Resistance, Synergism and clinical implications of Mupirocin against *S. aureus*, by Saeed Khoshnood, Mohsen Heidary, Arezoo Asadi, Saleh Soleimani, Moloudsadat Motahar, Mohammad savri, Morteza Saki, Mohtab abdi, Biomedicine and Pharmacotherapy109, 1809-1818, 2019

[57] The emergence of Mupirocin resistance: A challenge to infection control and antibiotic prescribing practice, by D D Cookson Journal of Antimicrobial Chemotherapy 1998.

[58] Nasal Carriage And Antibiogram of *Staphylococcus Aureus* Amidst Healthcare Personnel From A Teaching Hospital In Coastal Karnataka,India. By F.Raseena,S Bhat,A Bhat-European Journal of Molecular and Clinical Medicine 7 (2),4820-4826,2020.

[59] Fusidic acid resistance through changes in dynamics of drug target.By – J H Tomlinson, A P kalverda, Antonio N Calabrese. Proceedings of the national academy of sciences 117 (41),25523-25531,2020

[60] Resistance of Fusidic Acid, by JOHN TURNIDGE, Peter Collignon, International Journal of Antimicrobial agents 12, S35, S44, 1999

[61] Fusidic Resistance in Staphylococcal aureus, by D Dobie, J Gray, Archives of diseases in childhood 89(1), 74, 2004

[62] Lei J, Sun L, Huang S, et al. The antimicrobial peptides and their potential clinical applications. Am J Transl Res. 2019;11(7):3919-3931. Published 2019 Jul 15.

[63] Kościuczuk EM, Lisowski P, Jarczak J, Strzałkowska N, Jóźwik A, Horbańczuk J, Krzyżewski J, Zwierzchowski L, Bagnicka E. Cathelicidins: family of antimicrobial peptides. A review. Mol Biol Rep. 2012 Dec;39(12):10957-70. doi: 10.1007/s11033-012-1997-x. Epub 2012 Oct 14. PMID: 23065264; PMCID: PMC3487008.

[64] Muthuirulan Pushpanathan, Paramasamy Gunasekaran, Jeyaprakash Rajendhran, "Antimicrobial Peptides: Versatile Biological Properties", International Journal of Peptides, vol. 2013, Article ID 675391, 15 pages, 2013. https://doi.org/10.1155/2013/675391

[65] Yuchen Huan, Qing Kong, Haijin Mou and Huaxi Yi " Antimicrobial peptides: Classification, Design, Application and Research Progress in

Multiple fields" Front. Microbiol. 16 Oct 2020. Vol 11. https://doi.org/10.3389/fmicb.2020.582779

[66] Jun Lei, Lichun Sun, Siyu Huang et al " The Antimicrobial Peptides and their potential clinical applications" AM J Transl Res 2019; 11(7): 3919-3931.

[67] Akash Gupta, Shazia Mumtaz, Cheng-Husan Li, Irshad Hussain and Vincent M. Rotello " Combatting Antibiotic-Resistant Bacteria Using Nanomaterials" Chem Soc Rev. 2019 Jan 21; 48(2): 415-427.

[68] Torchilin VP, Nat. Rev. Drug Discov, 2014, 13, 813-827. [PubMed: 25287120]

[69] Hajipour M.J., Fromm, K.M., Ashkarran, A.A., Jimenez De Aberasturi, D., De Larramendi, I R., Roj, T., et al. "Antibacterial properties of Nanoparticles" Trends Biotechnolo. 2017, 30, 499-511.

[70] Hemeg, H.A. "Nanomaterials for alternative antibacterial therapy". Int. J Nanomed, 2017 12, 8211-8255

[71] Ouwehand AC, Forssten S, Hibberd AA, Lyra A, Stahl B. Probiotic approach to prevent antibiotic resistance. Ann Med. 2016;48(4):246-255. doi: 10.3109/07853890.2016.1161232. Epub 2016 Mar 26. PMID: 27092975.

[72] Ansari, Shamshul, Jha, Rajesh Kumar, Mishra, Shyam Kumar, Tiwari, Birendra Raj, Asaad, Ahmed Morad "Recent advances in *staphylococcus aureus* infection: Focus on vaccine development" Infection and Drug Resistance. 2019; 12: 1243-1255

Chapter 2

Genetic Diversity in *Staphylococcus aureus* and Its Relation to Biofilm Production

Furqan Awan, Muhammad Muddassir Ali, Muhammad Hassan Mushtaq and Muhammad Ijaz

Abstract

Staphylococcus aureus (*S. aureus*) has been a substantial economic problem due to its antibiotic resistance, persistence inside host and recurrence of disease. It escapes from immunity because of its intra-cellular growth. Moreover, it forms biofilm on both living and in-animate surfaces that leads to recurrent infections and growth in food industry, respectively. Further, *S. aureus* undergoes the vertical and horizontal evolution that has genetically diversified the bacterial population. All the factors such as point mutations, plasmids, phages etc. have played their roles in diversifying this bacterium. Many bacterial physiological characteristics have been affected by genetic diversity. Biofilm forming ability is also considered as a variable characteristic of *S. aureus* that can help the bacteria to survive in different environments with different levels of biofilm production. In adapting the environment, *S. aureus* also forms different types of biofilm for its better survival. How genetic diversity is playing its role in this division of *S. aureus* is yet to be revealed. This chapter focuses on the factors related to genetic diversity and biofilm formation of *S. aureus*.

Keywords: Genetic diversity, Non-synonymous mutations, ica-operon, biofilm production, agr-operon

1. Introduction

Staphylococcus aureus is a mammalian commensal [1] that colonizes mucosal membranes of its hosts around the world. The virulent *S. aureus* strains promote infections by producing potent protein toxins, colonizing factors and cell surface proteins that inactivate antibodies [2]. Contrastingly, genetic diversity in the *S. aureus* causes the variation in disease severity of the clinical strains [3]. This genetic diversity among *S. aureus* population around the world suggests the variation in spatial distribution. The development of different techniques such as multi-locus sequence typing (MLST) [4], Pulsed-field gel electrophoresis (PFGE) [5], and core genome phylogenetic reconstruction [6] have facilitated analysis of the genetic diversity in *S. aureus* population. MLST is commonly used to understand the *S. aureus* lineages [7]. It relies on the allelic profiles of housekeeping genes present throughout the core genome [8]. Previous studies showed that *S. aureus* population structure is composed of limited clonal complexes (CCs) that further comprises of new sequence types (STs) [9]. ST precisely defines a strain with a unique allelic profile that have descended from the same recent common ancestor. Such ST types indicate the evolution based on point mutations. Additionally, recombination also appears to have played a relatively minor role in shaping *S. aureus* population [10]. Such techniques and studies are well suited to undermine the global epidemiology and genetic diversity of *S. aureus* population [11].

S. aureus infections can be recurred and costs for a long-term treatment along with productivity losses [12]. This recurrence is the result of biofilm formation and persistence inside body. Similarly, *S. aureus* biofilms also poses a major problem in the device-related infections (DRIs) [13]. Biofilms provides a shelter to *S. aureus* that resist antibiotics and other cellular immunity defenses [14]. *S. aureus* biofilms are more potent as it can be formed on the fomites, pipelines in the food industry and on the skin [15]. In this way, biofilms can also act as source of spread for long term without being observed. Recent findings have shown that staphylococcal biofilm mechanisms are adaptable to the environmental changes and help the pathogen in adherence to the surfaces at any cost [12]. Genetic diversity could be one of the influencers among the biofilm production ability of this pathogen [16]. A deep understanding of mechanisms for such variation in biofilm production is yet to be discovered.

Here we will review how diversity has affected the *Staphylococcus aureus* population structure and its biofilm mechanisms.

2. Mechanism of genetic diversity in *S. aureus*

The architecture of *S. aureus* population is mainly based on its genetic markers. Its genome consists of a single chromosome of 2.7–3.1 Mbp [17]; mainly represents the core genome that undergoes the vertical evolution. While accessory genome is dominated by mobile genetic elements (MGE) that include plasmids, transposons, phages and insertion sequences (IS) [18]. Horizontal evolution in MGE is driving the genetic diversity in this fraction of genome. Therefore, diversity in *S. aureus* population include a highly varying accessory/disposable genome with variable distribution of antimicrobial resistance (AMR) genes, virulence factors (VF), sequence types (ST), and clonal complex (CC)-specific pathogenic potentials [19]. The causes of genetic diversity among *S. aureus* strains are: vertical evolution (mutation) [20] and horizontal evolution (transformation, conjugation, transduction, and transposition) [18].

2.1 Vertical evolution and genetic diversity

The majority of *Staphylococcus aureus* population has highly conserved core genome [21, 22] that has evolved mainly through mutations. This conserved core genome can further undergo to single nucleotide polymorphisms and SCV formation. Such mutations are detected by MLST of selected housekeeping genes (*arc, aroE, glpF, gmk, pta, tpi, yqiL*) or through whole-genome sequencing that helps the researchers to identify the phylogenetic relations in *S. aureus* populations. According to the pubmlst database, there are 632,297 allele sequences in the 35,804 isolates. Furthermore, there are total 6569 MLST types divided into 10 clonal complexes including the untypeable clonal complex [4]. However, mutations in core genome points at the continuous evolution of this bacterial pathogen.

Previous studies have mentioned the synonymous and non-synonymous mutations in bacterial genomes as two main types of mutations [23]. Synonymous mutations are mostly less diversifying and cause least impact due to presence of amino acids against different pairs of codons and introduction of amino acid from same groups [24]. Thus, these mutations are considered as mostly harmless for bacterial physiology. The other mutation type is non-synonymous mutation that causes gene rupturing by introducing a stop codon that further leads to significant changes in bacterial physiology [25]. Among *S. aureus* population, nonsynonymous mutations generate the irreversible small colony variants (SCVs) that play main role in this genetic diversity [26]. Irreversible mutations introduced in such variants are mainly shaped by parallel evolution and are generated due to environmental stress factors such as cationic peptides, oxidative stress, low pH, bacterial competition [27]. These SCVs have attributes of high biofilm formation, antibiotic resistance and low metabolism that reduce the cure rates [16, 28, 29]. Human joint infections, cystic fibrosis in lungs, and bovine chronic mastitis are some common examples [30]. Studying the underlying mechanisms is important to assess the physiological processes and genetic diversity.

Some recent reports have determined that *S. aureus* also undergo genome reduction similar to mycobacterium spp. [31]. Genome reduction is mainly caused by removal of the ruptured genes and pseudo genes that eventually shortens the genome size [31]. A recent example of such genome reduction in *S. aureus* is isolates from ST-228 that are believe to lose 522 genes in their history of evolution [21]. It can be estimated that persistence of *S. aureus* in an environment for very long time causes genome reduction. The possible reason behind this is the least utilization of genes that are not required in that particular environment [31]. In other words, these proteins could have evolved to fulfill specific nonessential innovations and hence could easily be lost in reductive evolutions. Such complex genetic diversity also points at the continuous evolution of this *S. aureus*. A deep understanding of the mechanisms behind this evolution and genetic diversity is required.

2.2 Horizontal evolution and genetic diversity

The accessory genome is highly diverse among *S. aureus* populations [9]. It mainly encodes proteins necessary for bacteria's adaptation to various environmental conditions via resistance genes or virulence factor [14]. Such exogenous genes are often shared by other bacteria/environment therefore containing different rate of G-C in as compared to the core genome [32]. Generally, these exogenous genes can be obtained through one or multiple ways of horizontal evolution such as transformation, conjugation, transduction, and transposition. The mobile genetic elements (MGEs) are responsible for such kind of genes transfer. MGEs prevalent in *S. aureus* population include plasmids, transposable elements, bacteriophages, and pathogenic islands [18]. A deep knowledge of these MGEs and their mobility methods are of great concern for understanding the horizontal evolution.

2.2.1 Plasmids and their role in genetic diversity

Plasmids are small self-replicating DNA molecules (ranging 1–60 kbp) that can be transferred from one bacterium to other [18]. *S. aureus* has three classes of plasmids based on their sizes and other properties. Class I plasmids include small sized (<4.6 kbp) but multicopy plasmids often with a single resistance determinant [33]. Such type of plasmids is never reported to bear transposons or prophages [34]. Class II plasmids are of intermediate size (15–46 kbp) with lesser number of copies as compared to class I [33]. But some of the plasmids included in this class are antibiotic resistance plasmids such as pencillinase and aminoglycoside resistance plasmids [35]. In addition, there are different resistances genes do present on this kind of plasmids. Class III consisted of large and complex plasmids with determinant of transfer (*tra*) by conjugation along with different combinations of resistant markers [36]. Such plasmids also possess few transposons and insertion sequences.

Staphylococcus aureus strains commonly resist against Penicillin and glycopeptides such as vancomycin [15]. The resistance to methicillin is commanded by the *mecA* gene, responsible of the 76 kDa penicillin binding protein (PBP) synthesis. This protein with a low affinity to β-lactams is called PBP 2′ or PBP 2a [37]. The *blaZ* gene encodes for β-lactamase in *S. aureus* strains and both the two adjacent regulatory genes *blaI* (repressor) and *blaR1* (antirepressor) control this gene [38]. There are five different phenotypes of resistance genes (*vanA*, *vanB*, *vanC*, *vanD* and *vanE*) to vancomycin in enterococci [39]. *vanA* and *vanB* resistance operons in the plasmids possess the Tn1546-like and Tn1547 transposon elements [40].

2.2.2 Transposable elements (Tn) and insertion sequences (IS)

The genome of *S. aureus* carries heterogeneous MGE. The mobile genetic elements contain insertion sequences (IS), transposons (Tn), and transposon-like elements [40]. These mobile genetic elements are involved in evolution of bacteria and these can be found on chromosomes as single or multiple copies. MGE can also be found in association of other genetic elements.

IS sequences are the segments of DNA which can be transposed from one site of genome to another [18]. The genetic information required for their transposition is carried by these transposable elements. They are responsible for the recombination and stabilization of some genes which are responsible for resistance, though they do not code for resistance. These IS sequences are responsible for inducing changes in the expression levels of chromosomal genes and thus are very important in the process of evolution of the bacterial genome [41]. IS sequences can affect the transcription of other genes which are nearby, either by direct insertion or by polar effect, in order to inactivate them. IS sequences which also contain some other genes are called as composite transposons i.e. Tn4001 and Tn4003 which are composite transposons are known to contain IS256 and IS257 respectively which mediate resistance to gentamycin (Gmr), kanamycin (Kmr), and tobramycin (Tmr) [18]. IS256 and IS257 on styphylococcal chromosome have been observed in both contiguous and independent form. It suggested that these genetic elements in the genome may have a role in molecular rearrangements. The circular chromosome of *S. aureus* contains two copies of IS257. The recombination of either of IS257s of the plasmid (pJ3356) mediating ertgromycin resistance, in the pOX7 has been observed.

Transoposons present in staphylococcal genome are relatively small and they carry genes for resistance. Tn552 carries 'bla' gene for pencillinase and Tn554 carries gene for resiatance against spectinomycin, erythromycin and mactolide-lincosamide-streptogramin B [18, 40]. These elements are present in staphylococal cassette chromosome, plasmids or on the chromosome in multiple copies. Two copies of transposon 554 (Tn544) are commonly observed in N315, Mu50 and MRSA252 genome, while three addition copies were reported in N315 genome [33]. A unique conjugative transposon i.e., Tn5801 that carries '*tetM*' gene mediating resistance to tetracycline and minocycline was found in Mu50 genome. The single copies of transposons which are larger than 18 kbp are rare to find relatively. They encode genes mediating resistance to tetracycline, trimethoprim, aminoglycosides, or vancomycin. A specific transposon is present on the penicillinase plasmid (pl524) which carries methicillin resistance gene.

2.2.3 Bacteriophages and S. aureus *diversity*

The presence of mobile genetic elements, especially prophages, help to determine the diversity of *S. aureus* species [34]. Both the horizontal and vertical evolutions are closely linked to phages. In horizontal evolution, the phages being a mobile genetic element can be transferred to the recipient bacterial cell present in the environment. The prophages carry the many accessory genes in their genomes that are responsible for staphylococcal virulence factors and help in the survival of certain *S. aureus* strains [34, 42, 43]. The phages aid in the genomic island induction and its transfer. Additionally, phage transduction also transfers plasmids and chromosomal markers. Phages, in this way, diversify the *S. aureus* population and directs the horizontal evolution.

Currently, *S. aureus* strains isolated from non-human mammals are being sequenced and studied. Such strains have been shown adaptation to different host species through mutations in the core genome and through potential phage-encoded virulence genes [34]. Recent examples are the cattle-associated strains that were shown to originate in humans [43]. Furthermore, isolates from birds were shown to possess Sa3int phages with unique genes [44]. Therefore, phages are believed to be the one of the tools for host-diversification.

The phages are often regarded as selfish elements even though bacteria are utilizing them for their own survival. In this context, lysogeny could only serve as a short-term strategy of evolution. There are many reports indicating that phages provide *S. aureus* with additional genes that allow them to survive and persist. Several genes are the examples of introduction such as Panton-Valentine leukocidin (*lukSF*), exfoliative toxin A (*eta*), cell wall anchored *SasX* protein and the immune evasion group (IEC) composed of enterotoxin S (*mar*), staphylokinase (*sak*), the chemotaxis inhibitor protein (*chp*) and the inhibitor of the staphylococcal complement (*scn*) [45]. Such gene transfers between species and between different strains is limited due to receptor modifications in restriction barrier and phage exclusion. These effects most likely play an important role in species diversification of staphylococci. Hence, deeper insights into phage biology will be beneficial in understanding bacterial evolution.

3. Biofilm formation in *S. aureus* population

Biofilm production in *S. aureus* is comprised of three-steps. In each step, there is distinct bacterial physiology with expression of different sets of genes [46]. These steps can be described as follows: (i) initial attachment; (ii) colonization; and (iii) dispersion [47, 48]. In the initial attachment step, bacterial cells attach to the surfaces (6 h–11 h). This step is characterized by active metabolism of the bacterial cells and higher production of adhesion factors. In maturation step, the biofilm production is increased due to bacterial multiplication (18 h). During this step, metabolically active cells and slow metabolism cells both are present and subject to QS signals gene expression changes. At this step, persister cells can be found here. In the third and last step, upon finding the favorable conditions, the metabolically active cells separate from the colonies and begin to function as free cells [49]. Gene expression changes also force the bacteria to decrease the biofilm production [50]. Biofilm production in *S. aureus* is a complex phenomenon that secures this pathogen from environmental stress factors.

3.1 Role of outer surface proteins

Outer surface proteins play a very important role in initial adhesion and helps bacteria to adhere any surface; playing an important part in beginning of biofilm formation. Previous studies have focused on human isolated bacteria and whole proteome comparison of biofilm and planktonic states of *S. aureus* [47, 51]. But recent studies have shown that MRSA can also form a varying form of protein based biofilm that is not present in other *S. aureus* bacteria [52]. This difference includes the biofilm components, outer surface protein expression and encoding operons. For example, *S. aureus* can produce two types of biofilms (i) ica-operon dependant/ Polysaccharide intercellular adhesion-based biofilm (ii) ica-operon independent biofilm [13, 53]. Ica-operon independent biofilm is important for persistence in Hospital Associated infections (HA-MRSA) that is structurally different to the former type of biofilm. Hence drugs designed for the former type of biofilm might be not suitable for this type. This implicates that the drugs designed for other *S. aureus* biofilms will not be effective for native or highly antibiotic resistant strains.

Surface proteins are mainly classified into structural based classified groups (i) microbial surface component recognizing adhesive matrix molecule (MSCRAMM) (ii) Near iron transporter (NEAT) motif proteins. (iii) Three-helical bundle proteins (iv) G5–E repeat family (v) Structurally uncharacterized proteins [54]. Among these the last group is least studied and has potentially important proteins such as biofilm associated protein (bap). In this group, SasL and SasD proteins are also included that are expected to have important role in pathogenicity and biofilm formation [55]. But there are still no studies regarding gene mutation and characterization. Furthermore, all the proteins in this fraction are never studied for their role in ica-independent biofilm formation.

3.2 Quorum-sensing regulation system and biofilm formation

In Staphylococci spp., accessory gene regulator (agr) system acts as a main quorum sensing (QS) regulating system. Another QS regulation system i.e., luxS regulating system is also present but its role is less significant in the physiology of this bacteria [56]. Autoinducing peptide (AIPs) forms basis of agr-mediated QS system and acts as main signal peptides that regulates the biofilm formation and virulence. The main functions of agr mediated QS system are to sense the bacterial cell density in the surrounding environment and to respond with genetic adaptations.

S. aureus possess four main genes in the agr-operon such as agrA, agrB, agrC, agrD and divergent transcriptional units, such as RNAII and RNAIII, with promoter-2 (P2) and promoter-3 (P3), respectively. agrD gene in this operon produces a small oligopeptide that further undergoes maturation and transported in extracellular environment via agrB [57, 58]. These mature oligopeptides act as AIs in the extracellular environments. After reaching a certain threshold value, these AIs interacts with extracellular segment of histidine kinase, agrC. This agrC acts as a transmembrane receptor which activates the kinase leading to phosphorylation of agrA response regulator; resulting in the expression of biofilm related genes [59]. This activated agrA regulates the promoters P2 and P3 that further activates or deactivates transcriptional units.

It has been determined to maintain a balance between production of virulence factors and biofilm formation. The *agr* based QS system plays a major role in the dispersion step of biofilm formation [60]. Because agr system activation supports the free-living and more mobile lifestyle. On the other hand, its deactivation supports the colonization and sessile lifestyle. Therefore, *agr* mutants are shown to form a higher biofilm production as compared to the wild type. As mentioned, this increased biofilm production and thickness is associated with the inability of cells in dispersion from the mature biofilm. Thus production of factors that stops the bacteria to enter into mobile phase and not due to cell growth or death [61]. However, this agr-QS system needs a deep understanding of pathways and mechanisms.

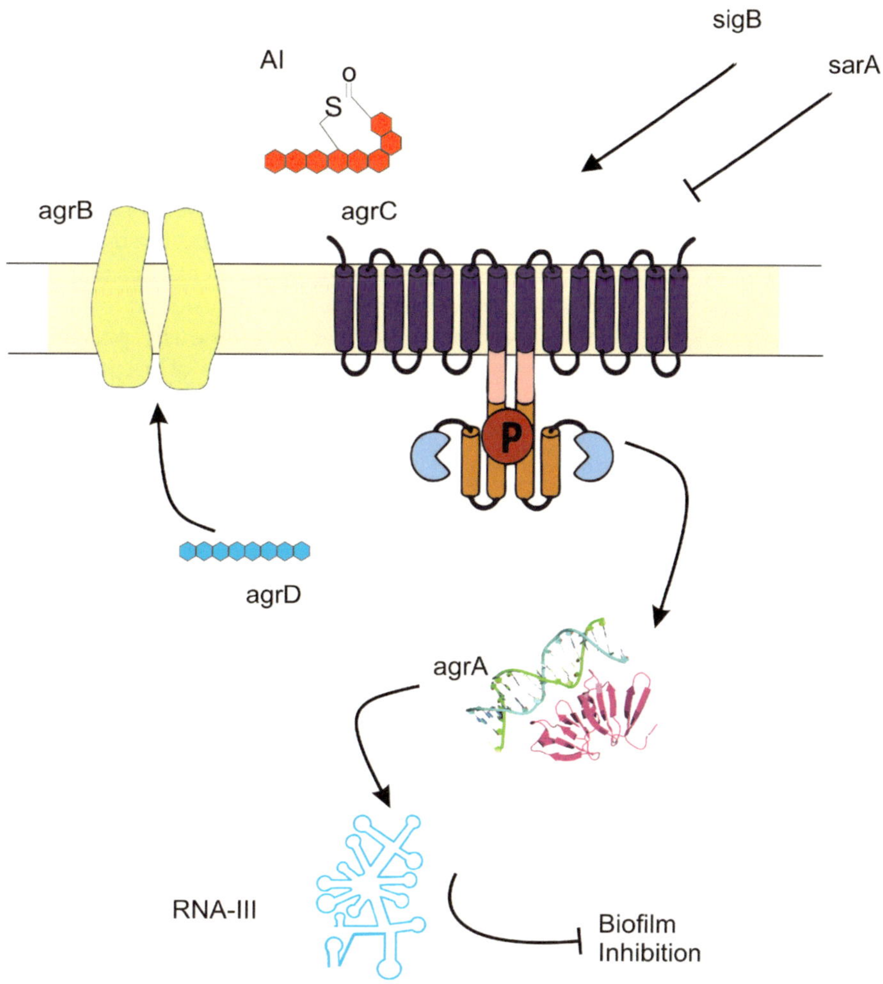

Figure 1.
Regulatory networks in biofilm formation. Sigma factor B (SigB) inhibits agr expression, while SarA has been shown to directly enhance it [62].

3.2.1 Role of alternative sigma B (sigB) operon and agr operon

Alternative sigma B (sigB) factor-regulated genes include those involved in general stress response, virulence, capsule formation, and biofilm formation (**Figure 1**) [62]. sigB operon is composed of *rsbU, rsbV, rsbW,* and *sigB* genes. It represses the agr operon that is important in depressing the biofilm production. Disruption of any gene from this operon could result in mal-function and enhance the biofilm production. Recently, this operon found to be playing an important role in counterfeiting the oxidation stress in *S. aureus* that are very important risk factors for mastitis infections.

4. How genetic diversity affects the biofilm production

Biofilm forming ability is a variable characteristic of Staph aureus that can categorize the bacteria into different categories such as level of biofilm formation, certain STs with high biofilm formation and types of biofilm formation (discussed earlier).

4.1 Relation of MLST with biofilm production

There is a proposal that genetic diversity could affect the biofilm production. A recent study has demonstrated that MLST types such as ST59 and ST188 isolated from human and canine sources were found to be associated with strong biofilm production [15]. This shows that the biofilm production capacity is strongly affected by evolutionary process that changed the biofilm production among different strain types. Parallel evolution could vary the biofilm production by introducing new mutations. But the genes and pathways in specific sequence types related to biofilm production affected by parallel evolution are not well understood. Further studies are underway to reveal this relation. As discussed previously, parallel evolution could help in emergence of new strains but its relation to biofilm production is still unknown.

4.2 Level of biofilm formation

Level of biofilm formation is another complex mechanism that shows the diversity among the strains and within the member of strains [46]. There are multiple estimations that can explain these variations [46, 50]. But most importantly these variations in expression of genes are associated with the environmental signals [63]. For instance, some bacterial cells in same colony can produce PNAG to capture water [13]. On the other hand, some pathways like c-di-AMP respond to external environmental chemicals such as glucose and drop in biofilm formation is measured [64]. Biofilm formation and eDNA release from bacterial cells are triggered by significant reduction in c-di-AMP levels and this reduction is related to low *agr* operon expression [65]. Importantly, *gdpP, xdrA* and *apt* genes also play important role in biofilm formation [66]. Although this pathway shifting is notified but environmental factors that drive this reduction in agr operon expression are still under study.

4.3 Types of biofilm

S. aureus biofilms can be classified as ica-dependent and ica-independent based on their matrix composition. Biofilm matrix composition in ica-dependent biofilms is synthesized by the icaADBC operon that is composed of polysaccharide intercellular adhesion (PIA) or polymeric N-acetylglucosamine (PNAG). On the other hand, ica-independent biofilms are further consisting of three types of biofilms based on their biofilm matrix. Protein/e-DNA biofilm, Fibrin biofilm, and Amyloid biofilm are included in this ica-independent classification (**Table 1**). There is an interesting comparison of biofilm types among MSSA and MRSA isolates also exists. It was reported that ica-dependant biofilm was more common in MSSA while ica-independent biofilms were more frequently observed among MRSA isolates [67]. It is possible that multiple types are present at same place [47]. *S. aureus* biofilms can be found everywhere in body after inoculation. These biofilms could of different types with different EPS, places of origin, and genes/operon controlling them.

5. Role of biofilm environment itself in SCV generation

Biofilm acts like a micro-environment with its own conditions and stressors. There are many studies demonstrated that chronic cases with biofilm formation for a certain period of time also cause the mutation in genomes via natural selection or parallel evolution [68–71]. This reshaping of genome could result in non-synonymous mutations or shortening of genome. In chronic mastitis, *S. aureus*

Characteristics	Polysaccharide-type biofilm	Protein/e-DNA biofilm	Fibrin biofilm	Amyloid biofilm	References
Extracellular Polymeric Substance (EPS)	Poly-N-acetylglucosamine (PNAG)/ Polysaccharide intercellular adhesin (PIA)	Autolysin-mediated release of cytoplasmic proteins and extracellular DNA	Coagulase-mediated fibrin production	Phenol-soluble modules and amyloid accumulation	[10, 64]
Gene/operon	Intracellular adhesion (icaADBC) operon	Surface proteins i.e. Bap, FnBPs, Aap/SasG etc.	Coagulase gene (*coa*) and von Willebrand factor binding protein (*vWbp*)	*psmα1-4*, *psmβ1-2*, *pmt* operon, SaeRS-two component system	[43, 48]
Location	Skin with higher NaCl concentrations and lower water availability	Low pH regions (e.g., urinary tract, vagina, mouth, and skin)	Inside blood or regions with fibrinogen	Iron- and nutrient-limiting conditions in blood.	[10, 65]

Table 1.
Comparison of different types of S. aureus *biofilms. Polysaccharide type biofilm is only considered as ica-dependent biofilm while all the remaining are considered as ica-independent biofilms.*

also form biofilm and remains sub-clinical for very long time that could be helpful in causing non-synonymous mutations. Non-synonymous mutations often also involve the introduction of stop codons that disrupt the gene leading to non-functional or pseudogene formation. Loss in gene function irreversibly changes the phenotype of bacterium. This newly formed phenotype could be more antibiotic resistant, highly biofilm forming or reduced metabolic form of persisters [72–74]. This phenotypic variation should be considered during therapeutic developments and treatment regimes. Hence, it is necessary to study and mimic those conditions to understand which genes undergo mutation formation.

6. Role of SCVs in persistence

Biofilm formation helps the *S. aureus* to persist and multiply sub-clinically in inhospitable environment. As mentioned earlier, the Small Colony Variants (SCV) phenotype are found potentially responsible for the sub-clinical and chronic infections. Such SCVs phenotypes share some common features of slow-growth and quasi-dormancy with low virulence potential [75]. SCVs further express some distinctive features such as small colony formation, a dormant metabolism, less enzymatic activities, and elevated antibiotic resistance [76]. Such SCVs are mostly point mutations in the important genes. Therefore, during proof-reading mechanisms, SCVs can be return to a wild-type (WT) or converted to a different phenotype. Later, clinically observed phenotypes are stable and permanent genetic changes showing irreversible SCVs. Such irreversible SCVs are examples of parallel evolution or evolution with-in population [77]. External environmental stress factors can also trigger the emergence of SCVs such as reactive oxygen species, low pH, cationic peptides, limited nutrition and bacterial biofilm competition [78, 79].

SCVs can be generated spontaneously under any sub-clinical and chronic disease condition. Considering bovine mastitis as an example, SCVs will be discussed now. The detection of mastitis origin SCVs, especially permanent genetic changes within population, in routine laboratories and their accurate studies in research laboratories are challenges not overcome yet. Among these mastitis studies, such isolates were also found positive for biofilm producing genes i.e., ica operon, adhesive proteins, bap operon [80]. According to a study based on different food samples, approximately 72% of the isolates produced biofilms. As discussed above, biofilm producing *S. aureus* are really important in chronic and sub-clinical mastitis infection. Moreover, a few studies have also studied the SCVs formed and found that SCVs formed can cause different level of mastitis based on their severity. Another study has also pointed out the isolation of *S. aureus* irreversible mutation variant from dairy cows in Yunnan province that was responsible for chronic mastitis [26]. This mutation was found in thymine related pathway that promotes the resistance against Sulfamethoxazole (SXT) and helps the bacterium to develop in fibrotic conditions. Similarly, a Beijing based study described the slow growth, antibiotic resistance and chronic mastitis as features of isolated irreversible thymidine SCV [81]. Most of the studies have focused on the antibiotic resistance profiles of *S. aureus* isolated from mastitis infection. On the other hand, there are very few studies that determined the SCVs and relation of chronic sub-clinical mastitis. Additionally, in Austria, a study related to chronic mastitis also revealed that irreversible mutations in rsbU, one of sigB genes, generated from SCVs caused the bacterium to persist and resist the therapy [16]. Further, SCVs related to regulatory circuits have also been revealed such as agr genes, hemin (hemB), menadione (menD), α-Toxin (hla), γ-Hemolysin (hld), Coagulase (coa), L-lactose dehydrogenase (ldh), Alcohol dehydrogenase (adh), Arginine deiminase (arcA), Capsular biosynthesis (capA) and Alkaline shock Proteins (Asp) [82]. Some experimental studies have reported the induction of SCVs by growing *S. aureus* with antimicrobial peptides, and magnesium ions (Mg^{+2}). Further these studies have also mentioned the need of in vivo experiments for complete understanding. This indicates that there is lack of animal experiments based comprehensive studies explaining the factors of this within population and parallel evolution.

7. Conclusions

Genetic diversity can generate new strains and ST types that behave like a different bacterium. Both horizontal and vertical evolutions are the ways to genetic diversity that can help the *S. aureus* to survive under various environments. Biofilm formation ability is also affected by the genetic diversity and can help our pathogen in not only surviving but also in pathogenesis. Plasmids, bacteriophages, Tn and IS elements are much more faster ways of evolution as compared to SCVs and point mutations. SCVs generation could be a slow phenomenon but once these are generated their characteristics can change the behavior of *S. aureus*. Understanding these mechanisms underlying these evolutions could help us in designing suitable strategies and anti-biofilm therapies against *S. aureus*.

Conflict of interest

The authors declare no conflict of interest.

Author details

Furqan Awan[1*], Muhammad Muddassir Ali[2], Muhammad Hassan Mushtaq[1] and Muhammad Ijaz[3]

1 Department of Epidemiology and Public Health, University of Veterinary and Animal Sciences, Lahore, Pakistan

2 Institute of Biochemistry and Biotechnology, University of Veterinary and Animal Sciences, Lahore, Pakistan

3 Department of Clinical Medicine and Surgery, University of Veterinary and Animal Sciences, Lahore, Pakistan

*Address all correspondence to: furqanvet@gmail.com

References

[1] Parlet CP, Brown MM, Horswill AR. Commensal Staphylococci Influence Staphylococcus aureus Skin Colonization and Disease. Trends Microbiol 2019; 27:497-507.

[2] Sieber RN, Skov RL, Nielsen J, et al. Drivers and Dynamics of Methicillin-Resistant Livestock-Associated *Staphylococcus aureus* CC398 in Pigs and Humans in Denmark. mBio 2018; 9:e02142-18.

[3] Collins A, Wakeland EK, Raj P, et al. The impact of Staphylococcus aureus genomic variation on clinical phenotype of children with acute hematogenous osteomyelitis. Heliyon 2018; 4:e00674.

[4] Jolley KA, Bray JE, Maiden MCJ. Open-access bacterial population genomics: BIGSdb software, the PubMLST.org website and their applications. Wellcome Open Res 2018; 3:124.

[5] Neoh H-m, Tan X-E, Sapri HF, et al. Pulsed-field gel electrophoresis (PFGE): A review of the "gold standard" for bacteria typing and current alternatives. Infection, Genetics and Evolution 2019; 74:103935.

[6] Stott CM, Bobay L-M. Impact of homologous recombination on core genome phylogenies. BMC Genomics 2020; 21:829.

[7] Stegger M, Wirth T, Andersen PS, et al. Origin and Evolution of European Community-Acquired Methicillin-Resistant *Staphylococcus aureus*. mBio 2014; 5:e01044-e01014.

[8] Leekitcharoenphon P, Lukjancenko O, Friis C, et al. Genomic variation in Salmonella enterica core genes for epidemiological typing. BMC Genomics 2012; 13:88.

[9] Planet PJ, Narechania A, Chen L, et al. Architecture of a Species: Phylogenomics of *Staphylococcus aureus* Trends in Microbiology 2017; 25:153-166.

[10] Ritchie SR, Thomas MG, Rainey PB. The Genetic Structure of Staphylococcus aureus Populations from the Southwest Pacific. PLOS ONE 2014; 9:e100300.

[11] David MZ, Daum RS. Community-Associated Methicillin-Resistant Staphylococcus aureus: Epidemiology and Clinical Consequences of an Emerging Epidemic. Clin Microbiol Rev 2010; 23:616-687.

[12] Dauros-Singorenko P, Wiles S, Swift S. Staphylococcus aureus Biofilms and Their Response to a Relevant in vivo Iron Source. Front Microbiol 2020; 11:

[13] M Z, E ON, JP OG. Untangling the Diverse and Redundant Mechanisms of *Staphylococcus aureus* Biofilm Formation. PLoS Pathog 2016; 12:e1005671.

[14] Otto M. Staphylococcal Biofilms. Microbiology spectrum 2018; 6:10.1128/microbiolspec.GPP3-0023-2018.

[15] Chen L, Tang Z-Y, Cui S-Y, et al. Biofilm Production Ability, Virulence and Antimicrobial Resistance Genes in *Staphylococcus aureus* from Various Veterinary Hospitals. Pathogens 2020; 9:264.

[16] Marbach H, Mayer K, Vogl C, et al. Within-host evolution of bovine Staphylococcus aureus selects for a SigB-deficient pathotype characterized by reduced virulence but enhanced proteolytic activity and biofilm formation. Scientific reports 2019; 9:13479.

[17] Jaillard M, Lima L, Tournoud M, et al. A fast and agnostic method for bacterial genome-wide association studies: Bridging the gap between

k-mers and genetic events. PLoS genetics 2018; 14:e1007758-e1007758.

[18] Alibayov B, Baba-Moussa L, Sina H, et al. *Staphylococcus aureus* mobile genetic elements Mol Biol Rep 2014; 41:5005-5018.

[19] Lebeurre J, Dahyot S, Diene S, et al. Comparative Genome Analysis of Staphylococcus lugdunensis Shows Clonal Complex-Dependent Diversity of the Putative Virulence Factor, ess/Type VII Locus. Front Microbiol 2019; 10:

[20] Ram Y, Liberman U, Feldman MW. Evolution of vertical and oblique transmission under fluctuating selection. Proc Natl Acad Sci U S A 2018; 115:E1174-E1183.

[21] Bosi E, Monk JM, Aziz RK, et al. Comparative genome-scale modelling of Staphylococcus aureus strains identifies strain-specific metabolic capabilities linked to pathogenicity. DNA Research 2016; 113:E3801-E3809.

[22] Xia G, Wolz C. Phages of Staphylococcus aureus and their impact on host evolution. Infection, Genetics and Evolution 2014; 21:593-601.

[23] Chu D, Wei L. Nonsynonymous, synonymous and nonsense mutations in human cancer-related genes undergo stronger purifying selections than expectation. BMC Cancer 2019; 19:359.

[24] BłaŻej P, Wnetrzak M, Mackiewicz D, et al. The influence of different types of translational inaccuracies on the genetic code structure. BMC Bioinformatics 2019; 20:114.

[25] Proctor RA, André Kriegeskorte, Barbara C. Kahl, et al. Staphylococcus aureus Small Colony Variants (SCVs): a road map for the metabolic pathways involved in persistent infections. Frontiers in Cellular and Infection Microbiology 2014; 4:1-8.

[26] Zhu LL, Zou FC, Yan YL, et al. The Characteristics of Staphylococcus aureus Small Colony Variant Isolated from Chronic Mastitis at a Dairy Farm in Yunnan Province, China. The Scientific World Journal 2016; 2016:9157605.

[27] García-Contreras R, Nuñez-López L, Jasso-Chávez R, et al. Quorum sensing enhancement of the stress response promotes resistance to quorum quenching and prevents social cheating. Isme j 2015; 9:115-125.

[28] Rom JS, Atwood DN, Beenken KE, et al. Impact of Staphylococcus aureus regulatory mutations that modulate biofilm formation in the USA300 strain LAC on virulence in a murine bacteremia model. Virulence 2017; 8:1776-1790.

[29] Uhlemann AC, McAdam PR, Sullivan SB, et al. Evolutionary Dynamics of Pandemic Methicillin-Sensitive Staphylococcus aureus ST398 and Its International Spread via Routes of Human Migration. MBio 2017; 8:

[30] Kahl BC, Becker K, Löffler B. Clinical Significance and Pathogenesis of Staphylococcal Small Colony Variants in Persistent Infections. Clin Microbiol Rev 2016; 29:401-427.

[31] Kurokawa M, Seno S, Matsuda H, et al. Correlation between genome reduction and bacterial growth. DNA Research 2016; 23:517-525.

[32] Bohlin J, Eldholm V, Pettersson JHO, et al. The nucleotide composition of microbial genomes indicates differential patterns of selection on core and accessory genomes. BMC Genomics 2017; 18:151.

[33] Malachowa N, DeLeo FR. Mobile genetic elements of Staphylococcus aureus. Cellular and molecular life sciences : CMLS 2010; 67:3057-3071.

[34] Xia G, Wolz C. Phages of Staphylococcus aureus and their impact on host evolution. Infect Genet Evol 2014; 21:593-601.

[35] Bukowski M, Piwowarczyk R, Madry A, et al. Prevalence of Antibiotic and Heavy Metal Resistance Determinants and Virulence-Related Genetic Elements in Plasmids of *Staphylococcus aureus*. 2019; 10:

[36] Virolle C, Goldlust K, Djermoun S, et al. Plasmid Transfer by Conjugation in Gram-Negative Bacteria: From the Cellular to the Community Level. 2020; 11:1239.

[37] Fishovitz J, Hermoso JA, Chang M, et al. Penicillin-binding protein 2a of methicillin-resistant Staphylococcus aureus. IUBMB life 2014; 66:572-577.

[38] Olsen JE, Christensen H, Aarestrup FM. Diversity and evolution of blaZ from Staphylococcus aureus and coagulase-negative staphylococci. Journal of Antimicrobial Chemotherapy 2006; 57:450-460.

[39] Mirzaei B, Babaei R, Asiabar APD, et al. Detection of both vanA & vanB genes in vanA phenotypes of Enterococci by Taq Man RT-PCR. Brazilian journal of microbiology : [publication of the Brazilian Society for Microbiology] 2015; 46:161-165.

[40] Hegstad K, Mikalsen T, Coque TM, et al. Mobile genetic elements and their contribution to the emergence of antimicrobial resistant Enterococcus faecalis and Enterococcus faecium. Clinical Microbiology and Infection 2010; 16:541-554.

[41] Yebra G, Haag AF, Neamah MM, et al. Massive genome decay and expansion of insertion sequences drive the evolution of a novel host-restricted bacterial pathogen. bioRxiv 2020; 2020.10.13.331058.

[42] Fitzgerald JR, Holden MT. Genomics of Natural Populations of Staphylococcus aureus. Annu Rev Microbiol 2016; 70:459-478.

[43] Kraushaar B, Hammerl JA, Kienöl M, et al. Acquisition of virulence factors in livestock-associated MRSA: Lysogenic conversion of CC398 strains by virulence gene-containing phages. Scientific reports 2017; 7:2004-2004.

[44] Yoon H, Yun J, Lim J-A, et al. Characterization and genomic analysis of two Staphylococcus aureus bacteriophages isolated from poultry/livestock farms. The Journal of general virology 2013; 94:2569-2576.

[45] van Wamel WJB, Rooijakkers SHM, Ruyken M, et al. The innate immune modulators staphylococcal complement inhibitor and chemotaxis inhibitory protein of Staphylococcus aureus are located on beta-hemolysin-converting bacteriophages. Journal of bacteriology 2006; 188:1310-1315.

[46] Kot B, Sytykiewicz H, Sprawka I. Expression of the Biofilm-Associated Genes in Methicillin-Resistant Staphylococcus aureus in Biofilm and Planktonic Conditions. Int J Mol Sci 2018; 19:3487.

[47] Resch A, Leicht S, Saric M, et al. Comparative proteome analysis of Staphylococcus aureus biofilm and planktonic cells and correlation with transcriptome profiling. Proteomics 2006; 6:1867-1877.

[48] Hennig S, Nyunt Wai S, Ziebuhr W. Spontaneous switch to PIA-independent biofilm formation in an ica-positive Staphylococcus epidermidis isolate. International Journal of Medical Microbiology 2007; 297:117-122.

[49] Archer NK, Mazaitis MJ, Costerton JW, et al. Staphylococcus aureus biofilms-Properties, regulation

and roles in human disease. Virulence 2011; 2:445-459.

[50] Chaffin DO, Taylor D, Skerrett SJ, et al. Changes in the Staphylococcus aureus Transcriptome during Early Adaptation to the Lung. PLOS ONE 2012; 7:e41329.

[51] Kim SJ, Chang J, Rimal B, et al. Surface proteins and the formation of biofilms by Staphylococcus aureus. Biochimica et Biophysica Acta (BBA) - Biomembranes 2018; 1860:749-756.

[52] McCarthy H, Rudkin JK, Black NS, et al. Methicillin resistance and the biofilm phenotype in Staphylococcus aureus. Frontiers in cellular and infection microbiology 2015; 5:

[53] Figueiredo AMS, Ferreira FA, Beltrame CO, et al. The role of biofilms in persistent infections and factors involved in ica-independent biofilm development and gene regulation in Staphylococcus aureus. Critical Reviews in Microbiology 2017; 43:602-620.

[54] Foster TJ, Geoghegan JA, Ganesh VK, et al. Adhesion, invasion and evasion: the many functions of the surface proteins of Staphylococcus aureus. Nature reviews. Microbiology 2014; 12:49-62.

[55] Joo H-S, Otto M. Molecular basis of in vivo biofilm formation by bacterial pathogens. Chemistry & biology 2012; 19:1503-1513.

[56] Rutherford ST, Bassler BL. Bacterial quorum sensing: its role in virulence and possibilities for its control. Cold Spring Harbor perspectives in medicine 2012; 2:a012427.

[57] Butterfield JM, Tsuji BT, Brown J, et al. Predictors of agr Dysfunction in Methicillin-Resistant Staphylococcus aureus (MRSA) Isolates among Patients with MRSA Bloodstream Infections. Antimicrob Agents Chemother 2011; 55:5433-5437.

[58] Choudhary KS, Mih N, Monk J, et al. The Staphylococcus aureus Two-Component System AgrAC Displays Four Distinct Genomic Arrangements That Delineate Genomic Virulence Factor Signatures. Front Microbiol 2018; 9:1082.

[59] Sikdar R, Elias M. Quorum quenching enzymes and their effects on virulence, biofilm, and microbiomes: a review of recent advances. Expert Rev Anti Infect Ther 2020; 18:1221-1233.

[60] Uruén C, Chopo-Escuin G, Tommassen J, et al. Biofilms as Promoters of Bacterial Antibiotic Resistance and Tolerance. Antibiotics (Basel, Switzerland) 2020; 10:3.

[61] Zhou L, Zhang Y, Ge Y, et al. Regulatory Mechanisms and Promising Applications of Quorum Sensing-Inhibiting Agents in Control of Bacterial Biofilm Formation. Frontiers in microbiology 2020; 11:589640-589640.

[62] Paharik AE, Horswill AR. The Staphylococcal Biofilm: Adhesins, Regulation, and Host Response. Microbiology Spectrum 2016; 4:

[63] Ackermann M, Sikora-Wohlfeld W, Beyer A. Impact of Natural Genetic Variation on Gene Expression Dynamics. PLOS Genetics 2013; 9:e1003514.

[64] Purcell EB, Tamayo R. Cyclic diguanylate signaling in Gram-positive bacteria. FEMS Microbiology Reviews 2016; 40:753-773.

[65] Syed AK, Vickery CR, Lenhart T, et al. Biofilm Formation by *Staphylococcus aureus* is Triggered by a Drop in the Levels of the Second Messenger cyclic-di-AMP. bioRxiv 2020; 2020.01.31.929125.

[66] DeFrancesco AS, Masloboeva N, Syed AK, et al. Genome-wide screen for genes involved in eDNA release during biofilm formation by Staphylococcus aureus. Proc Natl Acad Sci U S A 2017; 201704544.

[67] Ferreira FA, Souza RR, Bonelli RR, et al. Comparison of in vitro and in vivo systems to study ica-independent Staphylococcus aureus biofilms. Journal of Microbiological Methods 2012; 88:393-398.

[68] Leiman SA, Arboleda LC, Spina JS, et al. SinR is a mutational target for fine-tuning biofilm formation in laboratory-evolved strains of Bacillus subtilis. BMC Microbiology 2014; 14:301.

[69] DeFrancesco AS, Masloboeva N, Syed AK, et al. Genome-wide screen for genes involved in eDNA release during biofilm formation by Staphylococcus aureus. Proc Natl Acad Sci USA 2017; 114:E5969-E5978.

[70] Guérillot R, Kostoulias X, Donovan L, et al. Unstable chromosome rearrangements in Staphylococcus aureus cause phenotype switching associated with persistent infections. Proc Natl Acad Sci USA 2019; 116:20135-20140.

[71] Irvine S, Bunk B, Bayes HK, et al. Genomic and transcriptomic characterization of Pseudomonas aeruginosa small colony variants derived from a chronic infection model. Microbial Genomics 2019; 5:

[72] Lieberman TD, Michel J-B, Aingaran M, et al. Parallel bacterial evolution within multiple patients identifies candidate pathogenicity genes. Nature Genetics 2011; 43:1275-1280.

[73] Vogwill T, Kojadinovic M, Furió V, et al. Testing the role of genetic background in parallel evolution using the comparative experimental evolution of antibiotic resistance. Molecular biology and evolution 2014; 31:3314-3323.

[74] Victoria J. Savage, Ian Chopra, O'Neill* AJ. Population Diversification in *Staphylococcus aureus* Biofilms May Promote Dissemination and Persistence. PLOS ONE 2013; 8:e62513.

[75] Atalla H, Gyles C, Mallard B. Staphylococcus aureus small colony variants (SCVs) and their role in disease. Animal Health Research Reviews 2011; 12:33-45.

[76] Loss G, Simões PM, Valour F, et al. Staphylococcus aureus Small Colony Variants (SCVs): News From a Chronic Prosthetic Joint Infection. Frontiers in cellular and infection microbiology 2019; 9:363-363.

[77] Schleimer N, Kaspar U, Drescher M, et al. The Energy-Coupling Factor Transporter Module EcfAA'T, a Novel Candidate for the Genetic Basis of Fatty Acid-Auxotrophic Small-Colony Variants of Staphylococcus aureus. Frontiers in microbiology 2018; 9:1863-1863.

[78] Tuchscherr L, Medina E, Hussain M, et al. Staphylococcus aureus phenotype switching: an effective bacterial strategy to escape host immune response and establish a chronic infection. EMBO Mol Med 2011; 3:129-141.

[79] Koch G, Yepes A, Forstner KU, et al. Evolution of resistance to a last-resort antibiotic in Staphylococcus aureus via bacterial competition. Cell 2014; 158:1060-1071.

[80] Yang F, Zhang SD, Shang XF, et al. Detection and molecular characterization of methicillin-resistant Staphylococcus aureus isolated from subclinical bovine mastitis cases in China. J Dairy Sci 2020; 103:840-845.

[81] Alkasir R, Liu XQ, Zahra M, et al. Characteristics of Staphylococcus aureus Small Colony Variant and Its Parent Strain Isolated from Chronic Mastitis at a Dairy Farm in Beijing, China. Microbial Drug Resistance 2013; 19:138-145.

[82] Yang X, Dong F, Qian S, et al. Accessory gene regulator (agr) dysfunction was unusual in Staphylococcus aureus isolated from Chinese children. BMC Microbiol 2019; 19:95.

Chapter 3

Staphylococcus aureus and Virulence-Related Small RNA

Rudra Mishra Awdhesh Kumar Mishra, Bhama Mishra Awdhesh Kumar Mishra, Nalini Easwaran and Kodiveri Muthukaliannan Gothandam

Abstract

Staphylococcus aureus causes a wide range of diseases, including both community-associated and hospital-acquired infections such as abscesses, wound infections, osteomyelitis, endocarditis and septicemia. Regulation of the expression of various virulence factors is initiated through complex coordination between two-component systems, transcriptional regulatory proteins and regulatory small RNAs (sRNAs). *S.aureus* uses many sRNA and RNA–RNA interactions mediated the regulation of the expression of genes post-transcriptionally, but it uses few sigma factors to initiate the transcription function. sRNA transcripts are encoded within intergenic regions or in antisense orientation to mRNA transcripts, and sRNA regulation plays a central role in the response to stress stimuli encountered by pathogens during infection. One of the most intriguing examples of sRNA-mediated post-transcriptional regulation is RNAIII from *S.aureus*, which interacts with and regulates various RNA targets involved in virulence. Several genes known to be regulated by RNAIII have been demonstrated to be regulated by the *sarA* locus, independent of its effect on the expression of RNAIII. We discuss the potential role of small RNA (sRNA) in the pathogenesis and virulence factors production of *Staphylococcus aureus*.

Keywords: *Staphylococcus aureus*, regulatory small RNA (sRNA), virulence factors, RNA–RNA interactions

1. Introduction

Staphylococcus aureus is a human symbiotic microorganism that commonly colonizes in the anterior nasal regions and on the skin surface for 20–25% of the world population [1–3]. The distribution of multi-drug resistant strains among asymptomatic individuals is responsible for spreading the infections among the population very quickly [4]. Among the human populations, the carriage percentages of *Staphylococcus aureus* vary based on different factors. Broadly human carriers are classified into three categories: 20% non-carriers, 25% persistent carriers, and 60% population are intermediate carriers [5]. Usually, *Staphylococcus aureus* forms colonization in the nasal passage and axillae in humans and found its occurrence as flora in vaginal tracts and digestive tracts [6].

Among the various factors responsible for the regulation of virulence, small RNA (sRNA) has a major role in determining the virulence of the bacteria. sRNA are short 50–250 nucleotide long transcripts involving bacterial gene expression

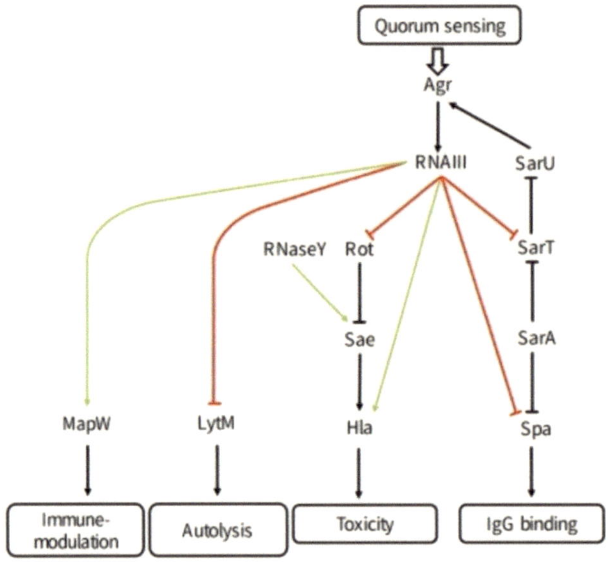

Figure 1.
Virulence factors regulation by RNAIII. RNAIII is regulated positively by the quorum-sensing agr operon. Post-transcriptional regulation is marked with colored lines, whereas up-regulation represented by green arrows and down-regulation by red cross bars. RNAIII in turn, positively regulates MapW and hla at a post-transcriptional level. MapW and hla prevents leucocyte attachment and promote dissemination by lysing host cells. RNAIII also negatively regulates LytM, rot, Spa and SarT, which will promote autolysis via LytM, blood cell toxicity by rot and expression of an IgG binding protein via SarT.

for rapid adaption to stress conditions. Small RNAs play a major role by pairing with bases of target mRNA or by interacting with the modulating proteins for both the positive and negative mechanism of biofilm formation. *Staphylococcus aureus* becomes more adherent resulting in increased biofilm formation when *agr* mediated mechanism is inhibited. Regulation of gene expression mediated by sRNAs is more beneficial when compared to proteins during a rapid response because it takes a short time for sRNAs to either synthesize or degrade. Various regulatory mechanism of sRNAs is similar to the regulation of quorum sensing in the bacteria. The quorum-sensing mechanism regulates the expression of virulence-related genes. Since the quorum sensing mechanism controls bacteria's virulence factor, it is considered a major target for finding out the new therapeutic methods [7]. We discuss the potential role of small RNA (sRNA) in the pathogenesis and virulence factors production of *Staphylococcus aureus* (**Figure 1**).

2. Bacterial small RNA

sRNAs mediate the regulation of mRNAs through direct binding interactions between the sRNA and the target. The sRNA usually binds to the 5′ end of the mRNA and blocks ribosomes binding. Although sRNAs often stimulate degradation of the target as well [8]. The interaction is initiated by a short sequence of perfect complementarity between the sRNA and target termed the seed region. Seed regions are generally 6–8 nt long, and a single sRNA can have one seed region that regulates all of its targets or multiple seed regions that each regulate a subset of targets. Additionally, seed regions are highly conserved, and mutations to the seed region lead to complete abrogation of target regulation. In order to facilitate intermolecular interactions with target mRNAs, seed regions are usually single-stranded in the folded sRNA and disruption of the sRNA secondary structure can drastically reduce sRNA function. However, seed regions alone are generally not sufficient to mediate target binding, most sRNA characterized to date rely on the assistance of an sRNA chaperone protein [9, 10].

The regulation mechanism for the SpoVG and SprX and their targets with interactions have been discussed below, which involves regulating virulence factors. Production of capsule, virulence factors, and the cell wall's metabolism is regulated by a transcription factor *SpoVG* also called a master regulator. It is also responsible for resistance against methicillin and glycopeptide antibiotics [11]. Synthesis of pentaglycine crosslinks between peptidoglycan strands carried out by *lytSR* operon and glycine glycyl transferases is positively regulated by SpoVG, whereas murein hydrolysate lytN regulated negatively. Base pairing of *sprX* (Highly conserved RNA) with the *SpoVG* mRNA during the translation process prevents loading of the ribosome. Small RNA *sprX* negatively regulated *SpoVG*, in four phases of exponential growth (lag, log, linear and late phase), but it decreases during the stationary growth phase. The SpoVG dependent process increases glycopeptides susceptibility and disrupts the cell membrane metabolism and other independent *SpoVG* mechanisms [12].

SpoVG and *SprX* both seem to contain extra regulatory targets, and antibiotic susceptibility through the *SprX*-dependant mechanism can be bound to susceptibility tied to extra phenotypic advantages that continue to be studied [13]. Various strains of *S.aureus* additionally show an antibiotic determination-related phenotypic variation called as small colony variants (SCVs), which stimulates the biofilm formation and reduced sensitivity to aminoglycosides [14]. The different variation form of small colony variants (SCV) of *S. aureus* has disturbed the expression of 18 sRNAs and increased regulation of the *RsaA*, which is a *sigB* dependent small RNA [15]. However, the network link among small colony variants, antibiotic resistance, and expression profiling of sRNAs has now no longer, but been delineated, those outcomes infer that regulatory sRNAs make contributions to antibiotic resistance through phenotypic maintenance of small colony variants [16].

2.1 RNAIII

RNAIII regulates the expression of genes encoding exoproteins and cell wall associated in *Staphylococcus aureus*. In the quorum sensing mechanism, RNAIII transcribed from the P3 operon, acts as an initiator for agr system in *Staphylococcus aureus*. It also contains the hld gene (delta haemolysin), which is 26 amino acid long sequences. By blocking the translation of transcription factor rot, it regulates its expression. It has been reported that binding of RNAIII with mRNA of transcriptional factor rot in an antisense manner, thus blocking the Shine-Dalgarno sequence [17, 18].

2.2 Teg49

It is a small RNA found in the extended promoter region of sarA, which is an accessory regulator of Staphylococcus bacteria. Confirmation and identification were performed by Northern blotting and RNA-sequencing method. Modulation of the expression of SarA it regulates the virulence factor of *Staphylococcus aureus* [19].

2.3 SprF1-SprG1

There are two types of Toxin-Antitoxin system, whereas Type I has two sub-type types, and Type II has three sub-types but remains uncharacterized. The first type I TA system was SprA1-SprAAS in, which the former denotes the toxin and the latter denotes the antitoxin in *Staphylococcus aureus.* Inhibition of translation and cell wall damage is done by toxin SprA1, a short peptide. txpA-ratA family, also referred to as SprF1-SprG1, is the second type I TA system, whereas SprG1 belongs to pore-forming toxin and antitoxin are SprF1. SprG1 consists of 44 amino acid sequence long peptide and 31 amino acid sequence of short peptide and they have cytotoxic properties [20].

It has been reported that a small RNA, which expresses from pathogenicity islands of SprD upon binding with antisense base pairing of sbi mRNA (encoding an immunoglobulin binding protein) will lead to an impaired host immune response [21]. Besides direct base-pairing with target mRNA, several other mechanisms, including dual-function sRNA that acts as an antisense molecule and codes for a small peptide (e.g., Hld in RNAIII), have been proposed to act on the same or other pathway genes, and also riboswitches that exhibit a structured receptor domain specifically recognized by a small molecule or metabolite [22].

3. Multifunctional small RNA couples QS to virulence

Regulation of virulence factors through quorum sensing mechanism involves the agr mediated pathway and the two-component system. RNAIII plays a major role in regulating the agr dependent transcriptional regulation in MRSA (Methicillin-Resistant *Staphylococcus aureus*). The significance of agr mediated regulations of *S. aureus* pathogenesis is the situation of an obvious paradox. By comparing with different *S. aureus* sRNAs, that has been discovered through bioinformatic strategies or RNA sequencing, RNAIII was the first predicted sRNA in transposon mutagenesis, which defines the epistasis outcomes for a point insertion [23]. The primary factor for virulence is agr and RNAIII, its effector molecule involved in producing virulence factors. Clinically isolated strains from acute infections of *S.aureus* have both virulence factor regulation through agr mediated along with RNAIII involvement. However, mutated strains of agr mediated pathway, which arose at some point of infection, also have been isolated from patients [24].

RNAIII as an effector regulates the expression of important virulence genes, including proteins associated with cell wall metabolism and exotoxins. Also involved in the expression of two-component systems, different global regulators such as *arl*, *sae*, *srr*, *rot* and other mechanisms in the formation of biofilm, synthesis of amino acid and peptidoglycan [25]. These factors vary quantitatively but not qualitatively in different *staphylococcal* strains.

Compared to UAMS-I (Virulent oxacillin susceptible clinical isolates) strain, the agr inactivation effect was observed more in the transcriptome of the *NCTC 8325* strain [26], but whether it exerts direct or indirect effect was studied only in certain genes from the structural prediction of RNAIII. Structurally *RNAIII* comprises 14 loop and two long helices aligned through the long-range base pairing, which blocked off self-reliant structural domains [27]. Some particular site-defined *RNAIII* domains are responsible for the regulation of various targets. The secondary structure of intramolecular RNA removes the hla ribosomal binding sites upon directly competing with the 59 ends of *RNAIII,* which positively induces translation of hla and alpha-hemolysin (**Figure 2**) [29, 30].

Production of various virulence determinants such as coagulase, protein A, and the rot (repressor of toxins) are repressed with minor variations by conserved regions or domains at the post-transcriptional level. These are repressed either individually or in combination by the H13 *RNAIII* hairpin and H14 terminator of the 39 domain, and central domain hairpin H7. The mechanism behind the repression of these virulence factors by the *RNAIII* is mediated through repression of the initiation process in translation mechanisms wherein the degradation of mRNA is initiated by *RNAIII* [31].

DOI: http://dx.doi.org/10.5772/intechopen.98520

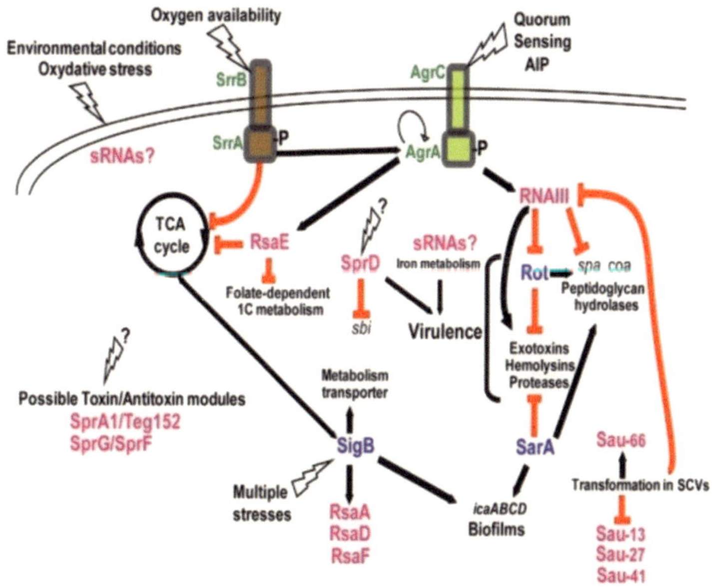

Figure 2.
Integration of sRNAs into gene cascades regulation. The "agr-RNAIII" auto activation circuits is indicated with two feed-forward loops involving RNAIII. The autoinducing peptide (AIP) activates the agr autocatalytic circuit, leading to RNAIII transcription on attaining optimal cell density. RNAIII represses the expression of rot, which activates spa transcription and represses that of hla. RNAIII also activates hla mRNA translation and represses spa mRNA translation. The white and broken lines indicate the direct or indirect gene activations. The red lines represent the down regulations through different RNAs. The black question marks above the see-sawing triangles point to the unknown triggering factors. The transcriptional regulatory proteins are in blue [28].

Complex structure was dependent on their target mRNA and included two factors (i) presence of an extended duplex between the mRNA of Ribosomal Binding Site (RBS) and *RNAIII* and (ii) an imperfect duplex which removes the finished RBS by the interaction between the loops in the coding region [32]. In the above two factors, an individual interaction between the loops is not enough for complete repression, accordingly proscribing the capability of *RNAIII* to behave as a repressor to the mRNA targets. Hence it will not have Shine Dalgarno (SD) series complementary to H7, H13, or H14 of RNAIII, however, it still show a further vicinity of communication or the potential to produce prolonged duplication. *Hfq* is an RNA binding protein and an important chaperone present in different staphylococcus species, but it does not play a role in the *RNAIII* dependent regulatory mechanisms. Whereas in the in-vitro assay, it binds to the *RNAIII* [33, 34].

The repression of all the target mRNA is carried out by the direct effects of *RNAIII* except the translational initiation of hla protein. The repression of Rot (a transcriptional regulatory protein) by RNAIII leads to indirectly regulating transcription for several genes, particularly the protein A repression and the alpha-toxin activation [35].

4. sRNA dependent mechanism of antibiotic resistance

Small RNAs play a major role in altering bacterial cell wall and hence would contribute to the antimicrobial-resistance mechanism. Small RNAs are present prominently on mobile genetic elements on which the resistance pattern for the AMR pathogens is found. SmallRNAs do not exert direct regulation on the resistance gene expression [36]. For example, Fudoh, a regulatory RNA present in

Staphylococcal species is encoded by the SCC mec family of methicillin resistance cassettes. SCCmec is a mobile element that is responsible for the antimicrobial resistivity of methicillin-resistant *Staphylococcus aureus* (MRSA). It also involves regulating the cell distribution process and the expression of alpha phenol soluble modulins, a catalytic peptide [28].

However, the resistance pattern of methicillin through fudoh is still not known. Regulatory small RNA is responsible for the expression of intrinsic antibiotic resistance and tolerance in different bacterial species. Since only some of the small RNA related research has been performed on the clinical strains, whereas most of the studies for RNA-dependent intrinsic antibiotic resistance were performed on the AMR-related pathogens [37].

5. sRNA and stress responses

Specific mechanisms and certain sRNAs involvement regulate the expression pattern of virulence factors under different stress conditions. Small RNA regulation can produce an immediate action to regulatory networks adapted to the acute stress induced by antibiotics. Emergency responders are referred to as Class I small RNAs because they enhance rapid stress responses and aids co-operative degradation of different mRNA targets. Class I sRNAs act in direct mode on the pre-existing mRNA clusters to alter the translation process or deterioration for the acute stress response. Mostly they are involved in disassociating the regulation of transcriptional responses and half-life kinetics of mRNA [38].

It has been reported that during the host infection, variations of temperature and pH, oxidative stress, quorum sensing, biofilm formation and nutrient starvation were related to the functional regulation of small RNAs in *Staphylococcus aureus* [39]. Such responses were controlled by alternative sB (sigma B factor). sB factor regulates several genes that regulate stress-mediated responses, biofilm formation, virulence factor expression, antibiotic resistance, and membrane transport mechanism [40].

Sigma B factor also represses several genes expression by an indirect pathway with the involvement of small RNA or sB-induced regulatory protein. RsaA has a typical sigma B factor promoter which detects its corresponding genes [41]. RsaA base pair with mRNAs repressed by sB like citM and involves in the encoding of Mg-citrate transport systems. sB-dependent sRNAs are the most conserved regions in *S.aureus*. It has been reported that among the three dependent sRNAs, two of them are expected to involve in the regulation of small, highly basic peptides [42].

Production of virulence factors has been regulated by sigma B factor under the stress-dependent activation process. SigB gets activated in the normal stress conditions, also during the growth phase transitions and in different physiological and biochemical changes in *S.aureus* [43]. Thus playing a major role for regulating several others downstream genes. Whereas rsaA are also regulated by a Sigma B-dependent promoter [44].

6. Regulatory sRNA network

Several sRNAs uses Hfq or ProQ chaperones to anneal with their respective mRNAs targets. *Hfq*, a RNA chaperone comprises a six-ring hexamer fostering annealing of RNAs by aligning to their distal and proximal surfaces [45]. The major function of small RNAs regulation is the suppression by base-pairing with the mRNA RBS to inhibit the initiation of translation. sRNA binding blocks binding of small ribosomal subunit [46]. They also regulate both positively and negatively various mechanisms involved in regulating gene expression [47]. The different mechanism includes the processing and stability of transcript process [48], transporting and localization of ribosomes, antisense sponging interactions and termination of transcription process [49, 50].

It has been reported that both small RNA and transcriptional mechanisms work together within interleaved feedback and feed-forward loops and regulate the expression of genes. 108 sRNAs were identified using RNA-seq analysis in the model organism *E.coli* [51], and similarly, around 1600–1900 sRNA-mRNA interactions were identified using interactome profiling analysis [52].

Therefore, it is hardly comparable with the 3446 sRNA-mRNA interactions being regulated by the 217 transcription factors with the chromosome [53]. Several transcriptional regulatory networks have an sRNA that integrates with the extra post-transcriptional networks. Small RNAs act similar to transcription factors as a regulatory centre and unevenly controls various RNAs targets. sRNAs are involved in antibiotic sensitivity by mRNAs interactions which take place in drug import, efflux pump regulation, cell membrane synthesis and enhancing antibiotic resistance pattern [54, 55].

7. sRNA expressions in infections

In *S.aureus*, some of the known sRNAs with their targets involve regulating major biochemical pathways that are further responsible for producing virulence factors [56]. *Staphylococcus aureus* sRNAs were identified using different techniques in various strains, and their expression profiling during the course of infections in humans was studied. Functions of around 250 sRNAs expressed under different conditions are yet unknown. But the expression profiling of *RNAIII* in clinical isolates from nasal cystic fibrosis patients was studied. In most of the clinical isolates of acute infections, *RNAIII* has been expressed in in-vivo conditions [57, 58]. Therefore these data infers that *RNAIII* majorly involves in the regulation of virulence factors and production of *agr*-defective mutants [59]. However, there has been a difference in the variation of agr-defective mutants in healthy and infected patients. Thus, agr regulation occurs during acute infections, whereas the agr mutants expression can only be observed during the stages of the chronic or dormant infection [60].

Expression profiling of five different small RNAs like *RNAIII*, *RsaE*, *RsaH*, *RsaG* and *RsaA* in *S. aureus* strains isolated from three conditions, including cutaneous infections, chronic cystic fibrosis and commensal nasal colonization [61]. Expression patterns of five small RNAs were strain-specific and do not have any correlations with respect to the variations of the infectivity pattern or colonization. However, it has been observed that there was a uniform expression pattern among the commensal strains in comparison to the infectious strains. Therefore, these results show that *S.aureus* was mainly a commensal strain and became an opportunistic pathogen [62, 63].

S. aureus regulatory RNA, SSR42, which modulates the expression of approximately 80 mRNA species, including several virulence factors, in *S.aureus* strains UAMS-1 and USA300 (LAC) during stationary-phase growth. Mutagenesis studies revealed that SSR42 codes for an 891-nucleotide RNA molecule and that the full-length transcript mediates the molecule's regulatory effects. Western blotting and functional assays indicated that the regulatory effects of SSR42 correlate with biologically significant changes in corresponding protein abundances. Further, in *S.aureus* strain LAC, SSR42 is required for wild-type levels of erythrocyte lysis, resistance to human polymorphonuclear leukocyte killing, and pathogenesis in a murine model of skin and soft tissue infection (**Figure 3**) [65].

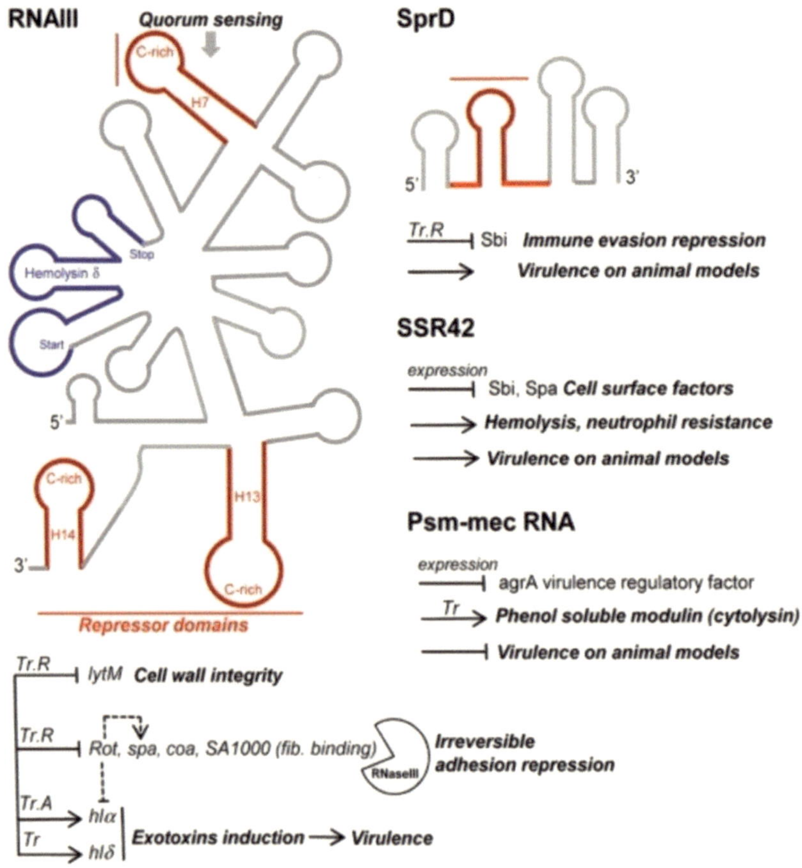

Figure 3.
S. aureus *sRNAs from the RNome implicated in bacterial virulence. Multitasking RNAIII is the effector of quorum sensing to perceive population density and regulates multiple targets involved in peptidoglycan synthesis, adhesions, exotoxins production and virulence. RNAIII internally encodes hemolysin represented in blue color. It contains three repressor domains which are represented in red color, containing accessible UCCC motifs that interact with antisense pairings, with the ribosome binding sites of numerous target mRNAs for translational repression (Tr.R), some triggering endoribonuclease III (RNase III) cleavages to induce target mRNA degradations and irreversible gene expression decay. Translation of at least two exotoxins is activated by RNAIII, one encoded (hld), and another (hla) by translation activation (Tr.A). SprD is expressed from the genome of a converting phage and interacts, by antisense pairings, with the 59 part of the sbi mRNA encoding an immune evasion molecule. SprD possesses an important role in* S. aureus *virulence, but the mechanism of its control is yet to be elucidated, with Sbi being only one player among others. The 891-nucleotide long SSR42 affects extracellular virulence expression, hemolysis, neutrophil virulence, and pathogenesis and contains a putative internal ORF. The mechanisms of target regulation remain to be elucidated. The SCCmec-encoded psm-mec RNA suppresses agrA translation and attenuates MRSA virulence, acting as a dual-function RNA regulator [64].*

8. Pathogenicity Island encoded RNAs

SCCmec (Staphylococcal Cassette Chromosome mec) is responsible for the regulation of antibiotic resistance genes, particularly for the methicillin resistance genes in facultative *S.aureus*. Thus it helps the pathogen to adapt under different stress conditions for survival in the hosts. Elements involved in these processes are genomic islands, transposons, plasmids, and the pathogenicity islands (PIs) acquired horizontally and encode various virulence factors like toxins and cell attachment factors, superantigens factors, invasion factors and two-component system [66]. Apart from the protein-coding genes, it pathogenicity islands also codes for phage-related genes and involves sRNA [67]. Several sRNAs are found in numerous copies distributed encircling the *S.aureus* genome and also some additional copies are present in the plasmids. Multiple copies are present due to either repeated events of gene duplication or horizontally gene transfer [68].

However, the sRNAs expressed from *S.aureus* Pathogenicity Islands (SaPIs) were involved in the regulation of gene expression present on the regions of cognate PIs (**Table 1**). Therefore it forms the functional linkage between the PIs and the genome of the organisms. Expression of SprD (Small Pathogenicity islands D) by PIw involves repression of sbi mRNAs during the initiation process of translation, which encodes an immune evasion molecule [69]. A central hairpin of SprD binds with the sbi mRNA RBS and thus prevents the initiation of the translation process. SprD sRNA has a prominent effect on virulence factors, it involves different pathways for regulating staphylococcal infectivity by altering the expression patterns of SprD. Several other sRNAs are also responsible for pathogenicity through regulatory networks by either direct or indirect way and other translational process regulatory networks. However, from the recently determined sRNAs, 4 are present in PIs and other 6 are in the SCCmec mobile element, with 54 to 400 nucleotides long in size [70].

Teg152 and SprF are two sRNAs that are completely complementary to other two sRNAs SprA1 and SprG. In type I TA (Toxins-Antitoxins) modules, the pairing of SprA1 with Teg152 and SprG with SprF sRNAs takes place. SprA and SprG encodes smaller hydrophobic peptides [53]. SprA1 is a multifunctional sRNA with pressumed antisense function. It's 3-end pairs with 39-UTRs region of three different mRNA targets. The independent transcriptional regulation is responsible for synthesizing appropriate expression levels of sRNAs for effective functional regulation [71].

Group	Examples of virulence factors	PAI
Iron uptake system	FyuA, acrobactin, Sit, Pit2ABCD	HPI, SPI-1, PPI-1, SHI-2,3, PAII-CFT073, PAI III, IV
Adhesins	Type 4 pili, P-pili, S- and P-fimbriae, sap adhesins, Hek adhesins, AfasE-III, Iha, TcpA	Major PAI,PAI I, II CFT 073,PAI I-IV, PAI-I AL863, TAI, VPI-I
Pore forming toxins	Listreiolysin, alpha-haemolysin, RTX-like exotoxins	aLIPI-I, PAI-I536
Second Messenger pathway toxins	CNF-I	PAI-I C5, PAI II J96
Protein causing apoptosis	SipB	SPI-I
Superantigens	TSST-I, ET	SAPI I, SAP I2, SAPIbov, etd
Secreted lipases	PlcA, plcB, SmlC	LIPI I, LIPI II
Secreted protease	EspC, SigA, Pic, ShetA1, Mop,	SHI-I, EspC, PAI-I, VPI-I, BFPAI
O antigens	GtrA, GtrB, Gtr	SHI-O
Proteins transported by type I, II, III, IV and V protein secretion system	Alpha -Hemolysin, EspI, EspC, SigA, Cag, Tir, EspB, G, F, map, SptP, Sae, SopD, SopE, SopE2, PipB, SifA, SifC, EspC, CagA	SHI-I, PAI-I, II536, PAI-I, PAI-II96, LPA, EspC, PAI, SPI-I, SPI-3, SPI-5, LEE, cag, PAI
Antibiotic resistance phenotypes	Pse-I, FloR, AadA2, Sull, TerR, G	SGI-I

Table 1.
Groups of virulence factors encoded by PAI (pathogenicity islands).

9. Phenotypes associated with sRNA expressions

The expression pattern of sRNAs is different in normal compared with SCV (small colony variants) phenotypes of *S.aureus* clinical isolates from the osteomyelitis patients [72]. Different characteristics of SCV strain are slow growth, low pigment production, lower hemolytic activity, lower susceptibility pattern to aminoglycosides, low production of toxins and improved intracellular persistence [73]. Usually, the normal phenotypes are considered as virulent strain and SCVs are considered as persister cells. RNA III expression is a phenotypic-specific, as it is detected in normal phenotypes but not in SCV phenotypes [74]. The absence of

Protein/Gene	Functions	References
FLIPr	Protein that inhibits leucocyte response mediated by activation of FPR-like protein 1. FPR is a high affinity receptor for N-formly-met-leu-phe signaling tripeptide.	[76]
CHIPS	Binds C5aR and the formyl peptide receptor FPR	[77]
Capsule	Polysaccharide capsule prevents phagocytosis and adherence	[78]
SCIN	Staphylococcal complement inhibitor interacts with C3 convertase, C4b2a and C3bBb	[79]
Ecb	Extracellular complement binding protein blocks C3 and C5 convertase	[80]
Efb	Extracellular fibrinogen binding protein, blocks complement and binding of neutrophils to fibrinogen, and platelet aggregation	[81]
Protease V8 (SspA)	Inhibition to complement pathway	[82]
Aureolysin (Aur)	Inhibition to complement pathway	[83]
Staphopain (SepA, SspB)	Cysteine protease cleaving CXCR2 chemokine receptor	[84]
Protein A	Interacts with Fc region of IgG	[85]
Sbi	Interacts with Fc region of IgG	[85]
Dismutases (SodA, SodM)	Conversion of superoxide to hydrogen peroxide	[86]
Catalase (KatA)	Conversion of hydrogen peroxide to water and oxygen	[86]
Staphyloxanthins	Antioxidant carotenoids	[87]
DNAses	Clears DNA in neutrophils extracellular traps, NETs	[88]
Dlt operon	Addition of D-alanyl esters to teichoic acids to protect against alpha defensins	[89]
Phenol soluble modulins	Small amphipathic alpha helical peptides	[90]
Alpha toxins, hla	Pore forming toxin, lyses human leucocyte, epithelial and endothelial cells, platelets	[91]
Panton-valentine leucocidin (PVL)	Pore forming bi-complement leucocidin	[91]
Gamma- haemolysin (HlgAB, HlgCB)	Pore forming bi-complement leukocidin	[91]
Coagulase	Activate prothrombin to induce blood coagulation	[92]
Von- willebrand factor binding protein	Activate prothrombin to induce blood coagulation	[93]
Staphylokinase	Plasminogen activator to form the active protease	[94]

Table 2.
Factors used by S.aureus *to counter host defense mechanism.*

RNAIII sRNA in SCV phenotypes may be the reason for the reduced production of toxins and less virulence. Several PI encoded sRNAs' expression pattern is switched off in the SCV phenotypes during the late growth phase. Also, the less expression profile of SprS in the SCV phenotypes may also be responsible for their less pathogenicity in comparison to the normal phenotypes [75] (**Table 2**).

It has been reported that there is an up-regulation of Sau-13 in normal phenotypes, whereas it is down-regulated in the SCV phenotypes. Sau-13 involve in ion transport and other metabolism by its antisense function against the precursor phoB. But Sau-66 sRNA up-regulated in SCV phenotypes only and down-regulated in normal phenotypes [95]. Sau-66 has antisense region on a gene encoding protein which is involved in folate biosynthesis. Sau-66 has a major impact on the formation of thymidine autotrophs in SCV phenotypes in purine biosynthesis pathway because folate is a carbon donor [96].

10. sRNAs as antimicrobial drug targets

The evolution of CA-MRSA (Community Associated-Methicillin Resistance *Staphylococcus aureus*) strains are major threats to healthcare. Currently available narrow-spectrum antibiotics target only particular functions of bacteria such as synthesis of peptidoglycans, DNA replication, and protein synthesis. Hence, a broad spectrum of antibiotics can target different cellular pathways, thus reducing the resistance pattern among the pathogens. Other methods to reduce antimicrobial resistance are by targetting the production of virulence factors causing the host damage and disease [97].

Since most of the currently used antibiotics bind to the ribosomal RNA, this influences the designing of new multi-targeted antibacterial drugs with respect to small RNAs. Riboswitches, which are termed as metabolites sensing mRNAs, are currently used as a structured receptor that binds with smaller metabolites with higher precision and thus regulates downstream genes. Riboswitches regulates 7 operons and 33 genes, which respond for intracellular concentration of SAM, TPP, FMN, Glc-6P, certain amino acids residues and 7- aminomethyl-7-deazaguanine (preQ1) [98]. Targeting any of these riboswitches would alter the gene's expression pattern even if the cells do not possess any natural compounds. Several synthetically designed analog of guanine upon binding with the purine riboswitches inhibits growth [99].

11. Conclusion

This review focuses on the functions of sRNA and their role in regulating genes in *S. aureus*. Combined application of High throughput screening (HTS), genomic analysis and phenotypic methods for the prediction and determination of sRNAs, functional proteins, RNA binding proteins and riboswitches would provide information on the mechanism of integration of proteins and regulatory RNAs into interwined regulatory networks responsible for adaptation to stress conditions and virulence production [100]. Further study is needed for the determination of signals that can initiate the regulation of sRNA transcription and their targets. Another point that needs to be focused on is host-virulence adaptation or interactions, then cell communication among the dense population of microorganisms and cell differentiation. The expression pattern of sRNAs will be different in a population, leading to adaptability in response to various environmental and stress variations. Furthermore, variations in sRNA expression and their regulatory networks due to host-microbiome interactions also need to be studied. Metagenomic studies, HTS approach, RNA-seq analysis and transcriptomics studies could help understand the mechanisms by which the commensal pathogens cause infections and disease.

Acknowledgements

We thank the Vellore Institute of Technology for providing the necessary facilities to carry out this work.

Conflict of interest

The authors declare no conflict of interest.

Author details

Rudra Mishra Awdhesh Kumar Mishra[1], Bhama Mishra Awdhesh Kumar Mishra[2], Nalini Easwaran[1] and Kodiveri Muthukaliannan Gothandam[1*]

1 School of Bio Sciences and Technology, Vellore Institute of Technology, Vellore, Tamil Nadu, India

2 Department of Biotechnology, Valliammal College for Women, Chennai, Tamil Nadu, India

*Address all correspondence to: gothandam@gmail.com

References

[1] Davoodabadi, F, Mobasherizadeh, S, Mostafavizadeh, K, Shojaei, H, Havaei, S. A, Koushki, A. M, Moghadasizadeh, Z, Meidani, M, & Shirani, K. Nasal colonization in children with community acquired methicillin-resistant *Staphylococcus aureus*. *Advanced biomedical research*, 2016;5, 86. DOI: 10.4103/2277-9175.182217.

[2] Bjarnsholt T, Jensen PØ, Fiandaca MJ, Pedersen J, Hansen CR, Andersen CB, Pressler T, Givskov M, Høiby N. Pseudomonas aeruginosa biofilms in the respiratory tract of cystic fibrosis patients. Pediatr Pulmonol. 2009;44(6):547-58. DOI: 10.1002/ppul.21011.

[3] Waters LS, Storz G. Regulatory RNAs in bacteria. Cell. 2009;20;136(4):615-28. DOI: 10.1016/j.cell.2009.01.043.

[4] Geissmann T, Possedko M, Huntzinger E, Fechter P, Ehresmann C, Romby P. Regulatory RNAs as mediators of virulence gene expression in bacteria. Handb Exp Pharmacol. 2006;(173):9-43. doi: 10.1007/3-540-27262-3_2.

[5] Svenningsen SL. Small RNA-Based Regulation of Bacterial Quorum Sensing and Biofilm Formation. Microbiol Spectr. 2018;6(4). DOI: 10.1128/microbiolspec.RWR-0017-2018.

[6] Eyraud A, Tattevin P, Chabelskaya S, Felden B. A small RNA controls a protein regulator involved in antibiotic resistance in *Staphylococcus aureus*. Nucleic Acids Res. 2014;42(8):4892-905. DOI: 10.1093/nar/gku149.

[7] Liu X, Zhang S, Sun B. SpoVG Regulates Cell Wall Metabolism and Oxacillin Resistance in Methicillin-Resistant *Staphylococcus aureus* Strain N315. Antimicrob Agents Chemother. 2016;23;60(6):3455-61. DOI: 10.1128/AAC.00026-16.

[8] Bohn C, Rigoulay C, Chabelskaya S, Sharma CM, Marchais A, Skorski P, Borezée-Durant E, Barbet R, Jacquet E, Jacq A, Gautheret D, Felden B, Vogel J, Bouloc P. Experimental discovery of small RNAs in *Staphylococcus aureus* reveals a riboregulator of central metabolism. Nucleic Acids Res. 2010;38(19):6620-36. DOI: 10.1093/nar/gkq462.

[9] Schu DJ, Zhang A, Gottesman S, Storz G. Alternative Hfq-sRNA interaction modes dictate alternative mRNA recognition. EMBO J. 2015;14;34(20):2557-73. DOI: 10.15252/embj.201591569.

[10] Xu KD, McFeters GA, Stewart PS. Biofilm resistance to antimicrobial agents. Microbiology (Reading). 2000;146(Pt 3):547-549. DOI: 10.1099/00221287-146-3-547.

[11] Abu-Qatouseh LF, Chinni SV, Seggewiss J, Proctor RA, Brosius J, Rozhdestvensky TS, Peters G, von Eiff C, Becker K. Identification of differentially expressed small non-protein-coding RNAs in *Staphylococcus aureus* displaying both the normal and the small-colony variant phenotype. J Mol Med (Berl). 2010;88(6):565-75. DOI: 10.1007/s00109-010-0597-2.

[12] Shimoni Y, Friedlander G, Hetzroni G, Niv G, Altuvia S, Biham O, Margalit H. Regulation of gene expression by small non-coding RNAs: a quantitative view. Mol Syst Biol. 2007;3:138. Doi: 10.1038/msb4100181.

[13] Benito Y, Kolb FA, Romby P, Lina G, Etienne J, Vandenesch F. Probing the structure of RNAIII, the *Staphylococcus aureus* agr regulatory RNA, and identification of the RNA domain involved in repression of protein A expression. RNA. 2000;6(5):668-79. Doi: 10.1017/s1355838200992550.

[14] Chao Y, Vogel J. The role of Hfq in bacterial pathogens. Curr Opin Microbiol. 2010;13(1):24-33. Doi: 10.1016/j.mib.2010.01.001.

[15] Huntzinger E, Boisset S, Saveanu C, Benito Y, Geissmann T, Namane A, Lina G, Etienne J, Ehresmann B, Ehresmann C, Jacquier A, Vandenesch F, Romby P. *Staphylococcus aureus* RNAIII and the endoribonuclease III coordinately regulate spa gene expression. EMBO J. 2005;23;24(4):824-35. Doi: 10.1038/sj.emboj.7600572.

[16] Chevalier C, Boisset S, Romilly C, Masquida B, Fechter P, Geissmann T, Vandenesch F, Romby P. *Staphylococcus aureus* RNAIII binds to two distant regions of coa mRNA to arrest translation and promote mRNA degradation. PLoS Pathog. 2010;12;6(3). Doi: 10.1371/journal.ppat.1000809.

[17] Boisset S, Geissmann T, Huntzinger E, Fechter P, Bendridi N, Possedko M, Chevalier C, Helfer AC, Benito Y, Jacquier A, Gaspin C, Vandenesch F, Romby P. *Staphylococcus aureus* RNAIII coordinately represses the synthesis of virulence factors and the transcription regulator Rot by an antisense mechanism. Genes Dev. 2007;1;21(11):1353-66. Doi: 10.1101/gad.423507. .

[18] Traber KE, Lee E, Benson S, Corrigan R, Cantera M, Shopsin B, Novick RP. Agr function in clinical *Staphylococcus aureus* isolates. Microbiology (Reading). 2008;154 (Pt 8):2265-2274. Doi: 10.1099/mic.0.2007/011874-0.

[19] Ellis MJ, Haniford DB. Riboregulation of bacterial and archaeal transposition. Wiley Interdiscip Rev RNA. 2016;7(3):382-98. Doi: 10.1002/wrna.1341.

[20] Fröhlich KS, Papenfort K. Interplay of regulatory RNAs and mobile genetic elements in enteric pathogens. Mol Microbiol. 2016;101(5):701-13. Doi: 10.1111/mmi.13428.

[21] Kaito C, Omae Y, Matsumoto Y, Nagata M, Yamaguchi H, Aoto T, Ito T, Hiramatsu K, Sekimizu K. A novel gene, fudoh, in the SCCmec region suppresses the colony spreading ability and virulence of *Staphylococcus aureus*. PLoS One. 2008;3(12):e3921. Doi: 10.1371/journal.pone.0003921.

[22] Kaito C, Saito Y, Nagano G, Ikuo M, Omae Y, Hanada Y, Han X, Kuwahara-Arai K, Hishinuma T, Baba T, Ito T, Hiramatsu K, Sekimizu K. Transcription and translation products of the cytolysin gene psm-mec on the mobile genetic element SCCmec regulate *Staphylococcus aureus* virulence. PLoS Pathog. 2011; 3;7(2):e1001267. Doi: 10.1371/journal.ppat.1001267.

[23] Rutherford ST, Valastyan JS, Taillefumier T, Wingreen NS, Bassler BL. Comprehensive analysis reveals how single nucleotides contribute to noncoding RNA function in bacterial quorum sensing. Proc Natl Acad Sci U S A. 2015;3;112(44):E6038-47. Doi: 10.1073/pnas.1518958112.

[24] Schu DJ, Zhang A, Gottesman S, Storz G. Alternative Hfq-sRNA interaction modes dictate alternative mRNA recognition. EMBO J. 2015;14;34(20):2557-73. Doi: 10.15252/embj.201591569.

[25] Howden BP, Beaume M, Harrison PF, Hernandez D, Schrenzel J, Seemann T, Francois P, Stinear TP. Analysis of the small RNA transcriptional response in multidrug-resistant *Staphylococcus aureus* after antimicrobial exposure. Antimicrob Agents Chemother. 2013;57(8):3864-74. Doi: 10.1128/AAC.00263-13.

[26] Jagodnik J, Chiaruttini C, Guillier M. Stem-Loop Structures within mRNA Coding Sequences Activate Translation Initiation and Mediate

Control by Small Regulatory RNAs. Mol Cell. 2017; 5;68(1):158-170.e3. Doi: 10.1016/j.molcel.2017.08.015.

[27] Soper T, Mandin P, Majdalani N, Gottesman S, Woodson SA. Positive regulation by small RNAs and the role of Hfq. Proc Natl Acad Sci U S A. 2010;25;107(21):9602-7. Doi: 10.1073/pnas.1004435107.

[28] Felden B, Vandenesch F, Bouloc P, Romby P. The *Staphylococcus aureus* RNome and its commitment to virulence. PLoS Pathog. 2011;7(3):e1002006. Doi: 10.1371/journal.ppat.1002006.

[29] Figueroa-Bossi N, Valentini M, Malleret L, Fiorini F, Bossi L. Caught at its own game: regulatory small RNA inactivated by an inducible transcript mimicking its target. Genes Dev. 2009;1;23(17):2004-15. Doi: 10.1101/gad.541609.

[30] Miyakoshi M, Chao Y, Vogel J. Cross talk between ABC transporter mRNAs via a target mRNA-derived sponge of the GcvB small RNA. EMBO J. 2015;3;34(11):1478-92. Doi: 10.15252/embj.201490546.

[31] Rabhi M, Espéli O, Schwartz A, Cayrol B, Rahmouni AR, Arluison V, Boudvillain M. The Sm-like RNA chaperone Hfq mediates transcription antitermination at Rho-dependent terminators. EMBO J. 2011;14;30(14):2805-16. Doi: 10.1038/emboj.2011.192.

[32] Göpel Y, Khan MA, Görke B. Domain swapping between homologous bacterial small RNAs dissects processing and Hfq binding determinants and uncovers an aptamer for conditional RNase E cleavage. Nucleic Acids Res. 2016;29;44(2):824-37. Doi: 10.1093/nar/gkv1161.

[33] Moon K, Gottesman S. A PhoQ/P-regulated small RNA regulates sensitivity of *Escherichia coli* to antimicrobial peptides. Mol Microbiol. 2009;74(6):1314-30. Doi: 10.1111/j.1365-2958.2009.06944.x.

[34] Vincent JL, Rello J, Marshall J, Silva E, Anzueto A, Martin CD, Moreno R, Lipman J, Gomersall C, Sakr Y, Reinhart K; EPIC II Group of Investigators. International study of the prevalence and outcomes of infection in intensive care units. JAMA. 2009; 2;302(21):2323-9. Doi: 10.1001/jama.2009.1754.

[35] Coyne S, Courvalin P, Périchon B. Efflux-mediated antibiotic resistance in Acinetobacter spp. Antimicrob Agents Chemother. 2011;55(3):947-53. doi: 10.1128/AAC.01388-10.

[36] Klobucar K, French S, Côté J-P, Howes JR, Brown ED. Genetic and chemical- genetic interactions map biogenesis and permeability determinants of the outer membrane of *Escherichia coli*. mBio, 2020. 11:e0016120. Doi : 10.1128/mBio.00161-20.

[37] Geissmann T, Chevalier C, Cros MJ, Boisset S, Fechter P, Noirot C, Schrenzel J, François P, Vandenesch F, Gaspin C, Romby P. A search for small noncoding RNAs in *Staphylococcus aureus* reveals a conserved sequence motif for regulation. Nucleic Acids Res. 2009;37(21):7239-57. Doi: 10.1093/nar/gkp668.

[38] Bouvier M, Sharma CM, Mika F, Nierhaus KH, Vogel J. Small RNA binding to 5' mRNA coding region inhibits translational initiation. Mol Cell. 2008;26;32(6):827-37. Doi: 10.1016/j.molcel.2008.10.027.

[39] Bandyra KJ, Said N, Pfeiffer V, Górna MW, Vogel J, Luisi BF. The seed region of a small RNA drives the controlled destruction of the target mRNA by the endoribonuclease RNase E. Mol Cell. 2012;28;47(6):943-53. Doi: 10.1016/j.molcel.2012.07.015.

[40] Papenfort K, Sun Y, Miyakoshi M, Vanderpool CK, Vogel J. Small RNA-mediated activation of sugar phosphatase mRNA regulates glucose homeostasis. Cell. 2013;11;153(2):426-37. Doi: 10.1016/j.cell.2013.03.003.

[41] Bossi L, Schwartz A, Guillemardet B, Boudvillain M, Figueroa-Bossi N. A role for Rho-dependent polarity in gene regulation by a noncoding small RNA. Genes Dev. 2012;15;26(16):1864-73. Doi: 10.1101/gad.195412.112.

[42] Rabhi M, Espéli O, Schwartz A, Cayrol B, Rahmouni AR, Arluison V, Boudvillain M. The Sm-like RNA chaperone Hfq mediates transcription antitermination at Rho-dependent terminators. EMBO J. 2011;14;30(14):2805-16. dDi: 10.1038/emboj.2011.192.

[43] Sedlyarova N, Shamovsky I, Bharati BK, Epshtein V, Chen J, Gottesman S, Schroeder R, Nudler E. sRNA-Mediated Control of Transcription Termination in E.coli. Cell. 2016;22;167(1):111-121. Doi: 10.1016/j.cell.2016.09.004.

[44] Kavita K, de Mets F, Gottesman S. New aspects of RNA-based regulation by Hfq and its partner sRNAs. Curr Opin Microbiol. 2018;42:53-61. Doi: 10.1016/j.mib.2017.10.014.

[45] Wong J., Pang I., Wilkins M., Tree J.J. Systems-Level Analysis of Bacterial Regulatory Small RNA Networks. Systems Biology. RNA Technologies. Springer, Cham. 2018; pp.97-127. Doi: 10.1007/978-3-319-92967-5_6.

[46] Li L, Huang D, Cheung MK, Nong W, Huang Q, Kwan HS. BSRD: a repository for bacterial small regulatory RNA. *Nucleic Acids Res*. 2013;41:D233-D238. Doi:10.1093/nar/gks1264.

[47] Iosub IA, van Nues RW, McKellar SW, Nieken KJ, Marchioretto M, Sy B, Tree JJ, Viero G, Granneman S. Hfq CLASH uncovers sRNA-target interaction networks linked to nutrient availability adaptation. Elife. 2020;1;9:e54655. Doi: 10.7554/eLife.54655.

[48] Sahar Melamed, Philip P. Adams, Aixia Zhang, Hongen Zhang, Gisela Storz. RNA-RNA Interactomes of ProQ and Hfq Reveal Overlapping and Competing Roles. Molecular Cell, 2020;77(2),411-425.e7. DOI: 10.1016/j.molcel.2019.10.022.

[49] Melamed S, Peer A, Faigenbaum-Romm R, Gatt YE, Reiss N, Bar A, Altuvia Y, Argaman L, Margalit H. Global Mapping of Small RNA-Target Interactions in Bacteria. Mol Cell. 2016;1;63(5):884-97. Doi: 10.1016/j.molcel.2016.07.026.

[50] Waters SA, McAteer SP, Kudla G, Pang I, Deshpande NP, Amos TG, Leong KW, Wilkins MR, Strugnell R, Gally DL, Tollervey D, Tree JJ. Small RNA interactome of pathogenic E.coli revealed through crosslinking of RNase E. EMBO J. 2017;1;36(3):374-387. Doi: 10.15252/embj.201694639.

[51] Kosmidis C, Schindler BD, Jacinto PL, Patel D, Bains K, Seo SM, Kaatz GW. Expression of multidrug resistance efflux pump genes in clinical and environmental isolates of *Staphylococcus aureus.* Int J Antimicrob Agents. 2012;40(3):204-9. Doi: 10.1016/j.ijantimicag.2012.04.014.

[52] Lamers RP, Stinnett JW, Muthukrishnan G, Parkinson CL, Cole AM. Evolutionary analyses of *Staphylococcus aureus* identify genetic relationships between nasal carriage and clinical isolates. PLoS One. 2011;21;6(1):e16426. Doi: 10.1371/journal.pone.0016426.

[53] Feng L, Rutherford ST, Papenfort K, Bagert JD, van Kessel JC, Tirrell DA, Wingreen NS, Bassler BL. A qrr

noncoding RNA deploys four different regulatory mechanisms to optimize quorum-sensing dynamics. Cell. 2015;15;160(1-2):228-40. Doi: 10.1016/j.cell.2014.11.051.

[54] Shopsin B, Drlica-Wagner A, Mathema B, Adhikari RP, Kreiswirth BN, Novick RP. Prevalence of agr dysfunction among colonizing *Staphylococcus aureus* strains. J Infect Dis. 2008;15;198(8):1171-4. Doi: 10.1086/592051.

[55] Song J, Lays C, Vandenesch F, Benito Y, Bes M, Chu Y, Lina G, Romby P, Geissmann T, Boisset S. The expression of small regulatory RNAs in clinical samples reflects the different life styles of *Staphylococcus aureus* in colonization vs. infection. PLoS One. 2012;7(5):e37294. Doi: 10.1371/journal.pone.0037294.

[56] Pichon C, Felden B. Small RNA genes expressed from *Staphylococcus aureus* genomic and pathogenicity islands with specific expression among pathogenic strains. Proc Natl Acad Sci U S A. 2005;4;102(40):14249-54. Doi: 10.1073/pnas.0503838102.

[57] Geissmann T, Chevalier C, Cros MJ, Boisset S, Fechter P, Noirot C, Schrenzel J, François P, Vandenesch F, Gaspin C, Romby P. A search for small noncoding RNAs in *Staphylococcus aureus* reveals a conserved sequence motif for regulation. Nucleic Acids Res. 2009;37(21):7239-57. Doi: 10.1093/nar/gkp668.

[58] Novick RP, Subedi A. The SaPIs: mobile pathogenicity islands of Staphylococcus. Chem Immunol Allergy. 2007;93:42-57. Doi: 10.1159/000100857.

[59] Fozo EM, Makarova KS, Shabalina SA, Yutin N, Koonin EV, Storz G. Abundance of type I toxin-antitoxin systems in bacteria: searches for new candidates and discovery of novel families. Nucleic Acids Res. 2010;38(11):3743-59. doi: 10.1093/nar/gkq054.

[60] Romilly C, Caldelari I, Parmentier D, Lioliou E, Romby P, Fechter P. Current knowledge on regulatory RNAs and their machineries in *Staphylococcus aureus*. RNA Biol. 2012;9(4):402-13. Doi: 10.4161/rna.20103.

[61] Proctor RA, von Eiff C, Kahl BC, Becker K, McNamara P, Herrmann M, Peters G. Small colony variants: a pathogenic form of bacteria that facilitates persistent and recurrent infections. Nat Rev Microbiol. 2006;4(4):295-305. Doi: 10.1038/nrmicro1384.

[62] Lannergård J, von Eiff C, Sander G, Cordes T, Seggewiss J, Peters G, Proctor RA, Becker K, Hughes D. Identification of the genetic basis for clinical menadione-auxotrophic small-colony variant isolates of *Staphylococcus aureus*. Antimicrob Agents Chemother. 2008;52(11):4017-22. doi: 10.1128/AAC.00668-08.

[63] Schmidt, Katherine & Manna, Adhar & Cheung, Ambrose. SarT Influences sarS Expression in *Staphylococcus aureus*. Infection and immunity. 2003;71. 5139-48. DOI: 10.1128/IAI.71.9.5139-5148.2003.

[64] Guillet J, Hallier M, Felden B. Emerging functions for the *Staphylococcus aureus* RNome. PLoS Pathog. 2013;9(12):e1003767. doi: 10.1371/journal.ppat.1003767.

[65] Gao J, Stewart GC. Regulatory elements of the *Staphylococcus aureus* protein A (Spa) promoter. J Bacteriol. 2004;186(12):3738-48. doi: 10.1128/JB.186.12.3738-3748.2004.

[66] Beaume M, Hernandez D, Farinelli L, Deluen C, Linder P, Gaspin C, Romby P, Schrenzel J,

Francois P. Cartography of methicillin-resistant *S. aureus* transcripts: detection, orientation and temporal expression during growth phase and stress conditions. PLoS One. 2010;20;5(5):e10725. Doi: 10.1371/journal.pone.0010725.

[67] Marchais A, Naville M, Bohn C, Bouloc P, Gautheret D. Single-pass classification of all noncoding sequences in a bacterial genome using phylogenetic profiles. Genome Res. 2009;19(6):1084-92. Doi: 10.1101/gr.089714.108.

[68] Kahl BC, Belling G, Becker P, Chatterjee I, Wardecki K, Hilgert K, Cheung AL, Peters G, Herrmann M. Thymidine-dependent *Staphylococcus aureus* small-colony variants are associated with extensive alterations in regulator and virulence gene expression profiles. Infect Immun. 2005;73(7):4119-26. Doi: 10.1128/IAI.73.7.4119-4126.2005.

[69] Anderson KL, Dunman PM. Messenger RNA Turnover Processes in *Escherichia coli*, Bacillus subtilis, and Emerging Studies in *Staphylococcus aureus.* Int J Microbiol. 2009;2009:525491. Doi: 10.1155/2009/525491.

[70] Prévost K, Desnoyers G, Jacques JF, Lavoie F, Massé E. Small RNA-induced mRNA degradation achieved through both translation block and activated cleavage. Genes Dev. 2011;15;25(4):385-96. Doi: 10.1101/gad.2001711.

[71] Papenfort K, Bouvier M, Mika F, Sharma CM, Vogel J. Evidence for an autonomous 5' target recognition domain in an Hfq-associated small RNA. Proc Natl Acad Sci. 2010;107(47):20435-20440. DOI: 10.1073/pnas.1009784107.

[72] Peterman N, Lavi-Itzkovitz A, Levine E. Large-scale mapping of sequence-function relations in small regulatory RNAs reveals plasticity and modularity. Nucleic Acids Res. 2014;29;42(19):12177-88. Doi: 10.1093/nar/gku863.

[73] Richter AS, Backofen R. Accessibility and conservation: general features of bacterial small RNA-mRNA interactions? RNA Biol. 2012;9(7):954-65. Doi: 10.4161/rna.20294.

[74] Vogel J, Luisi BF. Hfq and its constellation of RNA. Nat Rev Microbiol. 2011;15;9(8):578-89. Doi: 10.1038/nrmicro2615.

[75] Lalaouna D, Baude J, Wu Z, Tomasini A, Chicher J, Marzi S, Vandenesch F, Romby P, Caldelari I, Moreau K. RsaC sRNA modulates the oxidative stress response of *Staphylococcus aureus* during manganese starvation. Nucleic Acids Res. 2019;10;47(18):9871-9887. Doi: 10.1093/nar/gkz728.

[76] Manna AC, Kim S, Cengher L, Corvaglia A, Leo S, Francois P, Cheung AL. Small RNA teg49 Is Derived from a *sarA* Transcript and Regulates Virulence Genes Independent of SarA in *Staphylococcus aureus.* Infect Immun. 2018;22;86(2):e00635-17. Doi: 10.1128/IAI.00635-17.

[77] Rochat T, Bohn C, Morvan C, Le Lam TN, Razvi F, Pain A, Toffano-Nioche C, Ponien P, Jacq A, Jacquet E, Fey PD, Gautheret D, Bouloc P. The conserved regulatory RNA RsaE down-regulates the arginine degradation pathway in *Staphylococcus aureus*. Nucleic Acids Res. 2018;28;46(17):8803-8816. Doi: 10.1093/nar/gky584.

[78] Felden B, Vandenesch F, Bouloc P, Romby P. The *Staphylococcus aureus* RNome and its commitment to virulence. PLoS Pathog. 2011;7(3):e1002006. Doi: 10.1371/journal.ppat.1002006.

[79] Prat C, Bestebroer J, de Haas CJ, van Strijp JA, van Kessel KP. A new *staphylococcal* anti-inflammatory protein that antagonizes the formyl peptide

receptor-like 1. J Immunol. 2006;1;177(11):8017-26. Doi: 10.4049/jimmunol.177.11.8017.

[80] de Haas CJ, Veldkamp KE, Peschel A, Weerkamp F, Van Wamel WJ, Heezius EC, Poppelier MJ, Van Kessel KP, van Strijp JA. Chemotaxis inhibitory protein of *Staphylococcus aureus*, a bacterial antiinflammatory agent. J Exp Med. 2004;1;199(5):687-95. Doi: 10.1084/jem.20031636.

[81] Filkins LM, Graber JA, Olson DG, Dolben EL, Lynd LR, Bhuju S, O'Toole GA. Coculture of *Staphylococcus aureus* with *Pseudomonas aeruginosa* Drives *S. aureus* towards Fermentative Metabolism and Reduced Viability in a Cystic Fibrosis Model. J Bacteriol. 2015;197(14):2252-64. Doi: 10.1128/JB.00059-15.

[82] Rooijakkers SH, Ruyken M, Roos A, Daha MR, Presanis JS, Sim RB, van Wamel WJ, van Kessel KP, van Strijp JA. Immune evasion by a *staphylococcal* complement inhibitor that acts on C3 convertases. Nat Immunol. 2005;6(9):920-7. Doi: 10.1038/ni1235.

[83] Jongerius I, von Köckritz-Blickwede M, Horsburgh MJ, Ruyken M, Nizet V, Rooijakkers SH. *Staphylococcus aureus* virulence is enhanced by secreted factors that block innate immune defenses. J Innate Immun. 2012;4(3):301-11. Doi: 10.1159/000334604.

[84] Jusko M, Potempa J, Kantyka T, Bielecka E, Miller HK, Kalinska M, Dubin G, Garred P, Shaw LN, Blom AM. *Staphylococcal* proteases aid in evasion of the human complement system. J Innate Immun. 2014;6(1):31-46. Doi: 10.1159/000351458.

[85] Atkins KL, Burman JD, Chamberlain ES, Cooper JE, Poutrel B, Bagby S, Jenkins AT, Feil EJ, van den Elsen JM. *S. aureus* IgG-binding proteins SpA and Sbi: host specificity and mechanisms of immune complex formation. Mol Immunol. 2008;45(6):1600-11. Doi: 10.1016/j.molimm.2007.10.021.

[86] Indian Network for Surveillance of Antimicrobial Resistance (INSAR) group, India. Methicillin resistant *Staphylococcus aureus* (MRSA) in India: prevalence & susceptibility pattern. Indian J Med Res. 2013;137(2):363-9.

[87] Casey JA, Cosgrove SE, Stewart WF, Pollak J, Schwartz BS. A population-based study of the epidemiology and clinical features of methicillin-resistant *Staphylococcus aureus* infection in Pennsylvania, 2001-2010. Epidemiol Infect. 2013;141(6):1166-79. Doi: 10.1017/S0950268812001872.

[88] Clauditz A, Resch A, Wieland KP, Peschel A, Götz F. Staphyloxanthin plays a role in the fitness of *Staphylococcus aureus* and its ability to cope with oxidative stress. Infect Immun. 2006;74(8):4950-3. Doi: 10.1128/IAI.00204-06.

[89] Berends ET, Horswill AR, Haste NM, Monestier M, Nizet V, von Köckritz-Blickwede M. Nuclease expression by *Staphylococcus aureus* facilitates escape from neutrophil extracellular traps. J Innate Immun. 2010;2(6):576-86. Doi: 10.1159/000319909.

[90] Queck SY, Khan BA, Wang R, Bach TH, Kretschmer D, Chen L, Kreiswirth BN, Peschel A, Deleo FR, Otto M. Mobile genetic element-encoded cytolysin connects virulence to methicillin resistance in MRSA. PLoS Pathog. 2009;5(7):e1000533. Doi: 10.1371/journal.ppat.1000533.

[91] Seilie ES, Bubeck Wardenburg J. *Staphylococcus aureus* pore-forming toxins: The interface of pathogen and host complexity. Semin Cell Dev Biol. 2017;72:101-116. Doi: 10.1016/j.semcdb.2017.04.003.

[92] Friedrich R, Panizzi P, Fuentes-Prior P, Richter K, Verhamme I, Anderson PJ, Kawabata S, Huber R, Bode W, Bock PE. Staphylocoagulase is a prototype for the mechanism of cofactor-induced zymogen activation. Nature.2003;2,425(6957):535-9. Doi: 10.1038/nature01962.

[93] Kroh HK, Panizzi P, Bock PE. Von Willebrand factor-binding protein is a hysteretic conformational activator of prothrombin. Proc Natl Acad Sci U S A. 2009;106(19):7786-91. Doi: 10.1073/pnas.0811750106.

[94] McAleese F, Wu SW, Sieradzki K, Dunman P, Murphy E, Projan S, Tomasz A. Overexpression of genes of the cell wall stimulon in clinical isolates of *Staphylococcus aureus* exhibiting vancomycin-intermediate- *S. aureus*-type resistance to vancomycin. J Bacteriol. 2006;188(3):1120-33. Doi:10.1128/JB.188.3.1120-1133.2006.

[95] Tomasini A, François P, Howden BP, Fechter P, Romby P, Caldelari I. The importance of regulatory RNAs in *Staphylococcus aureus*. Infect Genet Evol. 2014;21:616-26. Doi: 10.1016/j.meegid.2013.11.016.

[96] Westermann AJ, Förstner KU, Amman F, Barquist L, Chao Y, Schulte LN, Müller L, Reinhardt R, Stadler PF, Vogel J. Dual RNA-seq unveils noncoding RNA functions in host-pathogen interactions. Nature. 2016;28;529(7587):496-501. Doi: 10.1038/nature16547.

[97] Eyraud A, Tattevin P, Chabelskaya S, Felden B. A small RNA controls a protein regulator involved in antibiotic resistance in *Staphylococcus aureus.* Nucleic Acids Res. 2014;42(8):4892-905. Doi: 10.1093/nar/gku149.

[98] Howden BP, Beaume M, Harrison PF, Hernandez D, Schrenzel J, Seemann T, Francois P, Stinear TP. Analysis of the small RNA transcriptional response in multidrug-resistant *Staphylococcus aureus* after antimicrobial exposure. Antimicrob Agents Chemother. 2013;57(8):3864-74. doi: 10.1128/AAC.00263-13.

[99] Carroll RK, Weiss A, Broach WH, Wiemels RE, Mogen AB, Rice KC, Shaw LN. Genome-wide Annotation, Identification, and Global Transcriptomic Analysis of Regulatory or Small RNA Gene Expression in *Staphylococcus aureus.* MBio. 2016;9;7(1):e01990-15. Doi: 10.1128/mBio.01990-15.

[100] Kim, S., Reyes, D., Beaume, M., Francois, P., and Cheung, A. Contribution of teg49 Small RNA in the 5′ upstream transcriptional region of sarA to virulence in *Staphylococcus aureus*. *Infect. Immun.* 2014;82, 4369-4379. Doi: 10.1128/IAI.02002-2014.

Chapter 4

Mechanistic Insights of Drug Resistance in *Staphylococcus aureus* with Special Reference to Newer Antibiotics

Atamjit Singh, Kirandeep Kaur, Pallvi Mohana, Avneet Kaur, Komalpreet Kaur, Shilpa Heer, Saroj Arora, Neena Bedi and Preet Mohinder Singh Bedi

Abstract

Staphylococcus aureus is the most ubiquitous microorganism in both environment as well as animals and exists as commensal and pathogenic bacterium. In past few years it has been emerged as a superbug causing serious burden on healthcare system. This bacterium has been found to be the most resistant one toward most of the antibiotics due to its rapid structural and genetic modifications. This chapter will shed light on various types of molecular mechanisms responsible for resistance of *Staphylococcus aureus* showcasing how it has been emerged as a superbug. Moreover, the recent approaches which include exploring of different drug targets keeping in view the structural and functional behavior of the *Staphylococcus aureus* has also been discussed.

Keywords: Antimicrobial resistance, *Staphylococcus aureus*, Superbug, Resistance Mechanism, Drug resistance, Bacterial resistance

1. Introduction

Staphylococcus aureus is a Gram-positive, catalase and coagulase positive strain of bacteria belongs to Micrococcaceae family. Staphylococcus spp. to which these bacteria belong is commonly found in nature and human flora. *Staphylococcus aureus* is generally isolated from community as well as hospital gained infections and have capability to cause superficial to life threatening infections [1–3]. However, the worst scenario in field of microbiology was observed in late 90's when resistance among several microbes including *Staphylococcus aureus* was reported for various antibiotics. *Staphylococcus aureus* was the most prominent threat among all other pathogens due to the rapid emergence of resistance in it. The inappropriate use of antimicrobials in clinical therapy and agriculture, extensive antimicrobial consumption and transfer of antimicrobial resistant genes due to increased anthropogenic activity are potential risk factors for development of antimicrobial resistance and considered as primary reasons responsible for the rapidly growing resistance in *Staphylococcus aureus* [4–6]. Moreover, the intrinsic virulence of *Staphylococcus aureus*, its nature to adapt to the corresponding environment are some other factors which makes it the foremost challenge for microbiology scientists. Even though, many potential therapeutics have been synthesized/approved by USFDA for the treatment of *Staphylococcus* infections but unfortunately besides this the mortality rate of *Staphylococcus* bacteraemia is 20-40% [7–9]. Furthermore, the clinical sample (blood samples) of patients with nosocomial infections/staphylococcus infections were investigated which confirmed the resistant strains of *Staphylococcus aureus* against various antibiotics that include first- and second-generation fluroquinolones, β-Lactam antibiotics, trimethoprim sulphamethoxazole and vancomycin etc. [7, 10, 11]. Surprisingly, the number of antibiotics emerging for treatment of this bacteria is directly proportionate to the rapidly evolving resistance mechanisms within *Staphylococcus aureus* to combat the therapeutic efficacy of these antibiotics. In year of 2002-2003 *Staphylococcus aureus* was found resistant to the highly efficient antibiotic vancomycin which left the physicians with no competent antibiotic for its treatment. Subsequently it urged the need to explore more drug targets and novel approaches for new antibiotics to treat staphylococcus infections. Conclusively, the rapid structural and genetic modifications of *Staphylococcus aureus* counterbalance the effect of even magnificent antibiotics. Therefore, various molecular mechanisms of *Staphylococcus aureus* have been deeply explored in the recent past to overcome the life-threatening implications of this resistant bacteria [12, 13]. This chapter enlightens the historical evolution of resistance in *Staphylococcus aureus*, molecular mechanism of resistance for various antibiotics and the modified approaches for its treatment.

2. Quorum sensing in *Staphylococcus aureus*

Quorum sensing is a well-known phenomenon used mainly by prokaryotes for communication among themselves [14]. Particularly in bacteria quorum sensing is monitored by a set of signaling molecules called autoinducers as density dependent variables. They are released by bacteria around their surrounding environment which up on reaching at particular concentration develop a well-coordinated response. Density of autoinducers is monitored by bacteria for tracking changes in cell number and to alter the gene expression pattern. This is also a factor that is responsible for resistance of bacteria against antibiotics [15, 16]. Quorum sensing in *Staphylococcus aureus* has been coordinated through modified oligopeptide

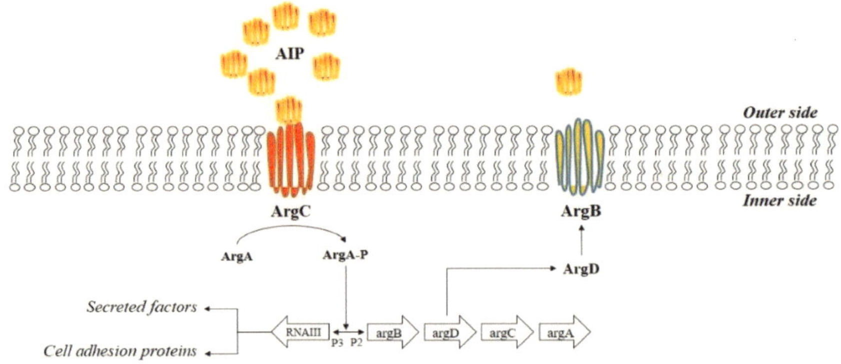

Figure 1.
Mechanistic insight of quorum sensing in Staphylococcus aureus.

known as autoinducing peptide (AID). In the pathophysiology of *Staphylococcus aureus* regarding quorum sensing, biphasic mechanism exist. At lower cell density, *Staphylococcus aureus* generally express protein factors i.e. Coagulase and fibronectin binding proteins A and B etc. which promote their attachment as well as colonization while at higher cellular density *Staphylococcus aureus* repress these traits and initiate secretion of toxins and proteases that needed for dissemination. The switching of this gene expression is controlled by Agr quorum sensing system that consist of autoinducing peptide (AID) encoded by agrD and two other sensor kinase-response regulators called AgrC and AgrA (**Figure 1**) [17–19].

3. Various resistance mechanisms of different classes of antibiotics in *Staphylococcus aureus*

3.1 Resistance to β-lactam antibiotics

In early 1940's introduction of penicillin improved the outcome cases due to *Staphylococcus* infections but soon penicillin resistance *Staphylococcus* were recognized in early 1942 [20] which among late 1960's reaches to 80% in both community and hospital-acquired staphylococcal isolates with well-established pattern of resistance [21]. Furthermore, blaZ gene is responsible for resistance in *Staphylococcus aureus*, that encodes for β-lactamase an enzyme which is synthesized when *Staphylococcus aureus* is exposed to β-lactam antibiotics by hydrolyzing the β-lactam ring, rendering the β-lactam inactive. blaZ is regulated by the two adjacent genes blaR1 and blaI. The gene blaR1 is anti-repressor and blaI is repressor [22]. For the synthesis of β-lactamase, the signaling pathway involves the sequential cleavage of these regulatory proteins such as blaR1 and blaI where on exposure to β-lactams, blaR1 which is a transmembrane sensor transducer cleaves itself [23, 24], cleaved protein acts as protease that directly or indirectly cleaves the repressor blaI and thus allowing the blaZ to synthesize enzyme [23]. Furthermore, Methicillin, the first semisynthetic penicillin which was resistance to penicillinase, introduced in 1961 and soon followed by the reporting of methicillin-resistance isolates [25]. The spread of Methicillin-resistant *Staphylococcus aureus* (MRSA) has been critical and the infections resulting from MRSA is worse than the infections outcome of methicillin ensitive strains [26]. MRSA isolates like the penicillin resistance strains too carried resistance genes for other antimicrobial agents [27]. For the resistance to methicillin, requires chromosomally localized mecA gene [28, 29], which is a part of large unique mobile genetic element, SCC mec found in all MRSA strains may contain additional genes for antimicrobial resistance [30, 31] is responsible for the synthesis of PBP2a/PBP2′ a 78-kDa protein which binds to penicillin (penicillin-binding protein 2a) [32–34]. Transpeptidation which is necessary for the cross-linkage of peptidoglycan chains is catalyzed by these membranes bound enzymes-PBPs, thought to have appeared and works similar as serine proteases. PBP2a blocks the binding of all β-lactams but allows transpeptidation and because of its low affinity it allows staphylococci to survive even in the high concentration exposure of β-lactam antibiotics. Isolates Resistance to methicillin shows resistance to all β-lactam agents, including cephalosporins [34–36]. In some MRSA strains its resistance mechanism by mecA via the mecI and mecR1 genes is regulated in the manner similar to the regulation of blaZ by the genes blaR1 and blaI when exposed to penicillin [37]. Fem genes (factor essential for resistance to methicillin resistance, also play a role in cross-linking the peptidoglycan strands and contribute in methicillin resistance [38]. Ceftaroline the fifth-generation cephalosporin according to the U.S. Food and Drug Administration (FDA) in 2010 has been considered superior among other comparator drugs for the treatment of complicated skin and soft tissue infections as well as pneumonia [39]. β -lactam antibiotics bind to other PBPs, named PBP1, −2, −3, and − 4 but in the presence of PBP2a they are unable to bind effectively to their PBP targets. Ceftaroline on other hand is active against MRSA strains because of its high binding affinity for PBP2a as comparison to other β -lactam [40]. Binding of PBPs by ceftaroline block these enzymes to catalyze the transpeptidase function that is important for the synthesis of staphylococcal cell wall [41]. Ceftaroline is generally considered safe and successfully used to treat wide infections alone and in combination with other active drugs often with daptomycin [42]. Several studied over MRSA clinal strains showed these were susceptible to ceftaroline in wide range such as >98.4% in North America [43], >83.3% in Latin America [44], >83% in Europe [45], 78.8% in Asia/South Pacific countries [46] the variation in resistance among MRSA may be due to the variation in geographical distribution of strains around the world [47, 48]. MRSA strains carry mobile genetic element known as SCCmec, which carries mecA gene [40]. Ceftaroline resistance is usually due to the nonsense mutations in mecA, resulting in amino acid sequence change in PBP2a hence a target protein mutation [49]. Glu447Lys mutation in mecA in presence of ceftaroline on SF8300 USA300 MRSA strain yields low level resistance isolates whereas COL common laboratory strain showed high ceftaroline resistance due to mutations in pbp2, pbp4 and gdpP not due to mecA [50]. There are strains developing resistance with no change in mecA [51].

3.2 Resistance to vancomycin

Vancomycin, a lipopeptide antibiotic approved by Food and Drug Administration of the United States in 1958 found in recent years that the MRSA isolates are resist to it [52]. Vancomycin works by binding to bacterial cell envelopes and inhibiting their cell wall synthesis instead of targeting protein like other antibiotics [53]. It binds to C-terminal D-Ala–D-Ala residue of the pentapeptide to inhibit the cross-bridge formation between pentapeptide and pentaglycine preventing cell wall synthesis [54]. MRSA strains shows different ranges of resistance against vancomycin according to their MIC and are named accordingly such as MRSA showing complete resistance to vancomycin is termed vancomycin-resistant *Staphylococcus aureus* (VRSA), showing medium resistance is termed as vancomycin intermediate-resistant *Staphylococcus aureus* (VISA) and least resistance as VSSA [55].

Failure in vancomycin treatment of MRSA results due to formation of intermediate-resistant isolates namely hetero resistant vancomycin-intermediate *Staphylococcus aureus* (hVISA) and vancomycin intermediate *Staphylococcus aureus* (VISA) [56] which includes features such as cell wall thickening, reduced autolytic activit and reduced growth rates [57]. Several studies found that the mutation in genes VraS(S329L), MsrR(E146K), GraR(N197S), RpoB(H481Y), Fdh2(A297V) and Sle1(67aa) were also responsible for vancomycin resistance in VISA strain Mu50 [58]. Other genes involving in high- and low-level resistance to vancomycin includes vanA, vanB, vanD, vanF, vanI, vanM, encodes for D-Ala:D-Lac ligases whereas vanC, vanE, vanG, vanL, and vanNgenes encoding D-Ala:D-Ser ligases (**Figure 2**) [59, 60].

3.3 Resistance to lipopeptide based antibiotic daptomycin

The only approved and available lipopeptide in the US in the year 2003 with in vitro bactericidal activity and an alternative to vancomycin for various MRSA infections, is daptomycin [61]. However, during the treatment, the emergence of non-susceptible MRSA strains for daptomycin has been reported [62, 63]. Even

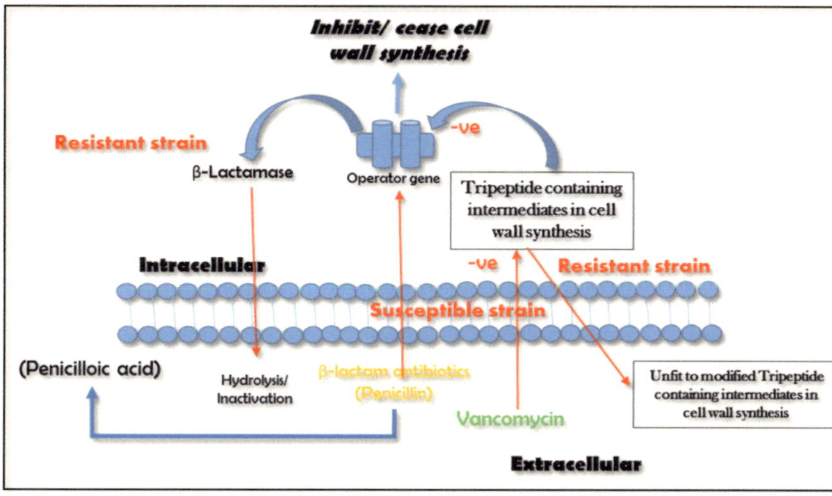

Figure 2.
Molecular mechanism of Staphylococcus aureus *resistance toward penicillin and vancomycin.*

before the approval of drug, Silverman et al. observed daptomycin non-susceptible mutants and identified number of changes such as increase in membrane fluidity, increase in net positive charge over the surface, decrease in susceptibility to daptomycin-induced depolarization and low in surface binding of daptomycin in the cytoplasmic membrane of non-susceptible strains [64, 65]. Though the basis for reduction in susceptibility to daptomycin in MRSA strains has not been fully clarified [66]. The transfer and addition of positively charged lysine molecules to phosphatidyl glycerol in the cell membrane associated with the activity of enzyme lysyl-phosphatidyl glycerol synthetase is encoded by mprF gene [67], Mutation in mprF gene causes an increase of lysyl-phosphatidyl glycerol in the outer layer of the cell membrane, leading to an increased positive charge resulting in reduced susceptibility to daptomycin [68]. mprF mutations are the most common type of mutation in MRSA strains with reduced susceptibility to daptomycin (**Figure 3**) [69]. Several more genes are also identified which are associated with the reduced susceptibility to daptomycin such as dsp1 or asp23. The inactivation of these genes leads to reduced daptomycin susceptibility and the overexpression of single or both of the genes leads increase in susceptibility [70] whereas expression of dltA gene contributes to the staphylococcal net positive surface charge [71]. Kanesaka et al. using transmission electron microscopy, found that the some of the strains which were exposed to daptomycin which shows resistance developed an increase in the thickness of their cell wall and their thickness decreases on revert to daptomycin susceptible [72].

3.4 Resistance to aminoglycosides

Aminoglycosides works by mistranslation and changing the conformation of tRNA during bacterial protein synthesis by binding to A-site present on 16S rRNA of the 30S ribosome. Some even acts by inhibiting initiation /or elongation phase thereby blocking bacterial protein synthesis [73]. Most common mechanism of resistance to aminoglycosides especially in *Staphylococcus aureus* includes Aminoglycoside modifying enzymes which works by acetylating, phosphorylating, or adenylating amino or hydroxyl groups therefore inactivating aminoglycosides. Hundreds of aminoglycosides modifying enzymes are known encoded by genes which are commonly found on plasmids and transposons [74]. On clinical practising with some

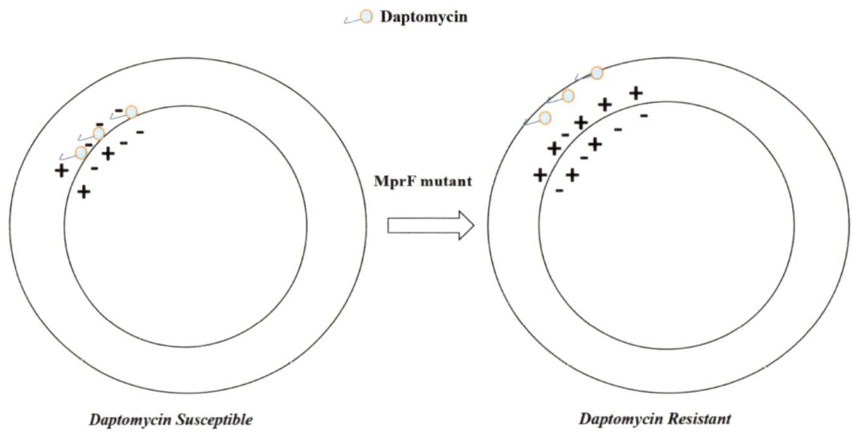

Figure 3.
Molecular mechanism of Staphylococcus aureus *resistance toward daptomycin via mprF.*

aminoglycosides such as gentamicin, tobramycin, and amikacin these three among Aminoglycoside modifying enzymes such as ANT(4=) nucleotide transferase, bidomain AAC(6=)le-APH(2=)la acetyltransferase and phosphotransferase, and APH(3=)IIIa phosphotransferase which are common in MRSA isolates with varied appearance, shows resistance [75]. Plazomicin, a synthetic aminoglycoside showed in vitro activity against 55 MRSA isolates that expressed one or more aminoglycoside-modifying enzymes [76] and has no protection against other resistance mechanism such as 16 s rRNA methyltransferases that modifies the aminoglycoside target site but these enzymes are not reported in S. aureus (**Figure 4**) [77].

3.5 Resistance to oxazolidinones

Oxazolidinones, the synthetic antibiotics blocks the formation of functional 70S initiation complex thereby preventing bacterial protein synthesis. Linezolid and tedizolid types of drugs from Oxazolidinones works interrupting transitional RNA positioning by binding to the bacterial 23S rRNA at the ribosomal peptide-transferase center. Even with the similarity in both of the structure tedizolid still

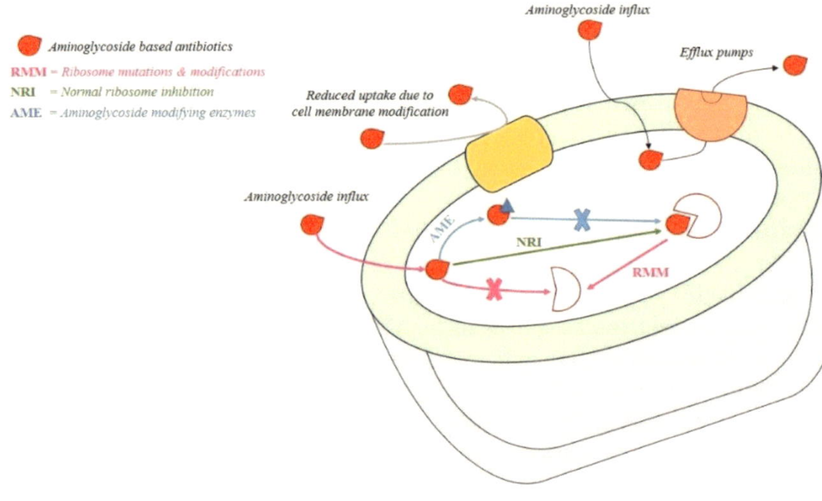

Figure 4.
Molecular mechanism of Staphylococcus aureus *resistance toward aminoglycosides.*

shows increased and better interactions at the binding site with increased potency [78]. All these resistance mechanisms make alteration to oxazolidinone binding site, most common are the point mutations occurring in the genes encoding for 23S rRNA mostly in the central loop of domain V [79]. S. aureus has four to seven copies of 23S rRNA gene collection of which determines the effect and degree of linezolid resistance [80, 81]. This kind of mutation, G2576T, in all five copies of its 23S rRNA gene has been found in the first clinical isolates of linezolid-resistant MRSA [82] are most common. Mutations in the genes which are encoding for L3 and L4 similar to mutation in 23S rRNA, induces a change in the linezolid binding site shows linezolid resistance. Studies showed structural rearrangement of the linezolid binding site due to deletion of one amino acid in L3 causing change in the position of several of the 23S rRNA bases as targeted by point mutations. Gene cfr (chloramphenicol-florfenicol resistance) linked with various mobile genetic elements also shows resistance to linezolid and other antibiotics by change in the drug binding site at the ribosomal peptide-transferase center by encoding a rRNA methyltransferase that causes change in position A2503 [83–85]. Several bacterial species port the cfr gene, a reservoir for drug resistance. MRSA isolates with cfr genes are more likely have additional antibiotic resistance genes as compared to non-cfr gene isolates. Another gene, optrA found commonly symbiosis with cfr gene in MRSA isolates also shows resistance to oxazolidinones [84]. Acts as an ATP-binding cassette transporter, which mediate the influx and efflux of drugs. Another optrA structurally similar gene poxtA first identified in MRSA isolates, shows in vitro resistance to oxazolones [86–89].

3.6 Resistance to quinolones with a focus on novel antibiotic delafloxacin

The fluoroquinolones (FQ) were first introduced into clinical practice in the year 1962 along with the development of Nalidixic acid. Fluoroquinolones (FQ) are class of fully synthetic antibiotics which are active against a broad range of gram positive and gram-negative bacteria and have a pivotal role in multidrug resistance therapy in Mycobacterial infection (Tuberculosis and non-tuberculosis). To treat acute bacterial skin and skin structure infections (ABSSSIs) with both enteral and intravenous preparations FDA approved non zwitter ionic FQ delafloxacin in 2017 [90]. Due slower MICs against S. aureus than other FQs delafloxacin has a higher barrier to resistance, it can serve as ant staphylococcal drug as monotherapy. Delafloxacin is found to be effective against multiple like Streptococcus pneumoniae, anaerobic bacteria Legionella, *Chlamydia pneumoniae*, *Neisseria gonorrhoeae*, Mycoplasma spp., in addition to *Staphylococcus aureus*. Its activity against the enterococci is variable [91]. Delafloxacin shows a property of "dual-targeting" in which it can form complexes with DNA and topoisomerase IV or DNA gyrase. Double strand break can be produced by the inhibiting the one or both the enzymes which results in the death of bacterial cell as they lack enzymes that can repair double strand break in DNA. Delafloxacin shows more potency against Gram positive bacteria as it shows anionic behavior at neutral pH due to the substitution of the R7 position (3-hydroxy-1-azetidinyl) [90, 92]. An anionic behavior of delafloxacin makes diffusion and accumulation of drug within the bacteria more readily as it is retained in bacterial cell for longer duration at neutral intracellular pH [93]. These characteristics makes antibiotics more effective in acidic environments [94]. Depending upon the ambient pH it shows activity against biofilm related infections and intracellular infections [91]. Estimated concentration of Delafloxacin selecting resistant mutant is 8 to 32 times lesser than for other Fluoroquinolones. This difference is due to the drugs dual targeting mechanism of action. Point mutations are method by which resistance is shown by bacteria, resistance occurs due to point mutations in target enzyme or by the action of efflux pump. Point mutation in ParC subunit of topoisomerase IV results in resistance in case of *Staphylococcus aureus*. Delfatoxin resistance occurs due to various mutations in the target regions of topoisomerase IV [92–95]. Resistance to the FQs, including delafloxacin, often involves point mutations in the target enzymes or the action of efflux pumps in bacterial cells. In S. aureus, resistance is usually mediated by point mutations in the ParC subunit of topoisomerase IV. Delafloxacin often retains potency against S. aureus resistant to other FQ drugs due to target gene mutations or modifications. This relative resistance seems related to the structure of delafloxacin (perhaps due to C-7 and C-8 substitutions); delafloxacin resistance occurs only with several mutations in the target regions of topoisomerase IV. NorA, NorB, NorC, MdeA, QacA, and QacB includes a resistant phenotype of Common S. aureus efflux pumps active against Fluoroquinolones. The antiseptic chlorhexidine gluconate is also removed from cells by the plasmid-encoded efflux pumps QacA and QacB, sometimes called antiseptic resistance genes and their acquisition in a S. aureus population is co-selected by use of chlorhexidine or FQs. Delafloxacin is not as active substrate for typical *Staphylococcus aureus* efflux pumps compared to other drugs in the class [96–99].

3.7 Resistance to new class of antibiotics: pleuromutilins

In 1951 a compound Pleuromutilin a class of antibacterial which is isolated from a fungus called Pleurotomariids. Pleuromutilin and its natural molecule found to be effective against Gram-positive bacteria. For veterinary use Tiamulin used in livestock for the treatment of gastrointestinal and respiratory disease. Valnemulin is a second veterinary systemic Pleuromutilin antimicrobial approves and widely use in Asia and Europe. For systemic human use lefamulin was synthesized in 2006, lefamulin is novel pleuromutilin drug effective against most MRSA strains [100]. In phase 2 lefamulin was non inferior to intravenous Vancomycin. Pleuromutilin interferes with the process of protein synthesis by inhibiting the 50s subunit of the ribosome binding at site called peptidyl transfer centre [101, 102]. They specifically target the inhibition of initiation of translation. The extensive use of tiamulin and valenemulin for decades in livestock leads to MRSA strains and their mechanism of resistance to pleuromutilin are well studied. One of the resistance mechanisms involves alteration of target site on the ribosome which may require three or more mutations to develop resistant phenotype [103–105]. Resistant clones may be formed when *Staphylococcus aureus* acquire new genes by horizontal gene transfer including transferable cfr gene methylation a specific site on 23S rRNA. This methylation by cfr gene product results in resistance to several class of antibiotics including pleuromutilin, linezolid, streptogramin, phenicol, and lincosamides. In *S. aureus* is the family of at least four vga genes with variants, including vga(A)v, vga(A), vga(C), and vga(E), as well as lsa(E), all result in ribosomal protection results in cause of pleuromutilin resistance in S. aureus. Plasmid or transposons can carry strains vga(A) may become transmissible among strains. In ST398 livestock-associated MRSA strains found vga(c) strain also be carried on plasmid. The spread of mobile genetic elements among animal and human S. aureus strains raises concern for the emergence of widespread pleuromutilin resistance among human strains if drugs in this class are widely used [106, 107].

3.8 Resistance to mupirocin

Mupirocin was used as a decolonizing agent. It is widely used in CA-MRSA epidemic United States in 1990. But it was discovered in in 1970. Resistance to mupirocin by MRSA developed [10, 108]. Mupirocin resistance is developed due to ileS-2 gene [109]. The mupA and mupB genes responsible for resistance to mupirocin these genes encode novel isoleucyl-tRNA synthetases and can be carried out by plasmids [110]. The threes aspect of REDUCE-MRSA study was cluster-randomized trial that evaluate screening, isolation, and decolonization with chlorhexidine and mupirocin in intensive care unit patients [111]. Mupirocin is best suitable option for MRSA nasal decolonization but shows some side effects. Development of novel decolonization agent should be our propriety. We can also develop agents that can act synergistically with mupirocin as recently described [112, 113].

3.9 Resistance to lipoglycopeptides

Dalbavancin, oritavancin, and telavancin, the semisynthetic derivatives of glycopeptides are the three lipoglycopeptides available in the US. Glycopeptides usually inhibits bacterial cell wall synthesis by binding to D-alanyl-D-alanine (D-Ala-D-Ala) terminal of growing peptidoglycan chains [114]. Due to their distinctiveness in structural modifications of each drugs heptapeptide core, lipoglycopeptides are more powerful than vancomycin which contains lipid side chain that helps in holding the drug to cell membrane providing stability and an increase in concentration of local drug. In case of oritavancin and telavancin their interaction with the cell wall promotes another mechanism of action as concentration-dependent depolarization of cell membrane leading to increase in permeability. Because of the structure of oritavancin it allows several other mechanisms of action which includes binding to the secondary site in peptidoglycan chains, pentaglycyl bridging segment of lipid II, transpeptidation inhibition and RNA synthesis inhibition [115, 116]. A survey study conducted from 2010 to 2014 in US and Europe showed 99.9% isolates of S. aureus susceptible to oritavancin and 98% isolates susceptible to dalbavancin in global survey during 2002 to 2012 [117] with rare Lipoglycopeptide resistance among S. aureus. Recently for dalbavancin, Resistance in some clinical isolates has been reported. On structural analysis showed an increase in the thickening of cell wall and abnormal cell wall construction in dalbavancin non-susceptible isolates [118, 119].

4. Evolution of *Staphylococcus aureus* as superbug

Alexander Flaming accidently discovered penicillin as fungal contaminant also having bactericidal effect against Staphylococcus aureus which in turn led to bulk production of this antibiotic [120]. Consequently, death rate due to bacterial pneumonia and meningitis fell down during World War II. Penicillin was discovered to act by breaking peptidoglycan assembly within bacterial cell wall followed by cell death due to osmotic fragility [121]. In early 1940's death rate of Staphylococcal infections was approximately 80%. However, resistance *Staphylococcus aureus* strains were observed after overuse of penicillin which got predominant in 1945 [122–124]. The major cause of this resistance was the eventual formation of plasmid encoded-lactamase which found to have ability of hydrolysing active moiety i.e. lactam ring of penicillin [124, 125]. The ability of plasmid encoded-lactamase to readily transfer which rises the penicillin against bacterial resistance rate up to 90-95%. Moreover, in 1950 a resistant clone of *Staphylococcus aureus* called phage 80/81 was responsible for the outbreak pandemic of skin infections, sepsis of skin and pneumonia. Initially it was concerned inside the premises of hospital but eventually it outspread within the public outside [126]. Australia, America and Canada were the majorly effected countries during this epidemic which lasted for almost 10 years until a methicillin came into market [127]. It was purposely designed in 1959 for the lactamase resistance strains of staphylococci and their treatment but surprisingly it worked efficiently for only one year because later on the methicillin resistance strain of Staphylococcus aureus was first observed in 1961 in United

Kingdom [128]. The major cause of acquired resistance was mecA gene at specific site of chromosome. mecA gene was reported to encode an alternative penicillin binding protein gene called PBR2a and PBR2 which possessed very little binding affinity against penicillin, methicillin, nafcillin and cephem derivatives [129]. However, this resistance was found to be different from penicillin acquired resistance as it included broad spectrum antibiotics i.e. almost entire class of lactams except ceftaroline and ceftobiprole [130]. Adding on, a genetic element was found to be the prime carrier of mecA gene and was responsible for the broad-spectrum resistance as well as outbreak of its infections in 1980 [131]. Few countries that had major impact were Ireland, United States and United Kingdom. Despite the fact that it was first observed in 1961 it was highly appeared in 1980 and responsible for pandemic. MRSA was major risk for people having low immunity therefore death rate was approximately 15 times and bacteraemia was observed to be 24-fold than earlier [132]. MRSA outspread in Europe in early 1970's was confirmed to be caused by one of the MRSA clones called 83 phages; an archaic clone which eventually became demolished and replaced by another five lineage clones of MRSA by 1980's. The foremost MRSA infection case was observed in Sydney in 1965 followed by sporadic nosocomial MRSA infections in Melbourne, Sydney and other cities of Australia [133, 134]. Western Australia was rather reported to be free from these infections until late 1980's when gentamicin susceptible Non-Multidrug Resistant (MDR) MRSA was observed first which later on outspread very fast [135, 136]. However, the quickest outbreak of MRSA was observed in Boston, United States of America in 1968 [137]. Number of cases increased drastically from 2.4–29% from 1968 to 1975 which rose to 56.1% till 2003 [138, 139]. Moreover, high rate of MRSA infections was observed in other parts across the world also [140–147]. In japan MRSA infections invaded in academic hospitals in 1980 which later become community spread in 1990 [148]. Number of MRSA infected patients were comparatively lower than observed in America however mild increase was observed in frequency of MRSA patients from 3.8% - 9.6% in 1990-1994. But when only the outpatients were considered the MRSA infection rate was observed to be drastically rose from 4.5-35% in 1994 [149, 150]. The first clinical isolate of MRSA known to carry PVL gene in CA-MRSA era was observed in 2003. Furthermore, according to the data given by National Infectious disease register in 10-fold increase in MRSA infectious cases i.e. 120-1458 has been found in 2004. Meanwhile the countries like Norway, Sweden, Denmark and Netherland were found to be free from these infections due to strict surveillance. In the period of six years (2000-2006), Eastern Australia and Queensland were reported to have an increase of 75-315 patients per million. MRSA strains prevalent in these countries were majorly non-MDR strains which have susceptibility to ciprofloxacin and resistant at least to one of the β-lactams. It was a period of high emergence of non-MDR strains of MRSA. In 2011, surveillance studies were carried out in Asian countries to find out the patients with MRSA infections [151–154]. Data revealed HA-MRSA prevalence was highest in Sri Lanka (86.5%) followed by Vietnam (74.1%), South Korea (65%), Thailand (57%) and Hong Kong (56.8%). However, the rate of infections in Indians and Philippines was quite low i.e. 22.6 and 38.1% approximately. Infected patients and staff were the major reason for the outbreak of MRSA across the countries and continents. With time and resistance MRSA had been found to be emerged, declined and modified accordingly. When initially observed, the MRSA strains were confined only to the hospitals and health care centres which later on becomes a pandemic via community spread. Moreover, livestock was also found to be affected by MRSA infections. According to last research report vancomycin was an antibiotic susceptible to MRSA however later on some investigations demonstrated Vancomycin Intermediate resistance *Staphylococcus aureus* (VISA) and Vancomycin Resistant *Staphylococcus aureus* (VRSA) in some clinical strains. If this trend gets continued to be followed further then MRSA will undoubtedly become completely resistant strain which is a serious topic of concern in field of infectious diseases [155–158].

5. Conclusion

The rapid evolution of resistance in *Staphylococcus aureus* toward almost every antibiotic makes it a most challenging threat for human health as well as for the microbiology scientists. This bacteraemia has been reported to possess resistance mechanisms on the exposure of antibiotics only. Staphylococcus aureus quickly develop the defense/survival mechanism for even the new antibiotics which probably due to their fast structural and genetical alterations. Keeping this in view, several novel compounds are in pipeline to combat the resistant strains of *Staphylococcus aureus*. Moreover, identification of additional drug targets, better stewardship and combination therapies are also in process for the treatment of resistant strains of *Staphylococcus aureus*.

Acknowledgements

Authors are grateful to the University Grants Commission for providing NFOBC to Atamjit Singh. The authors are also thankful to Guru Nanak Dev University, Amritsar for providing various facilities to carry out the work.

Conflict of interest

The authors declare no conflict of interest.

Author details

Atamjit Singh[1*†], Kirandeep Kaur[1†], Pallvi Mohana[2], Avneet Kaur[2], Komalpreet Kaur[1], Shilpa Heer[1], Saroj Arora[2], Neena Bedi[1] and Preet Mohinder Singh Bedi[1]

1 Department of Pharmaceutical Sciences, Guru Nanak Dev University, Amritsar, Punjab, India

2 Department of Botanical and Environmental Sciences, Guru Nanak Dev University, Amritsar, Punjab, India

*Address all correspondence to: atampanesar@yahoo.com

† Both sharing Co-first authorship.

References

[1] Ali, E. A., Alshuaibi, O. N., & Ali, K. S. (2021). Evaluation of some antibiotic resistance in staphylococcus aureus isolated by medical laboratories aden, yemen. Electronic Journal of University of Aden for Basic and Applied Sciences, 2(1), 49-53.

[2] Rağbetli, C., Parlak, M., Bayram, Y., Guducuoglu, H., & Ceylan, N. (2016). Evaluation of antimicrobial resistance in Staphylococcus aureus isolates by years. Interdisciplinary perspectives on infectious diseases, 2016.

[3] Ioannou, C. J., Hanlon, G. W., & Denyer, S. P. (2007). Action of disinfectant quaternary ammonium compounds against Staphylococcus aureus. Antimicrobial agents and chemotherapy, 51(1), 296.C. J. Ioannou,

[4] Cohen, M. L. (1992). Epidemiology of drug resistance: implications for a post—antimicrobial era. Science, 257(5073), 1050-1055.

[5] Tomasz, A. (1994). Multiple-Antibiotic-Resistant Pathogenic Bacteria--A Report on the Rockefeller University Workshop. New England journal of medicine, 330(17), 1247-1251.

[6] Swartz, M. N. (1997). Use of antimicrobial agents and drug resistance.

[7] Lowy, F. D. (1998). Staphylococcus aureus infections. New England journal of medicine, 339(8), 520-532.

[8] Mandell, G. L., Bennett, J. E., & Dolin, R. (2000). Staphylococcus aureus (including Staphylococcal toxic shock). Bennett's-Principles and Practice of Infectious Diseases.

[9] Mylotte, J. M., McDermott, C., & Spooner, J. A. (1987). Prospective study of 114 consecutive episodes of Staphylococcus aureus bacteremia. Reviews of infectious diseases, 9(5), 891-907.

[10] Diekema, D. J., Pfaller, M. A., Schmitz, F. J., Smayevsky, J., Bell, J., Jones, R. N., ... & SENTRY Participants Group. (2001). Survey of infections due to Staphylococcus species: frequency of occurrence and antimicrobial susceptibility of isolates collected in the United States, Canada, Latin America, Europe, and the Western Pacific region for the SENTRY Antimicrobial Surveillance Program, 1997-1999. Clinical Infectious Diseases, 32(Supplement_2), S114-S132.

[11] Hiramatsu, K., Hanaki, H., Ino, T., Yabuta, K., Oguri, T., & Tenover, F. C. (1997). Methicillin-resistant Staphylococcus aureus clinical strain with reduced vancomycin susceptibility. The Journal of antimicrobial chemotherapy, 40(1), 135-136.

[12] Centers for Disease Control and Prevention (CDC. (2002). Staphylococcus aureus resistant to vancomycin--United States, 2002. MMWR. Morbidity and mortality weekly report, 51(26), 565-567.

[13] Skinner, D., & Keefer, C. S. (1941). Significance of bacteremia caused by Staphylococcus aureus: a study of one hundred and twenty-two cases and a review of the literature concerned with experimental infection in animals. Archives of internal medicine, 68(5), 851-875.

[14] Rajput, A., Kaur, K. and Kumar, M., 2016. SigMol: repertoire of quorum sensing signaling molecules in prokaryotes. Nucleic acids research, 44(D1), D634-D639.

[15] Waters, C.M. and Bassler, B.L., 2005. Quorum sensing: cell-to-cell communication in bacteria. Annu. Rev. Cell Dev. Biol., 21, 319-346.

[16] Papenfort, K. and Bassler, B.L., 2016. Quorum sensing signal–response systems in Gram-negative bacteria. Nature Reviews Microbiology, 14(9), 576-588.

[17] Huang, J., Shi, Y., Zeng, G., Gu, Y., Chen, G., Shi, L., Hu, Y., Tang, B. and Zhou, J., 2016. Acyl-homoserine lactone-based quorum sensing and quorum quenching hold promise to determine the performance of biological wastewater treatments: an overview. Chemosphere, 157, 137-151.

[18] Queck, S.Y., Jameson-Lee, M., Villaruz, A.E., Bach, T.H.L., Khan, B.A., Sturdevant, D.E., Ricklefs, S.M., Li, M. and Otto, M., 2008. RNAIII-independent target gene control by the agr quorum-sensing system: insight into the evolution of virulence regulation in Staphylococcus aureus. Molecular cell, 32(1), 150-158.

[19] Queck, S.Y., Jameson-Lee, M., Villaruz, A.E., Bach, T.H.L., Khan, B.A., Sturdevant, D.E., Ricklefs, S.M., Li, M. and Otto, M., 2008. RNAIII-independent target gene control by the agr quorum-sensing system: insight into the evolution of virulence regulation in Staphylococcus aureus. Molecular cell, 32(1), 150-158.

[20] Rammelkamp, C. H., & Maxon, T. (1942). Resistance of Staphylococcus aureus to the Action of Penicillin. Proceedings of the Society for Experimental Biology and Medicine, 51(3), 386-389.

[21] Chambers, H. F. (2001). The changing epidemiology of Staphylococcus aureus?. Emerging infectious diseases, 7(2), 178.

[22] Kernodle, D. S. (2000). Gram-positive pathogens. Fischetti, VA, 609-620.

[23] Gregory, P. D., Lewis, R. A., Curnock, S. P., & Dyke, K. G. H. (1997). Studies of the repressor (BlaI) of β-lactamase synthesis in Staphylococcus aureus. Molecular microbiology, 24(5), 1025-1037.

[24] Zhang, H. Z., Hackbarth, C. J., Chansky, K. M., & Chambers, H. F. (2001). A proteolytic transmembrane signaling pathway and resistance to β-lactams in staphylococci. Science, 291(5510), 1962-1965.

[25] Jevons, M. P. (1961). Letter Br. Med J, 1, 124-125.

[26] Cosgrove, S. E., Sakoulas, G., Perencevich, E. N., Schwaber, M. J., Karchmer, A. W., & Carmeli, Y. (2003). Comparison of mortality associated with methicillin-resistant and methicillin-susceptible Staphylococcus aureus bacteremia: a meta-analysis. Clinical infectious diseases, 36(1), 53-59.

[27] Lyon, B. R., Iuorio, J. L., May, J. W., & Skurray, R. A. (1984). Molecular epidemiology of multiresistant Staphylococcus aureus in Australian hospitals. Journal of medical microbiology, 17(1), 79-89.

[28] Kernodle, D. S. (2000). Gram-positive pathogens. Fischetti, VA, 609-620.

[29] Chambers, H. F. (1997). Methicillin resistance in staphylococci: molecular and biochemical basis and clinical implications. Clinical microbiology reviews, 10(4), 781-791.

[30] Katayama, Y., Ito, T., & Hiramatsu, K. (2000). A new class of genetic element, staphylococcus cassette chromosome mec, encodes methicillin resistance in Staphylococcus aureus. Antimicrobial agents and chemotherapy, 44(6), 1549-1555.

[31] Ito, T., Katayama, Y., & Hiramatsu, K. (1999). Cloning and nucleotide sequence determination of the entire mec DNA of pre-methicillin-resistant

Staphylococcus aureus N315. Antimicrobial agents and chemotherapy, 43(6), 1449-1458.

[32] Hartman, B. J., & Tomasz, A. (1984). Low-affinity penicillin-binding protein associated with beta-lactam resistance in Staphylococcus aureus. Journal of bacteriology, 158(2), 513-516.

[33] Utsui, Y. U. K. I. O., & Yokota, T. A. K. E. S. H. I. (1985). Role of an altered penicillin-binding protein in methicillin-and cephem-resistant Staphylococcus aureus. Antimicrobial agents and chemotherapy, 28(3), 397-403.

[34] Song, M. D., Wachi, M., Doi, M., Ishino, F., & Matsuhashi, M. (1987). Evolution of an inducible penicillin-target protein in methicillin-resistant Staphylococcus aureus by gene fusion. FEBS letters, 221(1), 167-171.

[35] Ghuysen, J. M. (1994). Molecular structures of penicillin-binding proteins and β-lactamases. Trends in microbiology, 2(10), 372-380.

[36] Lim, D., & Strynadka, N. C. (2002). Structural basis for the β lactam resistance of PBP2a from methicillin-resistant Staphylococcus aureus. Nature structural biology, 9(11), 870-876.

[37] Archer, G. L., & Bosilevac, J. M. (2001). Signaling antibiotic resistance in staphylococci. Science, 291(5510), 1915-1916.

[38] Berger-Bächi, B. (1994). Expression of resistance to methicillin. Trends in microbiology, 2(10), 389-393.

[39] Saravolatz, L. D., Stein, G. E., & Johnson, L. B. (2011). Ceftaroline: a novel cephalosporin with activity against methicillin-resistant Staphylococcus aureus. Clinical infectious diseases, 52(9), 1156-1163.

[40] Chung, M., Antignac, A., Kim, C., & Tomasz, A. (2008). Comparative study of the susceptibilities of major epidemic clones of methicillin-resistant Staphylococcus aureus to oxacillin and to the new broad-spectrum cephalosporin ceftobiprole. Antimicrobial agents and chemotherapy, 52(8), 2709-2717.

[41] Biek, D., Critchley, I. A., Riccobene, T. A., & Thye, D. A. (2010). Ceftaroline fosamil: a novel broad-spectrum cephalosporin with expanded anti-Gram-positive activity. Journal of antimicrobial chemotherapy, 65(suppl_4), iv9-iv16.

[42] Sakoulas, G., Moise, P. A., Casapao, A. M., Nonejuie, P., Olson, J., Okumura, C. Y., Rybak, M.J., Kullar, R., Dhand, A., Rose, W.E., & Nizet, V. (2014). Antimicrobial salvage therapy for persistent staphylococcal bacteremia using daptomycin plus ceftaroline. Clinical therapeutics, 36(10), 1317-1333.

[43] Sader, H. S., Farrell, D. J., Flamm, R. K., & Jones, R. N. (2015). Activity of ceftaroline and comparator agents tested against Staphylococcus aureus from patients with bloodstream infections in US medical centres (2009-13). Journal of Antimicrobial Chemotherapy, 70(7), 2053-2056.

[44] Biedenbach, D. J., Hoban, D. J., Reiszner, E., Lahiri, S. D., Alm, R. A., Sahm, D. F., Bouchillon, S.K., & Ambler, J. E. (2015). In vitro activity of ceftaroline against Staphylococcus aureus isolates collected in 2012 from Latin American countries as part of the AWARE surveillance program. Antimicrobial agents and chemotherapy, 59(12), 7873-7877.

[45] Farrell, D. J., Flamm, R. K., Sader, H. S., & Jones, R. N. (2013). Spectrum and potency of ceftaroline tested against leading pathogens causing skin and soft-tissue infections in Europe (2010). International journal of antimicrobial agents, 41(4), 337-342.

[46] Biedenbach, D. J., Alm, R. A., Lahiri, S. D., Reiszner, E., Hoban, D. J., Sahm, D. F., Bouchillon, S.K., & Ambler, J. E. (2016). In vitro activity of ceftaroline against Staphylococcus aureus isolated in 2012 from Asia-Pacific countries as part of the AWARE surveillance program. Antimicrobial agents and chemotherapy, 60(1), 343-347.

[47] Abbott, I. J., Jenney, A. W. J., Jeremiah, C. J., Mirčeta, M., Kandiah, J. P., Holt, D. C., Tong, S.Y.C., & Spelman, D. W. (2015). Reduced in vitro activity of ceftaroline by Etest among clonal complex 239 methicillin-resistant Staphylococcus aureus clinical strains from Australia. Antimicrobial agents and chemotherapy, 59(12), 7837-7841.

[48] Mubarak, N., Sandaradura, I., Isaia, L., O'Sullivan, M., Zhou, F., Marriott, D., Iredell, J.R., Harkness, J., & Andresen, D. (2015). Non-susceptibility to ceftaroline in healthcare-associated multiresistant MRSA in Eastern Australia. Journal of Antimicrobial Chemotherapy, 70(8), 2413-2414.

[49] Lahiri, S. D., McLaughlin, R. E., Whiteaker, J. D., Ambler, J. E., & Alm, R. A. (2015). Molecular characterization of MRSA isolates bracketing the current EUCAST ceftaroline-susceptible breakpoint for Staphylococcus aureus: the role of PBP2a in the activity of ceftaroline. Journal of Antimicrobial Chemotherapy, 70(9), 2488-2498.

[50] Chan, L. C., Basuino, L., Diep, B., Hamilton, S., Chatterjee, S. S., & Chambers, H. F. (2015). Ceftobiprole- and ceftaroline-resistant methicillin-resistant Staphylococcus aureus. Antimicrobial agents and chemotherapy, 59(5), 2960-2963.

[51] Lahiri, S. D., & Alm, R. A. (2016). Potential of Staphylococcus aureus isolates carrying different PBP2a alleles to develop resistance to ceftaroline. Journal of Antimicrobial Chemotherapy, 71(1), 34-40.

[52] Sarkar, P., & Haldar, J. (2019). Glycopeptide Antibiotics: Mechanism of Action and Recent Developments. Antibiotic Drug Resistance, 73-95.

[53] Lin, L. C., Chang, S. C., Ge, M. C., Liu, T. P., & Lu, J. J. (2018). Novel single-nucleotide variations associated with vancomycin resistance in vancomycin-intermediate Staphylococcus aureus. Infection and drug resistance, 11, 113.

[54] Tan, X. E., Neoh, H. M., Looi, M. L., Chin, S. F., Cui, L., Hiramatsu, K., Hussin, S., & Jamal, R. (2017). Activated ADI pathway: the initiator of intermediate vancomycin resistance in Staphylococcus aureus. Canadian journal of microbiology, 63(3), 260-264.

[55] Werner, G., Strommenger, B., & Witte, W. (2008). Acquired vancomycin resistance in clinically relevant pathogens.

[56] Gomes, D. M., Ward, K. E., & LaPlante, K. L. (2015). Clinical Implications of Vancomycin Heteroresistant and Intermediately Susceptible Staphylococcus aureus. Pharmacotherapy: The Journal of Human Pharmacology and Drug Therapy, 35(4), 424-432.

[57] Chen, H., Xiong, Z., Liu, K., Li, S., Wang, R., Wang, X., ... & Wang, H. (2016). Transcriptional profiling of the two-component regulatory system VraSR in Staphylococcus aureus with low-level vancomycin resistance. International journal of antimicrobial agents, 47(5), 362-367.

[58] Katayama, Y., Sekine, M., Hishinuma, T., Aiba, Y., & Hiramatsu, K. (2016). Complete reconstitution of the vancomycin-intermediate Staphylococcus aureus phenotype of strain Mu50 in vancomycin-susceptible S. aureus. Antimicrobial agents and chemotherapy, 60(6), 3730-3742.

[59] Yoo, J. I., Kim, J. W., Kang, G. S., Kim, H. S., Yoo, J. S., & Lee, Y. S. (2013). Prevalence of amino acid changes in the yvqF, vraSR, graSR, and tcaRAB genes from vancomycin intermediate resistant Staphylococcus aureus. Journal of microbiology, 51(2), 160-165.

[60] Hollenbeck, B. L., & Rice, L. B. (2012). Intrinsic and acquired resistance mechanisms in enterococcus. Virulence, 3(5), 421-569.

[61] Humphries, R. M., Pollett, S., & Sakoulas, G. (2013). A current perspective on daptomycin for the clinical microbiologist. Clinical microbiology reviews, 26(4), 759-780.

[62] Murthy, M. H., Olson, M. E., Wickert, R. W., Fey, P. D., & Jalali, Z. (2008). Daptomycin non-susceptible meticillin-resistant Staphylococcus aureus USA 300 isolate. Journal of medical microbiology, 57(8), 1036-1038.

[63] Mammina, C., Bonura, C., di Carlo, P., Calà, C., Aleo, A., Monastero, R., & Palma, D. M. (2010). Daptomycin non-susceptible, vancomycin intermediate methicillin-resistant Staphylococcus aureus ST398 from a chronic leg ulcer, Italy. Scandinavian journal of infectious diseases, 42(11-12), 955-957.

[64] Silverman, J. A., Oliver, N., Andrew, T., & Li, T. (2001). Resistance studies with daptomycin. Antimicrobial Agents and Chemotherapy, 45(6), 1799-1802.

[65] Jones, T., Yeaman, M. R., Sakoulas, G., Yang, S. J., Proctor, R. A., Sahl, H.G., Schrenzel, J., Xiong, Y.Q. , & Bayer, A. S. (2008). Failures in clinical treatment of Staphylococcus aureus infection with daptomycin are associated with alterations in surface charge, membrane phospholipid asymmetry, and drug binding. Antimicrobial agents and chemotherapy, 52(1), 269-278.

[66] Bellido, J. L. M. (2017). Mechanisms of resistance to daptomycin in Staphylococcus aureus. Rev. Esp. Quimioter, 30, 391-396.

[67] Mishra, N. N., Yang, S. J., Sawa, A., Rubio, A., Nast, C. C., Yeaman, M. R., & Bayer, A. S. (2009). Analysis of cell membrane characteristics of in vitro-selected daptomycin-resistant strains of methicillin-resistant Staphylococcus aureus. Antimicrobial agents and chemotherapy, 53(6), 2312-2318.

[68] Ernst, C. M., Slavetinsky, C. J., Kuhn, S., Hauser, J. N., Nega, M., Mishra, N. N., Gekeler, C., Bayer, A.S., & Peschel, A. (2018). Gain-of-function mutations in the phospholipid flippase MprF confer specific daptomycin resistance. MBio, 9(6).

[69] Roch, M., Gagetti, P., Davis, J., Ceriana, P., Errecalde, L., Corso, A., & Rosato, A. E. (2017). Daptomycin resistance in clinical MRSA strains is associated with a high biological fitness cost. Frontiers in microbiology, 8, 2303.

[70] Barros, E. M., Martin, M. J., Selleck, E. M., Lebreton, F., Sampaio, J. L. M., & Gilmore, M. S. (2019). Daptomycin resistance and tolerance due to loss of function in Staphylococcus aureus dsp1 and asp23. Antimicrobial agents and chemotherapy, 63(1).

[71] Sabat, A. J., Tinelli, M., Grundmann, H., Akkerboom, V., Monaco, M., Del Grosso, M., Errico, G., Pantosti, A., & Friedrich, A. W. (2018). Daptomycin resistant Staphylococcus aureus clinical strain with novel non-synonymous mutations in the mprF and vraS genes: a new insight into daptomycin resistance. Frontiers in microbiology, 9, 2705.

[72] Kanesaka, I., Fujisaki, S., Aiba, Y., Watanabe, S., Mikawa, T., Katsuse, A. K., Takahashi, H., Cui, L., & Kobayashi, I. (2019). Characterization of compensatory mutations associated

with restoration of daptomycin-susceptibility in daptomycin non-susceptible methicillin-resistant Staphylococcus aureus and the role mprF mutations. Journal of Infection and Chemotherapy, 25(1), 1-5.

[73] Vakulenko, S. B., & Mobashery, S. (2003). Versatility of aminoglycosides and prospects for their future. Clinical microbiology reviews, 16(3), 430-450.

[74] Ramirez, M. S., & Tolmasky, M. E. (2010). Aminoglycoside modifying enzymes. Drug resistance updates, 13(6), 151-171.

[75] Krause, K. M., Serio, A. W., Kane, T. R., & Connolly, L. E. (2016). Aminoglycosides: an overview. Cold Spring Harbor perspectives in medicine, 6(6), a027029.

[76] Díaz, M. C. L., Ríos, E., Rodríguez-Avial, I., Simaluiza, R. J., Picazo, J. J., & Culebras, E. (2017). In-vitro activity of several antimicrobial agents against methicillin-resistant Staphylococcus aureus (MRSA) isolates expressing aminoglycoside-modifying enzymes: potency of plazomicin alone and in combination with other agents. International journal of antimicrobial agents, 50(2), 191-196.

[77] Shaeer, K. M., Zmarlicka, M. T., Chahine, E. B., Piccicacco, N., & Cho, J. C. (2019). Plazomicin: A Next-Generation Aminoglycoside. Pharmacotherapy: The Journal of Human Pharmacology and Drug Therapy, 39(1), 77-93.

[78] Rybak, J. M., & Roberts, K. (2015). Tedizolid phosphate: a next-generation oxazolidinone. Infectious diseases and therapy, 4(1), 1-14.

[79] Munita, J. M., Bayer, A. S., & Arias, C. A. (2015). Evolving resistance among Gram-positive pathogens. Clinical Infectious Diseases, 61(suppl_2), S48-S57.

[80] Pillai, S. K., Sakoulas, G., Wennersten, C., Eliopoulos, G. M., Moellering Jr, R. C., Ferraro, M. J., & Gold, H. S. (2002). Linezolid resistance in Staphylococcus aureus: characterization and stability of resistant phenotype. The Journal of infectious diseases, 186(11), 1603-1607.

[81] Livermore, D. M. (2003). Linezolid in vitro: mechanism and antibacterial spectrum. Journal of Antimicrobial Chemotherapy, 51(suppl_2), ii9-ii16.

[82] Belousoff, M. J., Eyal, Z., Radjainia, M., Ahmed, T., Bamert, R. S., Matzov, D., Bashan, A., Zimmerman, E., Mishra, S., Cameron, D., & Yonath, A. (2017). Structural basis for linezolid binding site rearrangement in the Staphylococcus aureus ribosome. MBio, 8(3).

[83] Gu, B., Kelesidis, T., Tsiodras, S., Hindler, J., & Humphries, R. M. (2013). The emerging problem of linezolid-resistant Staphylococcus. Journal of Antimicrobial Chemotherapy, 68(1), 4-11.

[84] Li, S. M., Zhou, Y. F., Li, L., Fang, L. X., Duan, J. H., Liu, F. R., Liang, H.Q., Wu, Y.T., Gu, W.Q., Liao, X.P., & Liu, Y. H. (2018). Characterization of the multi-drug resistance gene cfr in methicillin-resistant Staphylococcus aureus (MRSA) strains isolated from animals and humans in China. Frontiers in microbiology, 9, 2925.

[85] Wang, Y., Lv, Y., Cai, J., Schwarz, S., Cui, L., Hu, Z., Zhang, R., Li, J., Zhao, Q., He, T., & Shen, J. (2015). A novel gene, optrA, that confers transferable resistance to oxazolidinones and phenicols and its presence in *Enterococcus faecalis* and *Enterococcus faecium* of human and animal origin. Journal of Antimicrobial Chemotherapy, 70(8), 2182-2190.

[86] Foster, T. J. (2017). Antibiotic resistance in Staphylococcus aureus.

Current status and future prospects. FEMS microbiology reviews, 41(3), 430-449.

[87] Wang, Y., Li, X., Wang, Y., Schwarz, S., Shen, J., & Xia, X. (2018). Intracellular accumulation of linezolid and florfenicol in OptrA-producing *Enterococcus faecalis* and Staphylococcus aureus. Molecules, 23(12), 3195.

[88] Sharkey, L. K., Edwards, T. A., & O'Neill, A. J. (2016). ABC-F proteins mediate antibiotic resistance through ribosomal protection. MBio, 7(2).

[89] Antonelli, A., D'Andrea, M. M., Brenciani, A., Galeotti, C. L., Morroni, G., Pollini, S., Varaldo, P.E., & Rossolini, G. M. (2018). Characterization of poxtA, a novel phenicol–oxazolidinone–tetracycline resistance gene from an MRSA of clinical origin. Journal of Antimicrobial Chemotherapy, 73(7), 1763-1769.

[90] Saravolatz, L. D., & Stein, G. E. (2019). Delafloxacin: A New Anti–methicillin-resistant Staphylococcus aureus Fluoroquinolone. Clinical Infectious Diseases, 68(6), 1058-1062.

[91] Lemaire, S., Tulkens, P. M., & Van Bambeke, F. (2011). Contrasting effects of acidic pH on the extracellular and intracellular activities of the anti-gram-positive fluoroquinolones moxifloxacin and delafloxacin against Staphylococcus aureus. Antimicrobial agents and chemotherapy, 55(2), 649-658.

[92] Van Bambeke, F. (2015). Delafloxacin, a non-zwitterionic fluoroquinolone in phase III of clinical development: evaluation of its pharmacology, pharmacokinetics, pharmacodynamics and clinical efficacy. Future microbiology, 10(7), 1111-1123.

[93] Bauer, J., Siala, W., Tulkens, P. M., & Van Bambeke, F. (2013). A combined pharmacodynamic quantitative and qualitative model reveals the potent activity of daptomycin and delafloxacin against Staphylococcus aureus biofilms. Antimicrobial agents and chemotherapy, 57(6), 2726-2737.

[94] Siala, W., Mingeot-Leclercq, M. P., Tulkens, P. M., Hallin, M., Denis, O., & Van Bambeke, F. (2014). Comparison of the antibiotic activities of daptomycin, vancomycin, and the investigational fluoroquinolone delafloxacin against biofilms from Staphylococcus aureus clinical isolates. Antimicrobial agents and chemotherapy, 58(11), 6385-6397.

[95] Wassenaar, T., Ussery, D., Nielsen, L., & Ingmer, H. (2015). Review and phylogenetic analysis of qac genes that reduce susceptibility to quaternary ammonium compounds in Staphylococcus species. European Journal of Microbiology and Immunology, 5(1), 44-61.

[96] Costa, S. S., Falcão, C., Viveiros, M., Machado, D., Martins, M., Melo-Cristino, J., Amaral, L., & Couto, I. (2011). Exploring the contribution of efflux on the resistance to fluoroquinolones in clinical isolates of Staphylococcus aureus. BMC microbiology, 11(1), 1-12.

[97] Muñoz-Bellido, J. L., Manzanares, M. A., Andrés, J. M., Zufiaurre, M. G., Ortiz, G., Hernández, M. S., & García-Rodríguez, J. A. (1999). Efflux pump-mediated quinolone resistance in Staphylococcus aureus strains wild type for gyrA, gyrB, grlA, and norA. Antimicrobial agents and chemotherapy, 43(2), 354-356.

[98] Remy, J. M., Tow-Keogh, C. A., McConnell, T. S., Dalton, J. M., & DeVito, J. A. (2012). Activity of delafloxacin against methicillin-resistant Staphylococcus aureus: resistance selection and characterization. Journal of antimicrobial chemotherapy, 67(12), 2814-2820.

[99] Greer, E. L., Banko, M. R., & Brunet, A. (2009). AMP-activated protein kinase and FoxO transcription factors in dietary restriction–induced longevity. Annals of the New York Academy of Sciences, 1170, 688.

[100] Prince, W. T., Ivezic-Schoenfeld, Z., Lell, C., Tack, K. J., Novak, R., Obermayr, F., & Talbot, G. H. (2013). Phase II clinical study of BC-3781, a pleuromutilin antibiotic, in treatment of patients with acute bacterial skin and skin structure infections. Antimicrobial agents and chemotherapy, 57(5), 2087-2094.

[101] Paukner, S., & Riedl, R. (2017). Pleuromutilins: potent drugs for resistant bugs—mode of action and resistance. Cold Spring Harbor perspectives in medicine, 7(1), a027110.

[102] Schwarz, S., Shen, J., Kadlec, K., Wang, Y., Michael, G. B., Feßler, A. T., & Vester, B. (2016). Lincosamides, streptogramins, phenicols, and pleuromutilins: mode of action and mechanisms of resistance. Cold Spring Harbor perspectives in medicine, 6(11), a027037.

[103] Gentry, D. R., Rittenhouse, S. F., McCloskey, L., & Holmes, D. J. (2007). Stepwise exposure of Staphylococcus aureus to pleuromutilins is associated with stepwise acquisition of mutations in rplC and minimally affects susceptibility to retapamulin. Antimicrobial agents and chemotherapy, 51(6), 2048-2052.

[104] Kehrenberg, C., Schwarz, S., Jacobsen, L., Hansen, L. H., & Vester, B. (2005). A new mechanism for chloramphenicol, florfenicol and clindamycin resistance: methylation of 23S ribosomal RNA at A2503. Molecular microbiology, 57(4), 1064-1073.

[105] Van Duijkeren, E., Greko, C., Pringle, M., Baptiste, K. E., Catry, B., Jukes, H., Moreno, M.A., Pomba, M.C.M.F., Pyörälä, S., Rantala, M., & Törneke, K. (2014). Pleuromutilins: use in food-producing animals in the European Union, development of resistance and impact on human and animal health. Journal of Antimicrobial Chemotherapy, 69(8), 2022-2031.

[106] Mendes, R. E., Paukner, S., Doyle, T. B., Gelone, S. P., Flamm, R. K., & Sader, H. S. (2019). Low prevalence of gram-positive isolates showing elevated lefamulin MIC results during the SENTRY surveillance program for 2015-2016 and characterization of resistance mechanisms. Antimicrobial agents and chemotherapy, 63(4).

[107] Kadlec, K., & Schwarz, S. (2009). Novel ABC transporter gene, vga (C), located on a multiresistance plasmid from a porcine methicillin-resistant Staphylococcus aureus ST398 strain. Antimicrobial agents and chemotherapy, 53(8), 3589-3591.

[108] Miller, M. A., Dascal, A., Portnoy, J., & Mendelson, J. (1996). Development of mupirocin resistance among methicillin-resistant Staphylococcus aureus after widespread use of nasal mupirocin ointment. Infection Control & Hospital Epidemiology, 17(12), 811-813.

[109] Vasquez, J. E., Walker, E. S., Franzus, B. W., Overbay, B. K., Reagan, D. R., & Sarubbi, F. A. (2000). The epidemiology of mupirocin resistance among methicillin-resistant Staphylococcus aureus at a Veterans' Affairs hospital. Infection Control & Hospital Epidemiology, 21(7), 459-464.

[110] de Castro Nunes, E. L., dos Santos, K. R. N., Mondino, P. J. J., de Freire Bastos, M. D. C., & Giambiagi-deMarval, M. (1999). Detection of ileS-2 gene encoding mupirocin resistance in methicillin-resistant Staphylococcus aureus by multiplex PCR. Diagnostic microbiology and infectious disease, 34(2), 77-81.

[111] Patel, J. B., Gorwitz, R. J., & Jernigan, J. A. (2009). Mupirocin resistance. Clinical infectious diseases, 49(6), 935-941.

[112] Hayden, M. K., Lolans, K., Haffenreffer, K., Avery, T. R., Kleinman, K., Li, H., Kaganov, R.E., Lankiewicz, J., Moody, J., Septimus, E., & Huang, S. S. (2016). Chlorhexidine and mupirocin susceptibility of methicillin-resistant Staphylococcus aureus isolates in the REDUCE-MRSA trial. Journal of clinical microbiology, 54(11), 2735-2742.

[113] Lounsbury, N., Eidem, T., Colquhoun, J., Mateo, G., Abou-Gharbia, M., Dunman, P. M., & Childers, W. E. (2018). Novel inhibitors of Staphylococcus aureus RnpA that synergize with mupirocin. Bioorganic & medicinal chemistry letters, 28(6), 1127-1131.

[114] Zhanel, G. G., Calic, D., & Schweizer, F. (2010). Dalbavancin, oritavancin and telavancin: a comparative review. Drugs, 70, 859-886.

[115] Zeng, D., Debabov, D., Hartsell, T. L., Cano, R. J., Adams, S., Schuyler, J. A., McMillan, R., & Pace, J. L. (2016). Approved glycopeptide antibacterial drugs: mechanism of action and resistance. Cold Spring Harbor perspectives in medicine, 6(12), a026989.

[116] McCurdy, S. P., Jones, R. N., Mendes, R. E., Puttagunta, S., & Dunne, M. W. (2015). In vitro activity of dalbavancin against drug-resistant Staphylococcus aureus isolates from a global surveillance program. Antimicrobial agents and chemotherapy, 59(8), 5007-5009.

[117] Duncan, L. R., Sader, H. S., Smart, J. I., Flamm, R. K., & Mendes, R. E. (2017). Telavancin activity in vitro tested against a worldwide collection of Gram-positive clinical isolates (2014). Journal of global antimicrobial resistance, 10, 271-276.

[118] Kussmann, M., Karer, M., Obermueller, M., Schmidt, K., Barousch, W., Moser, D., Nehr, M., Ramharter, M., Poeppl, W., Makristathis, A., & Lagler, H. (2018). Emergence of a dalbavancin induced glycopeptide/lipoglycopeptide non-susceptible Staphylococcus aureus during treatment of a cardiac device-related endocarditis. Emerging microbes & infections, 7(1), 1-10.

[119] Werth, B. J., Jain, R., Hahn, A., Cummings, L., Weaver, T., Waalkes, A., Sengupta, D., Salipante, S.J., Rakita, R.M., & Butler-Wu, S. M. (2018). Emergence of dalbavancin non-susceptible, vancomycin-intermediate Staphylococcus aureus (VISA) after treatment of MRSA central line-associated bloodstream infection with a dalbavancin-and vancomycin-containing regimen. Clinical Microbiology and Infection, 24(4), 429.e1-429.e5.

[120] Fleming, A. (2001). On the antibacterial action of cultures of a penicillium, with special reference to their use in the isolation of B. influenzae. Bulletin of the World Health Organization, 79, 780-790.

[121] Lederberg, J. (1957). Mechanism of action of penicillin. Journal of bacteriology, 73(1), 144.

[122] Lowy, F. D. (2003). Antimicrobial resistance: the example of Staphylococcus aureus. The Journal of clinical investigation, 111(9), 1265-1273.

[123] Kirby, W. M. (1944). Extraction of a highly potent penicillin inactivator from penicillin resistant staphylococci. Science, 99(2579), 452-453.

[124] Rammelkamp, C. H., & Maxon, T. (1942). Resistance of Staphylococcus aureus to the Action of Penicillin.

Proceedings of the Society for Experimental Biology and Medicine, 51(3), 386-389.

[125] Bondi Jr, A., & Dietz, C. C. (1945). Penicillin resistant staphylococci. Proceedings of the Society for Experimental Biology and Medicine, 60(1), 55-58.

[126] Smith, I. M., & Vickers, A. B. (1960). Natural History of 338 Treated and Untreated Patients with Staphylococcal septicaemia (1936-1955.). Lancet, 1318-22.

[127] Jessen, O., Rosendal, K., Bülow, P., Faber, V., & Eriksen, K. R. (1969). Changing staphylococci and staphylococcal infections: a ten-year study of bacteria and cases of bacteremia. New England Journal of Medicine, 281(12), 627-635.

[128] Jevons, M. P. (1961). "Celbenin"-resistant staphylococci. British medical journal, 1(5219), 124.

[129] Katayama, Y., Ito, T., & Hiramatsu, K. (2000). A new class of genetic element, staphylococcus cassette chromosome mec, encodes methicillin resistance in Staphylococcus aureus. Antimicrobial agents and chemo therapy, 44(6), 1549-1555.

[130] Hiramatsu, K., Asada, K., Suzuki, E., Okonogi, K., & Yokota, T. (1992). Molecular cloning and nucleotide sequence determination of the regulator region of mecA gene in methicillin-resistant Staphylococcus aureus (MRSA). FEBS letters, 298(2-3), 133-136.

[131] Hartman, B. J., & Tomasz, A. (1984). Low-affinity penicillin-binding protein associated with beta-lactam resistance in Staphylococcus aureus. Journal of bacteriology, 158(2), 513-516.

[132] Reynolds, P. E., & Brown, D. F. (1985). Penicillin-binding proteins of β-lactam-resistant strains of Staphylococcus aureus: effect of growth conditions. FEBS letters, 192(1), 28-32.

[133] Rountree, P. M., & Beard, M. A. (1968). Hospital strains of Staphylococcus aureus, with particular reference to methicillin-resistant strains. Medical Journal of Australia, 2(26), 1163-8.

[134] Mäkelä, M. J., Puhakka, T., Ruuskanen, O., Leinonen, M., Saikku, P., Kimpimäki, M., Blomqvist, S., Hyypiä, T., & Arstila, P. (1998). Viruses and bacteria in the etiology of the common cold. Journal of clinical microbiology, 36(2), 539-542.

[135] Torvaldsen, S., Roberts, C., & Riley, T. V. (1999). The continuing evolution of methicillin-resistant Staphylococcus aureus in Western Australia. Infection control and hospital epidemiology, 20(2), 133-135.

[136] Barret, F. F. (1968). Methicillin resistant Staphylococcus aureus at Boston City Hospital. N Engl J Med, 279, 441-448.

[137] Panlilio, A. L., Culver, D. H., Gaynes, R. P., Banerjee, S., Henderson, T. S., Tolson, J. S., Martone, W.J., & National Nosocomial Infections Surveillance System. (1992). Methicillin-resistant Staphylococcus aureus in US hospitals, 1975-1991. Infection Control & Hospital Epidemiology, 13(10), 582-586.

[138] Meyer, E., Schwab, F., Gastmeier, P., Jonas, D., Rueden, H., & Daschner, F. D. (2006). Methicillin-resistant Staphylococcus aureus in German intensive care units during 2000-2003: data from Project SARI (Surveillance of Antimicrobial Use and Antimicrobial Resistance in Intensive Care Units). Infection Control & Hospital Epidemiology, 27(2), 146-154.

[139] Alcoceba, E., Mena, A., Perez, M. C., de Gopegui, E. R., Padilla, E., Gil, J.,

Ramirez, A., Gallegos, C., Serra, A., Perez, J.L., & Oliver, A. (2007). Molecular epidemiology of methicillin-resistant Staphylococcus aureus in Majorcan hospitals: high prevalence of the epidemic clone EMRSA-15. Clinical microbiology and infection, 13(6), 599-605.

[140] Conceicao, T., Aires-de-Sousa, M., Füzi, M., Toth, A., Paszti, J., Ungvári, E., ... & De Lencastre, H. (2007). Replacement of methicillin-resistant Staphylococcus aureus clones in Hungary over time: a 10-year surveillance study. Clinical Microbiology and Infection, 13(10), 971-979.

[141] Durmaz, B., Durmaz, R., & Şahin, K. (1997). Methicillin-resistance among Turkish isolates of Staphylococcus aureus strains from nosocomial and community infections and their resistance patterns using various antimicrobial agents. Journal of Hospital Infection, 37(4), 325-329.

[142] Peng, Q., Hou, B., Zhou, S., Huang, Y., Hua, D., Yao, F., & shu Qian, Y. (2010). Staphylococcal cassette chromosome mec (SCCmec) analysis and antimicrobial susceptibility profiles of methicillin-resistant Staphylococcus aureus (MRSA) isolates in a teaching hospital, Shantou, China. African Journal of Microbiology Research, 4(9), 844-848.

[143] Fluit, A. C., Wielders, C. L. C., Verhoef, J., & Schmitz, F. J. (2001). Epidemiology and susceptibility of 3,051 Staphylococcus aureus isolates from 25 university hospitals participating in the European SENTRY study. Journal of clinical microbiology, 39(10), 3727-3732.

[144] Lin, Y. C., Lauderdale, T. L., Lin, H. M., Chen, P. C., Cheng, M. F., Hsieh, K. S., & Liu, Y. C. (2007). An outbreak of methicillin-resistant Staphylococcus aureus infection in patients of a pediatric intensive care unit and high carriage rate among health care workers. Journal of Microbiology, Immunology, and Infection, 40(4), 325-334.

[145] Manzur, A., Dominguez, A. M., Pujol, M., González, M. P. M., Limon, E., Hornero, A., Martín, R., Gudiol, F., & Ariza, J. (2008). Community-acquired methicillin-resistant Staphylococcus aureus infections: an emerging threat in Spain. Clinical Microbiology and Infection, 14(4), 377-380.

[146] Oteo, J., Baquero, F., Vindel, A., & Campos, J. (2004). Antibiotic resistance in 3113 blood isolates of Staphylococcus aureus in 40 Spanish hospitals participating in the European Antimicrobial Resistance Surveillance System (2000-2002). Journal of Antimicrobial Chemotherapy, 53(6), 1033-1038.

[147] Tiemersma, E. W., Bronzwaer, S. L., Lyytikäinen, O., Degener, J. E., Schrijnemakers, P., Bruinsma, N., Monen, J., Witte, W., Grundmann, H., & European Antimicrobial Resistance Surveillance System Participants. (2004). Methicillin-resistant Staphylococcus aureus in Europe, 1999-2002. Emerging infectious diseases, 10(9), 1627.

[148] Kayaba, H., Kodama, K., Tamura, H., & Fuhwara, Y. (1997). The spread of methicillin-resistant Staphylococcus aureus in a rural community: will it become a common microorganism colonizing among the general population?. Surgery today, 27(3), 217-219.

[149] Piao, C., Karasawa, T., Totsuka, K., Uchiyama, T., & Kikuchi, K. (2005). Prospective surveillance of community-onset and healthcare-associated methicillin-resistant Staphylococcus aureus isolated from a university-affiliated hospital in Japan. Microbiology and immunology, 49(11), 959-970.

[150] Udo, E. E., Pearman, J. W., & Grubb, W. B. (1993). Genetic analysis of community isolates of methicillin-resistant Staphylococcus aureus in Western Australia. Journal of Hospital Infection, 25(2), 97-108.

[151] Ito, T., Iijima, M., Fukushima, T., Nonoyama, M., Ishii, M., Baranovich, T., Otsuka, T., Takano, T., & Yamamoto, T. (2008). Pediatric pneumonia death caused by community-acquired methicillin-resistant Staphylococcus aureus, Japan. Emerging infectious diseases, 14(8), 1312.

[152] Takizawa, Y., Taneike, I., Nakagawa, S., Oishi, T., Nitahara, Y., Iwakura, N., Ozaki, K., Takano, M., Nakayama, T., & Yamamoto, T. (2005). A Panton-Valentine leucocidin (PVL)-positive community-acquired methicillin-resistant Staphylococcus aureus (MRSA) strain, another such strain carrying a multiple-drug resistance plasmid, and other more-typical PVL-negative MRSA strains found in Japan. Journal of clinical microbiology, 43(7), 3356-3363.

[153] Kerttula, A. M., Lyytikäinen, O., Kardén-Lilja, M., Ibrahem, S., Salmenlinna, S., Virolainen, A., & Vuopio-Varkila, J. (2007). Nationwide trends in molecular epidemiology of methicillin-resistant Staphylococcus aureus, Finland, 1997-2004. BMC Infectious Diseases, 7(1), 1-9.

[154] Andersen, B. M., Rasch, M., & Syversen, G. (2007). Is an increase of MRSA in Oslo, Norway, associated with changed infection control policy?. Journal of Infection, 55(6), 531-538.

[155] Skov, R., Gudlaugsson, O., Hardardottir, H., Harthug, S., Jakobsen, T., Jørn Kolmos, H., Olsson-Liljequist, B., Peltonen, R., Tveten, Y., Vuopio-Varkila, J., & Åhrén, C. (2008). Proposal for common Nordic epidemiological terms and definitions for methicillin-resistant Staphylococcus aureus (MRSA). Scandinavian journal of infectious diseases, 40(6-7), 495-502.

[156] Stenhem, M., Örtqvist, Å., Ringberg, H., Larsson, L., Olsson-Liljequist, B., Hæggman, S., & Ekdahl, K. (2006). Epidemiology of methicillin-resistant Staphylococcus aureus (MRSA) in Sweden 2000-2003, increasing incidence and regional differences. BMC Infectious Diseases, 6(1), 1-7.

[157] Nimmo, G. R., Fong, J., Paterson, D. L., & McLaws, M. L. (2008). Changing epidemiology of meticillin-resistant S. aureus in Queensland, Australia, 2000-2006: use of passive surveillance of susceptibility phenotypes. Journal of Hospital Infection, 70(4), 305-313.

[158] Song, J. H., Hsueh, P. R., Chung, D. R., Ko, K. S., Kang, C. I., Peck, K. R., Yeom, J.S., Kim, S.W., Chang, H.H., Kim, Y.S., & Carlos, C. C. (2011). Spread of methicillin-resistant Staphylococcus aureus between the community and the hospitals in Asian countries: an ANSORP study. Journal of antimicrobial chemotherapy, 66(5), 1061-1069.

Chapter 5

Antimicrobial Resistance in *Staphylococcus aureus*

Riya Mukherjee, Anjali Priyadarshini, Ramendra Pati Pandey and Vethakkani Samuel Raj

Abstract

Staphylococcus aureus is a Gram-Positive bacteria that are responsible to cause skin infections and also shows toxic shock syndrome. Several antibiotics were given against the *S. aureus* infections but eventually, the prevalence of multidrug resistance of *Staphylococcus aureus* started emerging. Since then Methicillin-resistant *Staphylococcus aureus* strains (MRSA)were very common which causes nosocomial infections. Microorganisms for the need of the survival undergoes mutational changes either in their chromosomal DNA/RNA which confers the resistance. One of the famous examples is the resistance against methicillin in *Staphylococcus aureus*. The evolution of *S. aureus* is successful in developing multiple resistant strains. Plasmids are capable of carrying the resistant genes and also several toxic genes. In a recent study, it has been observed that drug resistance genes are located in the R plasmids and they are also responsible in conferring multi drug resistance and induce less utilization of multiple antimicrobial therapy. MRSA was not only resistant to methicillin, studies proved MRSA strains were resistant to macrolides, tetracyclines, chloramphenicol. Resistance to vancomycin was very evidently observed, and its transfer among the population and rising of resistant strains was becoming a major threat globally. The resistance of all these antimicrobial agents against the pathogenic microorganisms are taking a rise in some patients due to prolong use of the antimicrobial agents by these patients. The multi drug resistance has enhanced the mortality and morbidity rate which referred to the infecting agents as the "Super Bugs". Survival of the microorganisms has increased due to the gradual development of extensive resistance against varied antimicrobial drugs. Possible treatments with combinations are found to be the only hope for infections against *S. aureus*. Few drugs are in development such as Dalbavancin, Oritavancin, Tigecycline. These are the possible treatments upon which the work is going on to reduce the resistance against the invasive MRSA. This chapter highlights the profiles of *Staphylococcus aureus* and the resistance patterns along with transmission and the role of the plasmid in transmitting the resistance.

Keywords: multi-drug resistance, SaPIs, *mec A* gene, clinical MDR, daptomycin, dalbavancin

1. Introduction

Multi-Drug Resistance *of S. aureus* is a massive concern in the clinical world. Immunocompromised, diabetic, and weak immune systems are general medical problems but patients already suffering from these are more susceptible to the Staphylococcal infections and mainly by *S. aureus* which causes skin infections and soft tissue infections. The severity of the infections caused by *S. aureus* increases when there is overgrowth of the *S. aureus* on the infected part of the body which results in the secretion of toxins and causes a fatal condition known as toxic shock syndrome. Penicillin was used predominantly against infections caused by *S. aureus* but the organism started having resistant strains developed for fighting against Penicillin. Methicillin was the next approach that came up for *S. aureus* but the major failure of methicillin by forming MRSA strains made vancomycin the last hope for *S. aureus* infections. Methicillin is the synthetic antibacterial drug given to *S. aureus* widely. *S. aureus* is resistant to almost all antibiotic drugs that are so far used and among them Methicillin and Vancomycin are the two drugs that have shown resistance in *S. aureus*. In this, we will emphasize the genetic aspects of the resistance that is observed in *S. aureus*. The antibiotic resistance genes are generally present on plasmids, and nonessential for the survival of the organism but it provides the bacterial population with a means to reduce the genetic and physiological load on the majority of cells. Plasmid-borne genes can undergo more radical evolutionary changes without affecting the viability of the cell, as would changes to indispensable chromosomal genes, and established plasmid transfer mechanisms can provide recipient cells with new genetic material which has already been refined by selective pressures elsewhere. Besides plasmids, bacteriophages too have contributed towards development of resistance by transduction. Thus the continuous evolution of *S. aureus* strains was successful to bring forth the vancomycin-resistant strains as well (VRSA). New drug development and treatments are applied to the *S. aureus* mediated infections which have proved to be the immediate possible treatment for this. This chapter will help the readers to acquire a comprehensive knowledge regarding the Multi-Drug Resistance of *S. aureus* along with the resistance mechanism and possible treatments of *Staphylococcal* infections.

2. Multi-drug resistance

2.1 Overview of multi-drug resistance

Multi-Drug Resistance (MDR) is a global concern that is having a very bad impact on health care. Microbes are getting resistant to antibiotic therapies due to the constant exposure of antimicrobial drugs. In the past decade, microbial infections have raised enormously and this has led to an increased amount of resistance [1]. Multi drug resistance is the phenomenon in which pathogenic organisms are resistant to multiple chemotherapeutic agents [2]. The emergence of MDR rises the mortality and morbidity rates for which they are known as 'Superbugs'. It is said that MDR is a very natural process among microorganisms but the increasing amount of this process is due to several reasons like the use of undefined antimicrobial agents, unhygienic sanitary conditions, poor health care facilities. The omnipresent threat of antibiotic-resistant pathogens entails having very few antimicrobial agents for other infections [2, 3].

2.2 Classification of MDR

Many different definitions for multidrug-resistant (MDR), extensively drug-resistant (XDR) and pandrug-resistant (PDR) bacteria are being used to characterize the different patterns of resistance. Was defined as acquired non-susceptibility to at least one agent in three or more antimicrobial categories, XDR was defined as non-susceptibility to at least one agent in all but two or fewer antimicrobial categories (i.e. bacterial isolates remain susceptible to only one or two categories) and PDR was defined as non-susceptibility to all agents in all antimicrobial categories. MDR is a frequently encountered phenomenon in *S. aureus* which can be broadly classified as primary MDR, secondary MDR and clinical MDR (**Figure 1**) [1, 4–6]. Survival of the microorganisms has gradually developed extensive resistance against varied antimicrobial drugs. Also, there is a failure of many clinical trials which are not always due to the occurrence of resistance but all due to poor bioavailability of drugs, very poor immune system, excessive-high metabolism of drugs.

2.3 Mechanism of multi-drug resistance (MDR)

Before studying the resistance of *S. aureus*, it is very important to take a look upon all the possible biochemical mechanisms of resistance that the microbes show. Microorganisms have the ability to employ several ways to develop multi drug resistance [2]. The resistance of all these antimicrobial agents against the pathogenic microorganisms are taking a rise in some patients due to prolong use of the antimicrobial agents by these patients. Below, is the schematic diagram of all methods of resistance mechanism (**Figure 2**). Microorganisms for the need of the survival undergoes mutational changes either in their chromosomal DNA/RNA which confers the resistance. One of the famous examples is the resistance against methicillin in *Staphylococcus aureus*. The cell wall of the microbes plays a vital role as a barrier and helps in their survival but due to alteration in the chromosomal DNA or genetic mutations the compositions of the cell wall or the plasma membrane changes and this in turn encourage the resistance phenomenon.

Drug Efflux Pumps are one of the major ways for the MDR mechanism. ABC transporters (ATP Binding Cassette) are membrane proteins which are commonly defined as drug efflux pumps that specifically helps in the transport of the drugs in the cell. The P-glycoprotein or multi-resistant protein (MRP) damages

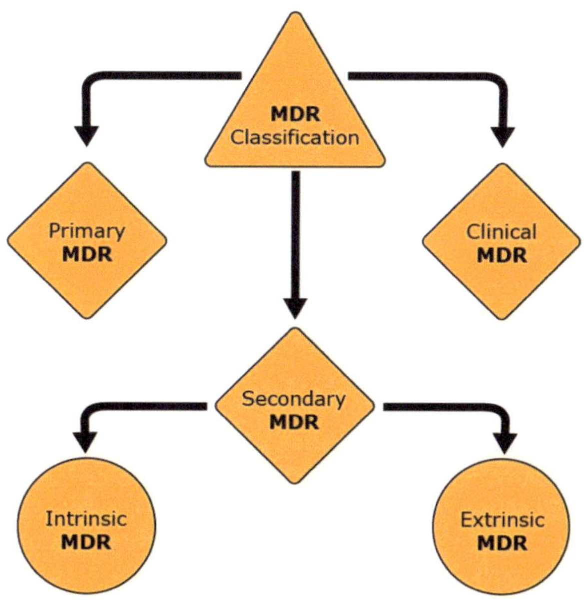

Figure 1.
Classification of MDR.

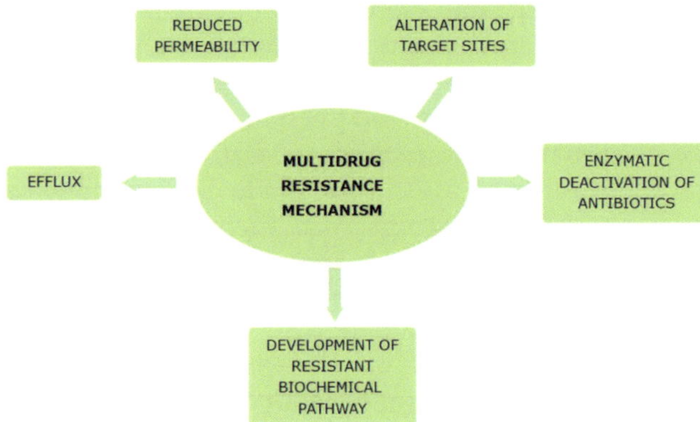

Figure 2.
Multi drug resistance mechanism.

the permeability and influences the ATP-dependent efflux of the drugs which is responsible for decreasing the intracellular concentrations [7–9].

3. Genetic aspect of resistance in *S. aureus*

The genetic determinants of resistance to many antimicrobial agents are believed to have evolved prior to the era of antibiotic chemotherapy. Processes such as phosphorylation, glycosylation, acetylation whose inactivation or chemical transformation is the major cause of the MDR. The schematic diagram shows the possible ways of causing antimicrobial resistance (**Figure 3**) [1, 4, 10–12].

Methicillin-Resistant *Staphylococcus aureus* (MRSA) came into the focus of attention when the Methicillin-Susceptible *Staphylococcus aureus* (MSSA) started adopting a specific gene (methicillin-resistant gene) named as *mecA* which is intervened by a genetic element called Staphylococcus cassette chromosome (SCC) and is transferred into the MSSA via either conjugation or transformation (Horizontal gene transfer). As SCC elements are carrying the gene *mecA* so, the complex is named *SCCmec.* The complex consists of the mecA and several other regulatory genes such as *mecR1*, *mecI*. (**Figure 4**), Demonstrate a schematic diagram of the SSC*mec* element. There is also the presence of a specific complex named Cassette Chromosome Recombinase (CCR) that helps in the integration and excision of the element from the chromosome of *Staphylococcal* species [13–16]. The region, origin of replication (oriC) in the *S. aureus* chromosomal element is accompanied by a special gene named as orfX towards the downstream of the oriC. The gene orfX is popular for encoding a specific enzyme called ribosomal RNA methyltransferase and this gene also has direct repeat sequences that help to protect the Staphylococcus cassette chromosome (SCC). In this way, multiple SCC elements are placed one after another in tandem which results in the formation of the cluster of foreign genes and forms a chromosomal region whose name is oriC environ [13, 17, 18]. Now, there are mainly two types of MRSA. One, the Community-Associated MRSA (CA-MRSA), and the other one is Hospital-Acquired MRSA (HA-MRSA). CA-MRSA has been found to get transmitted among the population from crowded places and the CA-MRSA isolates are highly resistant against methicillin and penicillin as well. Minor skin problems, redness, itchiness, and pain are the symptoms of the body affected by CA-MRSA. HA-MRSA is acquired from the hospital or any health care center. oriC environ has many transposons and insertion sequences (IS) which are capable to induce deletion, recombination, chromosomal

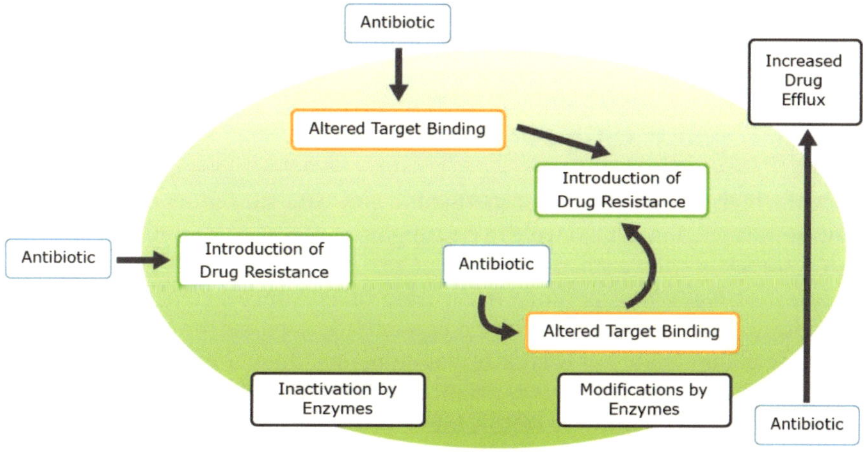

Figure 3.
Schematic diagram of antimicrobial resistance.

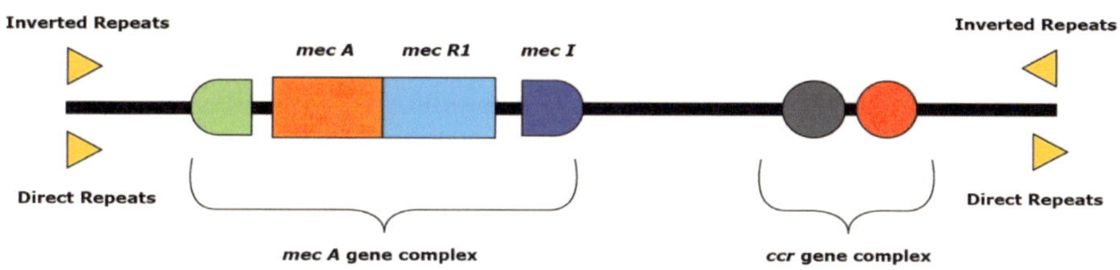

Figure 4.
*A schematic diagram of SCCmec element. The SCC*mec *consists of two components mec. A gene complex and* ccr *gene complex.* mec *gene complex helps to encode the methicillin resistance gene(*mec A*) and other two regulatory genes (*mecR1, mec1*).* ccr *gene complex takes care of the movement of the whole SCC element.*

inversion across oriC and this helps the *S. aureus* to maintain their survival strategy according to the environmental condition [18]. Horizontal gene transfer mediated by phage is one of the prime reason for the evolution of the *S. aureus*. It has been observed in the past studies that the Bacteriophages such as Staphylococcus Phage 80α is a specific helper bacteriophage that is required for the mobilization of SaPIs. This helps to carry the *Staphylococcus aureus* pathogenicity islands (SaPIs). SaPIs are known as mobile genetic elements which are the common residents in the genome of *S. aureus* and are transferred to other cells. These SaPIs are responsible for carrying several toxin genes and also superantigens [19, 20].

Plasmids are capable of carrying the resistant genes and also several toxic genes. In a recent study, it has been observed that when an *S. aureus* plasmid was sequenced which originated from a different bacterial environment, few trailblazing resistance genes named ampA and vgaC were discovered. The amp resistance gene is resistant to the antimicrobial drug named apramycin and the vgaC resistance gene is resistant against Streptogramin A, respectively. Along with these, many toxin genes are being carried on *S. aureus* plasmids such as exotoxin B (ETB) and enterotoxins (entA, entP, entG, entJ). R plasmids play a major role in mediating resistance among bacteria. Drug resistance genes are located in the R plasmids and they are also responsible in conferring multi drug resistance and induce less utilization of multiple antimicrobial therapy [21–23].

There is also support for the notion that some resistance determinants in staphylococci are derived from genes present in antibiotic-producing organisms. The *S. aureus* ermC methylase encoded on pE194 shares amino acid sequence homology with the analogous methylase encoded by erythromycin-producing organisms such as *Streptomyces erythraeus* (ermE) [24].

4. Resistance against antibiotics

Due to the high resistance against methicillin and after the failure of the drug, Vancomycin was playing a major role in treating most MRSA infections. Isolates of *S. aureus* were taken from a surgical wound of a Japanese baby and it was observed that the infection was not responding to the drug called Vancomycin. Vancomycin, is an antibiotic made up of glycopeptide and was initially used for the treatment of the MRSA strains as the efficacy of this drug was quite prominent but eventually because of prolong usage of the drug, it was resistant to MRSA infections. The resistance was not via the acquisition of vanA by MRSA infection-causing strain but this was because of unusual thickening of the cell wall which is rich in dipeptides and this results in the decreasing of the drug availability in the body. Despite the issues, in the year 2000, Vancomycin was considered to be one of the prominent drugs against the MRSA strains. The mechanism of the resistance is predicted to be a plasmid-mediated transfer among the species. The genes vraS, msrR, rpoB and graR were found to be mutated which was responsible for the resistance against the Vancomycin [13, 25–27]. Other than Methicillin and Vancomycin, Penicillin and Quinolones were also given to *S. aureus*.

In case of Penicillin, R plasmids encode the enzyme called as *penicillinase,* the plasmid gene that carries the enzyme is *blaz*, and the organisms that were resistant to penicillin were having this gene which inactivated the antibiotic by splitting the β-lactam ring. Slowly, this became a threat and major resistance towards penicillin antibiotic emerged world wide [28–30]. Use of Methicillin started when Penicillin failed to cure the Staphylococcal infections. After major failure of both these antibiotics, Quinolones were used. Quinolones destroy the bacteria by attacking and inhibiting their bacterial topoisomerases which generally ease the super coiling of DNA and also separates DNA strands. Moxifloxacin and Gemifloxacins are useful against the Gram-Positive bacteria but unfortunately *S. aureus* again developed resistance against quinolones [31, 32]. *S. aureus* developed resistance against fluoro-quinolones by overexpression of the NorA efflux pumps. Similarly, point mutation is another way by which this organism becomes resistant to quinolones. Point mutation in the subunits of topoisomerase takes place. Such as, point mutation at Gr1A in topoisomerase IV subunit and in GyrA, subunit of Gyrase [28].

4.1 Transmission pattern of resistance

Transmission of MRSA infections can take place from person to person who is contaminated with such infections. Proper hygienic condition is required to maintain infection from getting spread. Although the mode of transmission of infections mainly relies upon direct contact but contact with contaminated fomites can also transmit the infection. Several other factors of the host such as immunocompromised patients, defects in neutrophils, or destruction of the skin barriers can also give rise to the infections. *Staphylococcus aureus* has shown evolutionary changes in it and this phenomenon completely relies on the plasmid gene transfer mechanisms. The conventional mechanisms such as horizontal gene transfer popularly conjugation and transformation are followed by the strains to spread the resistance among the population or community but there is a very unique mechanism of *Staphylococcus* named SaPI-helper phage [33, 34]. Through all the studies it is quite evident that plasmids are the fundamental element that is helping in mediating the virulence and the resistance genes among the population of the *S. aureus* [35–37].

5. Treatment and future aspects

Drugs that are discussed to be used for MRSA infections are Daptomycin and Linezolid. Daptomycin is a synthetic drug that is the class of antibiotics that destroy the cell membrane ability by a calcium-dependent binding phenomenon which leads to bactericidal activity in a concentration-dependent way. So, one of the widely used antibiotics and which shows good efficacy even more than methicillin and vancomycin. Therefore, for any MRSA bacteremia, Daptomycin is considered to be very effective [38–40]. There were many topical drugs used against the MRSA strains. These anti MRSA drugs were quite effective. Mupirocin, is one of the anti MRSA topical drug which is applied on the skin for curing skin infections caused by *S. aureus* [41]. The mechanism of Mupirocin is, it binds to the isoleucyl t-RNA synthetase which inhibits the protein synthesis of the organisms resulting in the destruction of the organism [42]. Fusidic acid is another topical drug used against staphylococcal infections and it was reported effective as well. Fusidic acid binds to the elongation factor G of bacteria and interferes with the translocation process resulting in the inhibition of the protein synthesis [28].

Similarly, Linezolid which belongs to the oxazolidinones class predominantly inhibits the protein synthesis in the 50S ribosome of the cell. Linezolid shows a good amount of efficacy against several toxin-producing strains such as toxic shock syndrome toxin, Panton-Valentine leukocidin, α-hemolysin [38]. But the resistance against Linezolid was also observed. So, the combinatorial theory was taken into account. Combinatorial theory helps to mix multiple compounds to balance the inadequate conditions of other compounds and increase efficacy of drugs. The combinatorial theory started with Vancomycin and it shows synergistic interaction with β-lactams widely. Studies cleared that the capacity of clearing the MRSA infection-causing strains was not high in amount when the patients were only subjected to Vancomycin but in combination with β-lactams the clearance efficiency was much higher in amount. Combination with Vancomycin shows a specific effect named as Sea-Saw Effect where if the susceptibility of the vancomycin is decreased which results in decrease of transcription of the *mec A* gene and this increases the susceptibility of the β- lactams [43–46]. Combination with the Daptomycin has also been applied to check the outcome. This combination was to some extent very much successful as it enhanced the destruction of both Daptomycin-susceptible as well as Daptomycin-non-susceptible strains of MRSA. This combination showed high efficacy against the clearance of the bacteremia from the patient's body [47, 48].

Few drugs are in development such as Dalbavancin, Oritavancin, Tigecycline. Tigecycline inhibits protein synthesis and it shows broad-spectrum antibiotic activity. These are the possible treatments upon which the work is going on to reduce the resistance against the invasive MRSA. The prospect of the medication for *S. aureus* infections also lies in traditional medicines. The traditional herbal medicines are believed to have anti-MRSA activity. The bioactive phytoconstituents present in the plants such as Mansonone *F* from *Ulmus davidiana*, β-asarone from *Acorus calamus* rhizome, Prenylated flavonoids from *Desmodium caudatum* root, galloylated flavonol rhamnosides from *Calliandra tergemina* leaves, eupomatenoid-5 from *Piper regnellii* leaves are important for the MRSA treatment as they constitute anti-MRSA activity [49]. Some of the new relevant information regarding the treatment of AMR in *S. aureus* has come forward. Quinopristin-dalfopristin and Linezolid are another set of antimicrobial agents which have come up with activity against the resistance in *S. aureus*. Both these agents are protein inhibiting agents and Quinopristin-dalfopristin mainly exhibits bactericidal effects and Linezolid is bacteriostatic. Current studies against the treatment of this disease deal with the various combinations of antimicrobial agents [50]. Several compounds are known to inhibit the synthesis of fatty acid in bacteria and with this, two antibacterial agents have shown greater efficiency against *S. aureus*. Triclosan and Isoniazid are the two antimicrobial agents which target the FabI in the *S. aureus.* Fab I is one of the essential enzymes utilized in fatty acid elongation and it plays a major role in *S. aureus.* High throughput screening of the FabI inhibitors has led to come up with a new molecule AFN-1252 also called Affinium Pharmaceuticals was identified and proved to be efficient against the MRSA strains [51]. Multiple combinations were analyzed and several limitations emerged from those. Vancomycin and Rifampicin were in great demand for diagnosing MRSA infections but later on, Rifampicin proved not to be a better option for treating the disease as this drug is the primary drug given against one of the concerned diseases named Tuberculosis. This combination has exhibited higher possibilities of rising the resistance against Rifampicin and this was the major reason for the failure of the Vancomycin-Rifampicin combination against *S. aureus*. Similarly, Trimethoprim/Sulfamethoxazole and Rifampicin was a major failure because of the poor efficacy along with multiple side effects. Also, it was found to be resistant to infections. Among all this, Vancomycin is the only drug that is still either used in combinations or as monotherapy for treating MRSA infections but some of the new antibiotics such as Ceftaroline, Tedizolid, Plazomicin are proved to be successful among other antibiotics and are under research and development for further studies of treating the MRSA infections [52]. Other explored combinations with vancomycin have shown adverse nephrotoxicity. So, it is said that intensive research is required for novel approaches against the treatment of resistance to *S. aureus*. Above all the discussed conventional therapies for the treatment, either majority of them were proved to be ineffective or have shown severe side effects in the patients.

According to the future perspective, there is an immense need for an alternative strategy for treating the resistance against *S. aureus*. Treatment methods such as using nanoparticles are one of the efficient ways of delivering the drug directly to the patients. Under the nanoparticle treatment strategy, there is a unique feature of using ligands that are target specific for certain receptors in bacteria. AuNPs were surface modified by Vancomycin helps in reducing the bacterial growth and also the iron oxide nanoparticles are modified with the porphyrin platinum and Vancomycin which results in thermal degradation of the resistance strain of *S. aureus*. Another very interesting aspect is the usage of SiRNA therapy which enhances the MRSA inhibition. Vancomycin nanocomplexes are proved to have effective anti-MRSA effects which are very new to the study of alternative strategies [53].

The major limitation or failure that rises is intrinsic mechanisms of bacterial resistance and the target-specific antibiotics or drugs have disappointed to come up with any useful product. Another unique novel approach has come forth which combines the genomic information on the drug target and undergo chemical modifications along with efficacy testing [50].

6. Conclusion

Staphylococcus aureus is a major cause of bacterial infection in humans, which has been able to acquire resistance to a variety of antibiotics. MSRA is an emerging issue globally because apart from causing nosocomial infection also emerged as one of the key causative agents of community-acquired infections. Antibiotic resistance in *S. aureus* involves various mechanisms which are drug efflux, expression, or mutation of target proteins, leading to its rapid evolution which requires innovative approaches to develop novel treatment methodologies. A very limited amount of

DOI: http://dx.doi.org/10.5772/intechopen.96888

treatments are available for MRSA and this has become the reason for increasing the mortality rates. Appropriate use of the antimicrobial agents as the MDR is a very natural phenomenon and handling this type of phenomenon needs extra care to minimize the growth rate of resistant MRSA isolates further in the future. The development of new drugs is also in progress so that the resistance can be reduced. Anti MRSA topical drugs are extensively in use for treating skin infections. The new approaches have been initiated by the use of Fusidic acid, Linozolid against *Staphylococcal* infections.

Acknowledgements

We acknowledge the support of SRM University and C4D of SRM University for the help.

Conflict of interests

There is no Conflict of Interest in working with this chapter.

Author details

Riya Mukherjee, Anjali Priyadarshini, Ramendra Pati Pandey*
and Vethakkani Samuel Raj
Centre for Drug Design Discovery and Development (C4D), SRM University, Delhi-NCR, Rajiv Gandhi Education City, Sonepat, Haryana, India

*Address all correspondence to: ramendra.pandey@gmail.com

References

[1] Tanwar J, Das S, Fatima Z, Hameed S. Multidrug resistance: An emerging crisis. Vol. 2014, Interdisciplinary Perspectives on Infectious Diseases. Hindawi Limited; 2014.

[2] Nikaido H. Multidrug resistance in bacteria [Internet]. Vol. 78, Annual Review of Biochemistry. Annu Rev Biochem; 2009 [cited 2020 Dec 2]. p. 119-46. Available from: https://pubmed.ncbi.nlm.nih.gov/19231985/

[3] Vivas R, Barbosa AAT, Dolabela SS, Jain S. Multidrug-Resistant Bacteria and Alternative Methods to Control Them: An Overview. Microb Drug Resist [Internet]. 2019 Jul 1 [cited 2020 Dec 2];25(6):890-908. Available from: https://pubmed.ncbi.nlm.nih.gov/30811275/

[4] Loeffler J, Stevens DA. Antifungal drug resistance [Internet]. Vol. 36, Clinical Infectious Diseases. Oxford Academic; 2003 [cited 2020 Dec 2]. p. S31-41. Available from: https://academic.oup.com/cid/article/36/Supplement_1/S31/302495

[5] Marks SM, Flood J, Seaworth B, Hirsch-Moverman Y, Armstrong L, Mase S, et al. Treatment practices, outcomes, and costs of multidrug-resistant and extensively drug-resistant tuberculosis, United States, 2005-2007. Emerg Infect Dis [Internet]. 2014 [cited 2020 Dec 2];20(5):812-21. Available from: http://dx.doi.org/10.3201/eid2005.131037

[6] C Reygaert W. An overview of the antimicrobial resistance mechanisms of bacteria. AIMS Microbiol [Internet]. 2018 [cited 2020 Dec 2];4(3):482-501. Available from: /pmc/articles/PMC6604941/?report=abstract

[7] Orozco E, López C, Gómez C, Pérez DG, Marchat L, Bañuelos C, et al. Multidrug resistance in the protozoan parasite *Entamoeba histolytica*. Parasitol Int [Internet]. 2002 Dec [cited 2020 Dec 2];51(4):353-9. Available from: https://pubmed.ncbi.nlm.nih.gov/12421633/

[8] Ouellette M, Légaré D, Papadopoulou B. MDR in Parasitic Protozoa [Internet]. Vol. 3, J. Mol. Microbiol. Biotechnol. 2001 [cited 2020 Dec 2]. Available from: www.caister.com/bacteria-plant

[9] Hiramatsu K, Katayama Y, Matsuo M, Sasaki T, Morimoto Y, Sekiguchi A, et al. Multi-drug-resistant *Staphylococcus aureus* and future chemotherapy [Internet]. Vol. 20, Journal of Infection and Chemotherapy. Japanese Society for Cancer Chemotherapy; 2014 [cited 2020 Dec 2]. p. 593-601. Available from: https://pubmed.ncbi.nlm.nih.gov/25172776/

[10] Abbas A, Naz SS, Syed SA. Antimicrobial activity of silver nanoparticles (AgNPs) against Erwinia carotovora subsp. atroseptica & *Alternaria alternata*. Pakistan J Agric Sci. 2019;56(1):113-7.

[11] He X, Li S, Kaminskyj SGW. Using Aspergillus nidulans to identify antifungal drug resistance mutations. Eukaryot Cell [Internet]. 2014 Feb [cited 2020 Dec 2];13(2):288-94. Available from: https://pubmed.ncbi.nlm.nih.gov/24363365/

[12] Bansal D, Sehgal R, Chawla Y, Malla N, Mahajan RC. Multidrug resistance in amoebiasis patients. 2006 Aug.

[13] Ito T, Katayama Y, Hiramatsu K. Cloning and nucleotide sequence determination of the entire mec DNA of pre-methicillin-resistant *Staphylococcus aureus* N315. Antimicrob Agents Chemother [Internet]. 1999 [cited 2020 Dec 2];43(6):1449-58. Available

from: https://pubmed.ncbi.nlm.nih.gov/10348769/.

[14] Katayama Y, Ito T, Hiramatsu K. A new class of genetic element, staphylococcus cassette chromosome mec, encodes methicillin resistance in *Staphylococcus aureus*. Antimicrob Agents Chemother [Internet]. 2000 [cited 2020 Dec 2];44(6):1549-55. Available from: https://pubmed.ncbi.nlm.nih.gov/10817707/

[15] Ito T, Katayama Y, Asada K, Mori N, Tsutsumimoto K, Tiensasitorn C, et al. Structural comparison of three types of staphylococcal cassette chromosome mec integrated in the chromosome in methicillin-resistant *Staphylococcus aureus*. Antimicrob Agents Chemother [Internet]. 2001 [cited 2020 Dec 2];45(5):1323-36. Available from: /pmc/articles/PMC90469/?report=abstract

[16] Boundy S, Safo MK, Wang L, Musayev FN, O'Farrell HC, Rife JP, et al. Characterization of the *Staphylococcus aureus* rRNA methyltransferase encoded by orfx, the gene containing the staphylococcal chromosome cassette mec (SCCmec) insertion site. J Biol Chem [Internet]. 2013 Jan 4 [cited 2020 Dec 2];288(1):132-40. Available from: /pmc/articles/PMC3537007/?report=abstract

[17] Takeuchi F, Watanabe S, Baba T, Yuzawa H, Ito T, Morimoto Y, et al. Whole-genome sequencing of Staphylococcus haemolyticus uncovers the extreme plasticity of its genome and the evolution of human-colonizing staphylococcal species. J Bacteriol [Internet]. 2005 Nov [cited 2020 Dec 2];187(21):7292-308. Available from: /pmc/articles/PMC1272970/?report=abstract

[18] Novick RP, Christie GE, Penadés JR. The phage-related chromosomal islands of Gram-positive bacteria [Internet]. Vol. 8, Nature Reviews Microbiology. Nat Rev Microbiol; 2010 [cited 2020 Dec 2]. p. 541-51. Available from: https://pubmed.ncbi.nlm.nih.gov/20634809/

[19] Uchiyama J, Takemura-Uchiyama I, Sakaguchi Y, Gamoh K, Kato SI, Daibata M, et al. Intragenus generalized transduction in Staphylococcus spp. by a novel giant phage. ISME J [Internet]. 2014 [cited 2020 Dec 2];8(9):1949-52. Available from: /pmc/articles/PMC4139722/?report=abstract

[20] McCarthy AJ, Lindsay JA. The distribution of plasmids that carry virulence and resistance genes in *Staphylococcus aureus* is lineage associated. BMC Microbiol [Internet]. 2012 [cited 2020 Dec 2];12. Available from: https://pubmed.ncbi.nlm.nih.gov/22691167/

[21] Kadlec K, Schwarz S. Novel ABC transporter gene, vga(C), located on a multiresistance plasmid from a porcine methicillin-resistant *Staphylococcus aureus* ST398 strain. Antimicrob Agents Chemother [Internet]. 2009 Aug [cited 2020 Dec 2];53(8):3589-91. Available from: /pmc/articles/PMC2715595/?report=abstract

[22] Feßler AT, Kadlec K, Schwarz S. Novel apramycin resistance gene apmA in bovine and porcine methicillin-resistant *Staphylococcus aureus* ST398 isolates. Antimicrob Agents Chemother [Internet]. 2011 Jan 27 [cited 2020 Dec 2];55(1):373-5. Available from: http://intl-aac.asm.org/cgi/content/full/55/1/373

[23] Kumar M. Multidrug-resistant *Staphylococcus aureus*, India, 2013-2015 [Internet]. Vol. 22, Emerging Infectious Diseases. Centers for Disease Control and Prevention (CDC); 2016 [cited 2020 Dec 2]. p. 1666-7. Available from: http://dx.doi.org/10.1093/cid/ciu946http://dx.doi.org/10.3201/eid2109.150097

[24] Uchiyama, H., and B. Weisbium. 1985. N-Methyl transferase of

Streptomyces erythraeus that confers resistance to the macrolide-lincosamide-streptogramin B antibiotics: amino acid sequence and its homology to cognate r-factor enzymes from pathogenic bacilli and cocci. Gene 38:103-110.

[25] Methicillin-Resistant *Staphylococcus aureus* (MRSA).

[26] Matsuo M, Cui L, Kim J, Hiramatsu K. Comprehensive identification of mutations responsible for heterogeneous vancomycin-intermediate *Staphylococcus aureus* (hVISA)-to-VISA conversion in laboratory-generated VISA strains derived from hVISA clinical strain Mu3. Antimicrob Agents Chemother [Internet]. 2013 [cited 2020 Dec 2];57(12):5843-53. Available from: https://pubmed.ncbi.nlm.nih.gov/24018261/.

[27] Miller LG, Diep BA. Colonization, fomites, and virulence: Rethinking the pathogenesis of community-associated methicillin-resistant *Staphylococcus aureus* infection [Internet]. Vol. 46, Clinical Infectious Diseases. Clin Infect Dis; 2008 [cited 2020 Dec 2]. p. 752-60. Available from: https://pubmed.ncbi.nlm.nih.gov/18220477/

[28] Gnanamani A, Hariharan P, Paul-Satyaseela M. Staphylococcus aureus: Overview of Bacteriology, Clinical Diseases, Epidemiology, Antibiotic Resistance and Therapeutic Approach. In: Frontiers in *Staphylococcus aureus* [Internet]. InTech; 2017 [cited 2021 Jan 15]. Available from: http://dx.doi.org/10.5772/67338

[29] Hooper DC. Mechanisms of action and resistance of older and newer fluoroquinolones. In: Clinical Infectious Diseases [Internet]. Clin Infect Dis; 2000 [cited 2021 Jan 15]. Available from: https://pubmed.ncbi.nlm.nih.gov/10984324/

[30] Hooper DC. Mode of action of fluoroquinolones. In: Drugs [Internet]. Drugs; 1999 [cited 2021 Jan 15]. p. 6-10. Available from: https://pubmed.ncbi.nlm.nih.gov/10553698/

[31] Emmerson AM, Jones AM. The quinolones: Decades of development and use [Internet]. Vol. 51, Journal of Antimicrobial Chemotherapy. J Antimicrob Chemother; 2003 [cited 2021 Jan 15]. p. 13-20. Available from: https://pubmed.ncbi.nlm.nih.gov/12702699/

[32] Chambers HF. The changing epidemiology of *Staphylococcus aureus*? In: Emerging Infectious Diseases [Internet]. Centers for Disease Control and Prevention (CDC); 2001 [cited 2021 Jan 15]. p. 178-82. Available from: https://pubmed.ncbi.nlm.nih.gov/11294701/

[33] Chambers HF, DeLeo FR. Waves of resistance: *Staphylococcus aureus* in the antibiotic era [Internet]. Vol. 7, Nature Reviews Microbiology. NIH Public Access; 2009 [cited 2020 Dec 2]. p. 629-41. Available from: /pmc/articles/PMC2871281/?report=abstract

[34] McCarthy AJ, Witney AA, Gould KA, Moodley A, Guardabassi L, Voss A, et al. The distribution of mobile genetic elements (MGEs) in MRSA CC398 Is associated with both host and country. Genome Biol Evol [Internet]. 2011 [cited 2020 Dec 2];3(1):1164-74. Available from: https://pubmed.ncbi.nlm.nih.gov/21920902/

[35] Choo EJ, Chambers HF. Treatment of methicillin-resistant *Staphylococcus aureus* bacteremia [Internet]. Vol. 48, Infection and Chemotherapy. Korean Society of Infectious Diseases, Korean Society for Chemotherapy; 2016 [cited 2020 Dec 3]. p. 267-73. Available from: https://pubmed.ncbi.nlm.nih.gov/28032484/

[36] Lowy FD. Antimicrobial resistance: The example of *Staphylococcus aureus* [Internet]. Vol. 111, Journal of Clinical

Investigation. The American Society for Clinical Investigation; 2003 [cited 2021 Jan 15]. p. 1265-73. Available from: https://pubmed.ncbi.nlm.nih.gov/12727914/

[37] Rammelkamp CH, Maxon T. Resistance of *Staphylococcus aureus*> to the Action of Penicillin. Proc Soc Exp Biol Med. 1942;51(3):386-9.

[38] Fowler VG, Boucher HW, Corey GR, Abrutyn E, Karchmer AW, Rupp ME, et al. Daptomycin versus Standard Therapy for Bacteremia and Endocarditis Caused by *Staphylococcus aureus* . N Engl J Med [Internet]. 2006 Aug 17 [cited 2020 Dec 3];355(7):653-65. Available from: https://pubmed.ncbi.nlm.nih.gov/16914701/

[39] Carpenter CF, Chambers HF. Daptomycin: Another novel agent for treating infections due to drug-resistant gram-positive pathogens [Internet]. Vol. 38, Clinical Infectious Diseases. Clin Infect Dis; 2004 [cited 2020 Dec 3]. p. 994-1000. Available from: https://pubmed.ncbi.nlm.nih.gov/15034832/

[40] Park HJ, Kim SH, Kim MJ, Lee YM, Park SY, Moon SM, et al. Efficacy of linezolid-based salvage therapy compared with glycopeptide-based therapy in patients with persistent methicillin-resistant *Staphylococcus aureus* bacteremia. J Infect [Internet]. 2012 Dec [cited 2020 Dec 3];65(6):505-12. Available from: https://pubmed.ncbi.nlm.nih.gov/22902942/

[41] Dobie D, Gray J. Fusidic acid resistance in *Staphylococcus aureus* [Internet]. Vol. 89, Archives of Disease in Childhood. Arch Dis Child; 2004 [cited 2021 Jan 15]. p. 74-7. Available from: https://pubmed.ncbi.nlm.nih.gov/14709515/

[42] Ward A, Campoli-Richards DM. Mupirocin: A Review of Its Antibacterial Activity, Pharmacokinetic Properties and Therapeutic Use. Drugs. 1986;32(5):425-44.

[43] Sánchez García M. Clinical Outbreak of Linezolid-Resistant <emph type="ital">*Staphylococcus aureus*</emph> in an Intensive Care Unit. JAMA [Internet]. 2010 Jun 9 [cited 2020 Dec 3];303(22):2260. Available from: http://jama.jamanetwork.com/article.aspx?doi=10.1001/jama.2010.757

[44] Dilworth TJ, Ibrahim O, Hall P, Sliwinski J, Walraven C, Mercier RC. β-Lactams enhance vancomycin activity against methicillin-Resistant *Staphylococcus aureus* bacteremia compared to vancomycin alone. Antimicrob Agents Chemother [Internet]. 2014 Jan [cited 2020 Dec 3];58(1):102-9. Available from: https://pubmed.ncbi.nlm.nih.gov/24145519/

[45] Davis J, Sud A, O'Sullivan MVN, Robinson JO, Ferguson PE, Foo H, et al. Combination of Vancomycin and β-Lactam Therapy for Methicillin-Resistant *Staphylococcus aureus* Bacteremia: A Pilot Multicenter Randomized Controlled Trial. Clin Infect Dis [Internet]. 2016 Jan 15 [cited 2020 Dec 3];62(2):173-80. Available from: https://pubmed.ncbi.nlm.nih.gov/26349552/

[46] Chambers HF, Basuino L, Hamilton SM, Choo EJ, Moise P. Daptomycin-β-lactam combinations in a rabbit model of daptomycin-nonsusceptible methicillin-resistant *Staphylococcus aureus* endocarditis. Antimicrob Agents Chemother [Internet]. 2016 Jul 1 [cited 2020 Dec 3];60(7):3976-9. Available from: /pmc/articles/PMC4914634/?report=abstract

[47] Sakoulas G, Moise PA, Casapao AM, Nonejuie P, Olson J, Okumura CYM, et al. Antimicrobial salvage therapy for persistent staphylococcal bacteremia using daptomycin plus ceftaroline. Clin Ther [Internet]. 2014 Nov 10 [cited 2020 Dec 3];36(10):1317-33. Available from: https://pubmed.ncbi.nlm.nih.gov/25017183/

[48] Tong SYC, Davis JS, Eichenberger E, Holland TL, Fowler VG. Staphylococcus aureus infections: Epidemiology, pathophysiology, clinical manifestations, and management. Clin Microbiol Rev. 2015;

[49] Kali A. Antibiotics and bioactive natural products in treatment of methicillin-resistant *Staphylococcus aureus*: A brief review [Internet]. 9, Pharmacognosy Reviews. Medknow Publications; 2015 [cited 2020 Dec 3]. p. 29-34. Available from: /pmc/articles/PMC4441159/?report=abstract

[50] Franklin D. Lowy. 2003. Antimicrobial resistance: the example of *Staphylococcus aureus*, Science in Medicine, doi:10.1172/JCI200318535. 111:1265-1273.

[51] Krishnan Kumar, Sidharth Chopra, 2013, New drugs for methicillin-resistant *Staphylococcus aureus*: an update, J Antimicrob Chemother, 68(7):1465-70.

[52] Rahul Kashyap, Aditya Shah, 2019, Treatments and limitations for methicillin-resistant *Staphylococcus aureus*: A review of current literature, 9(1): 1-10, doi: 10.5495/wjcid.v9.i1.1.

[53] Vanamala K, Tatiparti K, Bhise K, Sau S, Scheetz MH, Rybak MJ, Andes D, Iyer AK. Novel approaches for the treatment of methicillin-resistant *Staphylococcus aureus*: Using nanoparticles to overcome multidrug resistance. Drug Discov Today. 2021 Jan;26(1):31-43. doi: 10.1016/j.drudis.2020.10.011. Epub 2020 Oct 20. PMID: 33091564; PMCID: PMC7855522.

Chapter 6

Extracellular Vesicles and Their Role in *Staphylococcus aureus* Resistance and Virulence

Brenda Silva Rosa da Luz, Vasco Azevedo, Yves Le-loir and Eric Guedon

Abstract

Staphylococcus aureus is a pathogen of great importance to clinical and veterinary medicine. Recently, there has been a growing interest in *S. aureus* extracellular vesicles (EVs) in the pathogenesis of this bacterium. Released by living cells into the extracellular milieu, EVs are membranous structures carrying macromolecules such as proteins, nucleic acids, and metabolites. These structures play several physiological roles and are, among others, considered a mechanism of intercellular communication within *S. aureus* populations but also in *trans* kingdom interactions. *S. aureus* EVs were shown to transport important bacterial survival and virulence factors, such as β-lactamases, toxins, and proteins associated with bacterial adherence to host cells, and to trigger the production of cytokines and promote tissue inflammation. In this chapter, we will review the main studies regarding *S. aureus* EVs, including their composition and roles in host-pathogen interactions, and the possible applications of EVs for vaccines and therapy development against staphylococcal infections.

Keywords: EV, membrane vesicles, composition, bacterial survival, cargo delivery, immunomodulation, host-pathogen interactions, immunization, vaccine, therapy

1. Introduction

1.1 EVs characteristics

The release of extracellular vesicles (EVs) is a long-known phenomenon widely reported, mainly in eukaryotes [1–4]. Archaea and Bacteria also release EVs, making their occurrence an evolutionally conserved feature among all three kingdoms [5]. They can be referred as membrane vesicles, microvesicles, ectosomes, exosomes, apoptotic bodies, outer membrane vesicles (OMVs), and others, depending on their origin and characteristics [5, 6]. The study of these particles is of great interest, as they are considered a mechanism of cell-free intercellular communication and *trans* kingdom interactions [7]. They are composed of a lipid bilayer and range from 20 to 1000 nm. They carry several bioactive molecules, such as proteins, lipids, metabolites, and nucleic acids, and were shown to modulate the metabolism and physiology of local or distant target cells [8]. Recently, the study of bacterial EVs has gained attention since they can affect pathogen-host interactions and contribute to bacterial pathogenesis.

1.2 History of bacterial EVs

The first study regarding bacterial EVs dates back to 1966, when lipid-like structures purified from culture supernatants of *Escherichia coli* were observed under electron microscopy [9]. In Gram-negative bacteria, vesiculation occurs from the budding out of the outer membrane (OM) that captures components present in the periplasm. This process forms nanoparticles called outer membrane vesicles (OMVs), which are released in the extracellular milieu [10]. Gram-positive bacteria lack an outer membrane and have a thicker peptidoglycan (PGN) cell wall, which was regarded as a barrier to EV release. This might explain why the first observations of EV release in Gram-positive bacteria were reported much later, in 2009,

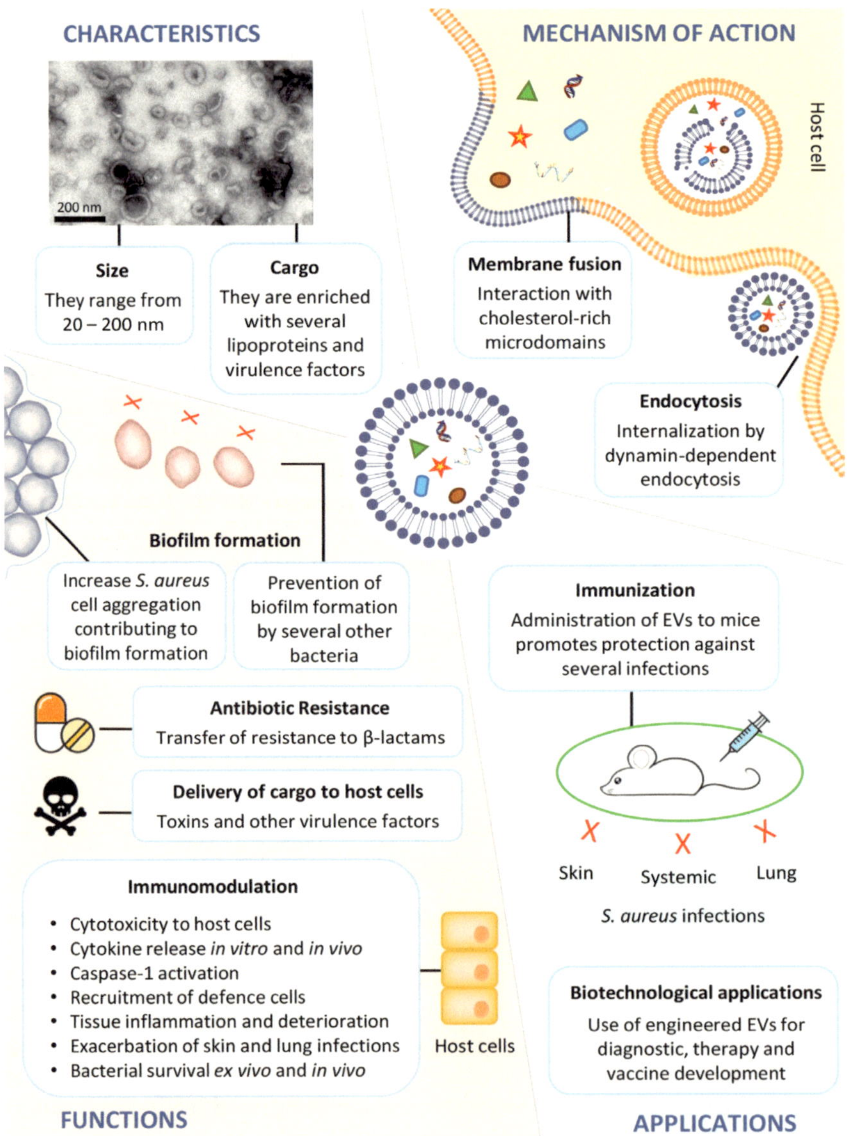

Figure 1.
General features of S. aureus *EVs.*

when Lee and collaborators demonstrated the production of EVs by *Staphylococcus aureus* [11]. Ever since, other studies confirmed EVs release by other Gram-positive bacteria belonging to various genera such as *Bacillus sp*, *Bifidobacterium sp*, *Cutibacterium sp*, *Clostridium sp*, *Enterococcus sp*, *Lactobacillus sp*, *Mycobacterium sp*, *Propionibacterium sp*, and *Streptococcus sp*, among others [12–22].

1.3 *S. aureus* and its derived EVs

S. aureus is a bacterium that asymptomatically colonizes the nasal track of 20–80% of the human population without causing disease [23]. *S. aureus* is also a major opportunistic pathogen in humans, being a common cause of nosocomial infections [24]. It is a causative agent of life-threatening diseases such as sepsis, endocarditis, pneumonia, and minor infections in soft tissues [25]. *S. aureus* is also an important pathogen in veterinary medicine. It is one of the main etiological agents of mastitis, an inflammation of the mammary gland that affects dairy herds and causes vast economic losses worldwide [26]. The type and severity of infections depend on strain-specific virulence factors, mostly expressed from accessory genetic elements [27]. Secreted and surface-exposed *S. aureus* virulence factors are responsible for weakening the host immune response, immune evasion, damage to host tissues, and infection onset [28].

One emerging field of great interest is the involvement of EVs in the infections caused by *S. aureus*. Recent studies have shown that *S. aureus* EVs carry important bacterial survival and virulence factors, such as β-lactamases, superantigens, toxins, coagulases, and proteins associated with bacterial adherence to host cells [11, 29–34]. In some cases, they trigger production of cytokines and promote tissue inflammation [35–38]. As EVs are also regarded as potential vehicles for biotechnological and clinical applications, such as the development of vaccines [39–42], their study is an attractive area in microbiology and the future development of new strategies against bacterial infections. Here, we will address the main studies regarding *S. aureus* EVs, their biogenesis, composition, and roles in bacterial resistance, virulence, host-pathogen interactions, and the possible applications of EVs for diagnostic, therapy, and vaccine development against diseases caused by this bacterium (see **Figure 1**).

2. Biogenesis of bacterial EVs

Several models have been proposed to elucidate how bacteria release EVs. Since the study of Gram-negative bacteria OMVs dates to the '60s, this phenomenon is better established and documented. Several hypotheses are proposed to explain EVs production, which include one or a combination of many processes [43]. It has been proposed that the accumulation of molecules in the periplasm space alters turgor pressure, promoting OMV release [44, 45]. In another model, alterations in lipid structure and topology could lead to modifications in the membrane curvature, resulting in vesicle bubbling from the outer membrane [46]. On the contrary, EVs biogenesis is still poorly understood in Gram-positive bacteria [47] due to the recent discovery of EV release by these microorganisms [11]. Notably, efforts have been made to better understand how EVs can get through the thick PGN layer present in the Gram-positive bacteria's cell wall structure.

In *S. aureus*, phenol-soluble modulins (PSMs) were shown to be associated with EVs release. These small proteins have surfactant-like properties and are considered crucial staphylococcal virulence factors since they can play various biological roles [48–50]. The staphylococcal PSMs were reported to have cytolytic and membrane-damaging activities, be proinflammatory, participate in biofilm formation, and be responsible for mobilizing lipoproteins from the staphylococcal cytoplasmic membrane, and the export of cytoplasmic proteins [51–55]. Since *S. aureus* EVs are generally enriched for both lipoproteins and cytoplasmic proteins, some studies investigated the role of PSMs in EV biogenesis. Wang et al. showed that deletion of *psmα* genes in *S. aureus* strain JE2 resulted in a significant decrease in size and number of EVs recovered from the culture supernatant [40]. Similarly, another study with strain USA300 revealed striking differences in EV production between the wild-type and a *Δpsmα3* mutant [56], supporting a conserved process in *S. aureus* species. It was shown that PSMα3 promotes EVs release by an increase in membrane fluidity, and that bacterial turgor under hypotonic osmotic conditions could be an important driving force for EV release in *S. aureus* [56]. Likewise, lipoproteins can also play a role in EV biogenesis since their absence resulted in an increase in membrane fluidity of *S. aureus*, as well as alterations in the protein content, the yield, and the size of EVs [57].

In addition to the importance of PSMs and lipoproteins in staphylococcal EV biogenesis, it was demonstrated that penicillin-binding proteins (PBPs) and autolysins also influence *S. aureus* EV release in acting likely on cell wall porosity to allow EVs to cross the cell wall. PBPs are involved in PGN cross-linking, a crucial EV release factor [40]. The autolysins Atl and Sle1 are PGN hydrolases that play an important role in cell division, modifying, therefore, cell wall integrity. Accordingly, a *pbp4* mutant, which was shown to significantly reduce PGN cross-linking [58], presents an increased EV production, whereas isogenic mutants for both Atl and Sle1 showed a significant decrease in EV size and release, consistent with their roles in peptidoglycan metabolism [40]. In another Gram-positive bacteria, *B. subtilis*, Toyofuku et al. evidenced that prophage-encoded endolysins create holes in the PGN, allowing, therefore, the protruding of biological components to form EVs that are released in the extracellular environment [59].

3. *S. aureus* vesicle cargo composition

3.1 *S. aureus* vesicle protein cargo

Different molecules may be incorporated into EVs during their biogenesis: nucleic acids, proteins, lipids, and metabolites [5, 8, 60, 61]. Most studies on *S. aureus* EV cargo composition, however, focused mainly on their proteome. The first study characterizing the proteome of *S. aureus* EVs identified with high confidence 90 proteins, distributed in cytoplasmic (56.7%), membrane (16.7%), and extracellular (23.3%) locations [11]. They included N-acetylmuramoyl-L-alanine amidase, which could have a predatory role in competing with other bacteria, transporters (SecD/SecF), and proteins related to antibiotic resistance, such as penicillin-binding proteins PBP1, PBP2 and PBP3, and β-lactamase [11]. They also found that *S. aureus* EVs comprise key virulence factors, such as superantigens (SSaA1 and SSaA2), toxins that disrupt host cell wall (α- and δ-hemolysins), coagulase factors, and immunomodulatory proteins, such as staphylococcal protein A (Spa), and immunoglobulin-binding protein (Sbi). Since then, several studies characterized the EV protein content of other *S. aureus* strains, revealing from 90 to 617 identified proteins, including numerous virulence factors (**Table 1**).

Strain	No. of proteins	Function	Ref.
01ST93		Non-cytotoxic to host cells (Hep-2)	[31]
03ST17	143	Non-cytotoxic to host cells (Hep-2, HaCaT)	[31, 38]
		Cytotoxic to host cells (HaCaT)	[62]
		Immunomodulation *in vitro* and *in vivo* (e.g., ↑ IL-1β, IL-6, IL-8, TNF-α, and MCP-1)	[38, 62]
		Mast cell recruitment and exacerbation of skin inflammation	
06ST1048		Cytotoxic to host cells (Hep-2)	[29, 31]
	143	Delivery of Spa protein through EVs (Hep-2)	[29]
8325–4		Induction of the MAPK pathway (THP-1 and MLE-12)	[63]
		Cytotoxicity to host cells (HeLa)	[64]
		Hemolytic activity	[63, 64]
8325-4Δ*hla*		Low cytotoxic to host cells (HeLa)	[64]
		Weaker induction of MAPK pathway (THP-1 and MLE-12)	[63]
ATCC 14458	90	ND	[11]
		Cytotoxic to host cells (HaCaT)	[30]
		Immunomodulation *in vivo* (↑ IL-1β and IL-6, ↓ TNF-α)	
		Immunomodulation *in vitro* and *in vivo* (e.g., ↑ IL-6, INF-γ, MIP-1α, eotaxin)	[37]
		Immunomodulation *in vitro* and *in vivo* (e.g., ↑ IL-6, TNF-α, IL-12, INF-γ)	[35]
		Induce skin inflammation in mice	[30, 37]
		Promote lung inflammation in mice	[35]
		Protective against lung infections	[42]
		Transfer of resistance to β-lactams	[32]
ATCC 25923		Cytotoxic to host cells (HaCaT)	[65]
		Immunomodulation *in vitro* (↑ IL-1β, IL-6, TNF-α, IL-8, and MCP-1)	
		Prevention of biofilm formation by other bacteria	[66]
ATCC 6538		Non-cytotoxic to host cells (HDMECs)	[36]
		Induce recruitment of monocytes (THP-1)	
		Immunomodulation *in vitro* (e.g., ↑ E-selectin, ICAM1 and VCAM1, IL-6)	
BWMR22		Exogenous EVs from vancomycin treated culture promote *S. aureus* aggregation	[67]
CI1449		Exogenous EVs confer bacterial resistance to whole blood killing	[68]
JE2	180	Cytotoxic to host cells (human leukocytes, THP-1 cells, human macrophages MΦ)	[40, 57]
		Immunomodulation *in vitro* (↑ IL-1β, IL-18, and caspase-1 activation)	

Strain	No. of proteins	Function	Ref.
JE2 Δ*arg*, Δ*sae*, Δ*lukAB*, Δ*lukSF-PV*, Δ*hla*		Decreased cytotoxicity and immunomodulation (THP-1 cells)	[57]
JE2-Δ*agr*-Δ*spa*	212	Non-cytotoxic to host cells (human leukocytes, A549, HL60, and rabbit erythrocytes)	[40]
		Non-protective against lethal sepsis	
JE2Δ*agr*Δ*spa* pHla$_{H35L}$-LukE		Non-cytotoxic to host cells (human leukocytes, A549, HL60, and rabbit erythrocytes)	[40]
		Protective against lethal sepsis	
JE2Δ*lgt*	198	Decreased cytotoxicity to host cells (human macrophages)	[57]
		Defective in the induction of IL-1β, IL-18, and IL-6, and caspase-1 activation *in vitro*	
M060	153	Cytotoxic to host cells (Hep-2, COS-7 and HaCaT)	[31, 65]
	153	Immunomodulation *in vitro* (↑ IL-1β, IL-6, TNF-α, IL-8, and MCP-1)	[65]
MSSA476	LB[1]: 131 BHI[2]: 617	Exogenous EVs promotes bacterial survival *ex vivo* and *in vivo* (human whole blood and neutrophils)	[69]
MW2	168	ND	[34]
N305*	222	Non-cytotoxic to host cells (PS and MAC-T)	[33]
		Immunomodulation *in vitro* and *in vivo* (e.g., ↑ IL-8, IL-1β, TNF-α, DEFβ1, MIP-2, BAFF)	
		Induction of neutrophil recruitment *in vivo*	
		ND	[34]
Newman		Immunomodulation *in vitro* (↑ IFN-β mRNA)	[70]
O11*	164	ND	[34]
O46*	171	ND	[34]
RF122*	160	ND	[34]
RN4220	92	ND	[41]
RN4220 Δagr	119	Engineered EVs protect mice against viral infections	[41]
ST692	[3]: 137 [4]: 156	Transfer of resistance to β-lactams	[71]
USA300		Immunomodulation *in vivo* (↑ IGM, total IgG, IgG1, IgG2a, and IgG2b)	[56]
		Protective against systemic and skin infections	[69]

*Note: Production of EVs was also demonstrated for S. aureus strains ATCC 35556 [72], ATCC 700699 [29], NRS135 [68], NRS77$_{phage}$ [68], RN4220$_{phage}$ [68], RN6390 [32], and TSST-1 103D [29], however, proteomic or functional characterization were not performed. *Animal isolates; ND, not determined.*
[1]*Luria-Bertani Medium.*
[2]*Brain Heart Infusion Medium.*
[3]*Optimal condition.*
[4]*Sub-inhibitory concentration of ampicillin.*

Table 1.
S. aureus-*EVs characterization and functions.*

As shown in **Table 1**, *S. aureus* EVs comprise several proteins. The numbers of proteins vary from one study to another because of the proteomic approaches used and the growth conditions. Sometimes EV proteome comprises up to 24% of the whole bacterial predicted proteome. It is expected that different methods of protein detection may give divergent results, and, indeed, some studies have evidenced such variations. Lee et al. identified 41 and 84 proteins with In-gel and In-solution digestion methods, respectively, with only 35 proteins shared by both sets of proteins identified [11]. In another study, Askarian et al. demonstrated that 43 and 286 proteins are exclusively identified when using either In-solution and Lipid-Based Protein Immobilization (LPI) methods, respectively [69]. These results highlight the impact of detection methods for EVs characterization. Therefore, comparison of EVs produced by different *S. aureus* strains should be done carefully, like other comparative proteomic analysis.

In this regard, a recent study characterized and compared the proteome of EVs derived from several *S. aureus* strains using the same experimental approach [34]. This work was carried out on EVs produced by five *S. aureus* strains of diverse host origins (human, bovine, and ovine). A total of 253 proteins were identified (from 160 to 218 EV proteins according to the strain), 119 of which were common to EVs derived from all strains. This conserved EV proteome included several proteins related to nutrient uptake, antibiotic resistance, virulence, and pathogenesis, reinforcing the importance of EV cargo for bacterial survival and staphylococcal infections [34]. Numerous of these core EV proteins are also present within EVs produced by phylogenetically distant species supporting the existence of specific and conserved rules for protein loading into EVs that remain to be uncovered [34].

3.2 Selective protein cargo sorting into EVs

Since EVs bud out of the cytoplasmic membrane, it is natural that their composition mainly reflects the physiological state of the producing cells, as it has been shown by several studies characterizing the EV cargo [73, 74]. However, several studies showed strong evidence that protein cargo sorting is a selective regulated process in both Gram-negative and Gram-positive bacteria [8, 34, 75, 76]. As mentioned before, OMV biogenesis involves the capture of components associated with the periplasm and the OM. Interestingly, OMVs derived from *Serratia marcescens* lack proteins abundant in the OM and, in contrast, can be enriched with proteins that are absent in this compartment [77]. As another example, *Porphyromonas gingivalis* OMVs also exclude proteins abundant in the OM and are enriched with several virulence factors [78]. Regarding Gram-positive bacteria, studies demonstrated that the non-pathogenic *B. subtilis* secretes EVs enriched with lipoproteins and siderophore-binding proteins, which are essential to survival [13]. *Mycobacterium bovis* and *Mycobacterium tuberculosis* were also shown to be enriched with several lipoproteins, some of which can modulate the host response in a TLR2-dependent fashion, contributing to mycobacterial virulence [21].

Several studies demonstrated that *S. aureus* EV cargo comprises secreted, cell wall-anchored, membrane, and cytoplasmic proteins. The latter are their most abundant component [11, 33, 34, 69]. This feature is interesting since it is the unique known pathway of a Gram-positive bacteria to secrete cytoplasmic proteins, which lack any export signals. Moreover, compared to whole-cell proteome, *S. aureus* EVs were also enriched with virulence-factors, extracellular proteins, and lipoproteins [11, 34]. For instance, Lee *et al*. demonstrated that Sbi is highly enriched in *S. aureus* EVs and is localized at the vesicle surface, enhancing its ability to bind to host cells [11]. Furthermore, secreted virulence factors such as coagulases, β-lactamase, and hemolysins were also enriched [11]. Finally, comparative proteomics revealed that lipoproteins of five *S. aureus* clinical and animal isolates accounted for approximately 20% of the EV content, while they corresponded to only 2.5% of the whole predicted proteome [34]. These data show that some protein populations are enriched in *S. aureus* EVs, and they reinforce the hypothesis that the selection of protein cargo occurs through a dynamic mechanism common to the strains of *S. aureus* species. To date, the molecular mechanisms that drive the recruitment of proteins into EVs remain unclear. Nevertheless, it was proposed that abundance, charge, and subcellular location of proteins could influence their availability and packing into *S. aureus* EVs [34].

3.3 *S. aureus* vesicle cargo: other components

As mentioned earlier, data regarding the characterization of the other components of staphylococcal EVs apart from proteins are scarce. Although some studies demonstrated that lipids, carbohydrates, or nucleic acids are also associated with *S. aureus* EVs, they did not perform an extensive characterization of these components. Schlatterer et al. used a fluorescent membrane dye (FM4–64) to quantify lipids present in the membrane of *S. aureus*-derived EVs and demonstrated that lipid release is also dependent on PSMs [56]. In another study, the Fourier Transform InfraRed spectroscopy (FTIR) approach showed that administration of the antibiotic vancomycin induced chemical changes on *S. aureus* EVs, including the reduction of carbohydrate yield in comparison to untreated cells [67]. Regarding nucleic acids, in the study by Andreoni et al., quantification with PicoGreen dsDNA kit revealed the association of DNA molecules to *S. aureus* EVs [68]. Finally, Rodriguez and Kuehn recently demonstrated that *S. aureus* Newman strain secrets EVs containing DNAs of ~500 base-pair long and RNAs with sizes of <300 nucleotides in length [70]. However, further investigations are necessary to better characterize the nucleic acid content of *S. aureus* EVs.

4. *S. aureus*-EVs functions

First considered "trash bags" to remove unwanted molecules from cells, nowadays, it is well-established that EVs play essential roles for bacterial fitness. Several described biological functions of OMVs and EVs include offensive and defensive mechanisms, such as quorum sensing, competition, delivery of toxins, resistance to antibiotics, horizontal DNA transfer, and transfer of regulatory RNAs (sRNAs), which can hijack the host immune response altering host-pathogen interactions. *S aureus* EVs were shown to participate in several metabolic and infectious processes, exhibiting several functions (**Table 1**).

4.1 *S. aureus*-EVs in cell toxicity

Studies demonstrated that *S. aureus* EVs can be cytotoxic and can induce cell death by delivering their toxin content. For example, δ-hemolysin (*hld*) and the exfoliative toxin A (ETA) were shown to be delivered to HEp-2 cells, inducing cytotoxicity [31]. Moreover, exposition of human macrophages THP-1 to *S. aureus* JE2 EVs during 24 h also occasioned significant cellular cytotoxicity, a result that was sharply decreased when EVs were isolated from mutant lacking several pore-forming toxins (PFTs) [57]. In another study, Thay et al. showed that *S. aureus* EVs contributed to HeLa cell cytotoxicity and erythrocyte lysis in a dose-dependent manner [64]. These results were tightly associated with biologically active α-hemolysin within EVs since their cytolytic and cytotoxic effects were significantly attenuated when EVs were isolated from an isogenic *hla* mutant [64]. Furthermore, *in vivo* experiments conducted by Hong et al. revealed that only *S. aureus* EVs could disrupt the skin barrier and cause dermal inflammation, which was not observed in the presence of purified α-hemolysin or EVs from strains that lack this protein [30]. More interestingly, they showed that EV-associated α-hemolysin was more cytotoxic than the purified toxin itself, and while the first induced necrosis, soluble α-hemolysin induced apoptotic cell death [30]. Together, these findings highlight the critical role of EVs in host cell death during staphylococcal toxicity.

4.2 *S. aureus*-EVs in antibiotic resistance and biofilm formation

Besides delivering toxins to host cells, *S. aureus* EVs were shown to play an important role in antibiotic resistance. Lee et al. demonstrated that biologically active BlaZ, a β-lactamase protein, is present inside *S. aureus* EVs [32]. EVs containing BlaZ were able to confer a transient resistance against ampicillin to susceptible surrounding Gram-negative and Gram-positive bacteria, including different strains of *E. coli*, *Salmonella enterica* serovar Enteritidis, *Staphylococcus epidermidis,* and *S. aureus* [32]. In a more recent report by Kim et al., the protective effect of EVs derived from the methicillin-resistant *S. aureus* (MRSA) strain ST692 grown in the presence of ampicillin was evaluated. Accordingly, ST692 EVs were shown to protect susceptible ATCC29213 strain against six different β-lactam antibiotics in a dose-dependent manner [71]. In another study, the addition of exogenous EVs purified from the culture supernatant of strain BWMR22 grown in the presence of a sub-inhibitory concentration of vancomycin was able to increase *S. aureus* adhesion and cell aggregation, contributing to biofilm formation [67]. Finally, it was shown that application of *S. aureus* EVs to polystyrene surfaces reduces biofilm formation by several other pathogenic bacteria, including *Acinetobacter baumannii*, *Enterococcus faecium*, and *Klebsiella pneumonia* [66]. This can be explained by the ability of *S. aureus* EVs to increase the hydrophilicity of surfaces, a key parameter for the initiation of biofilm formation [66]. This conversion of surface properties confers a vital competitive advantage that could explain the prevalence of *S. aureus* as a nosocomial pathogen.

4.3 *S. aureus*-EVs in immunomodulation

Various studies also demonstrated the role of *S. aureus* EVs on immunomodulation and their contribution to the induction or exacerbation of pulmonary and skin inflammations. Detection of *S. aureus* EVs in house dust led Kim et al. to investigate their role in lung infection models. Repeated airway exposure of mice to these particles resulted in a local increase in cytokine production and neutrophilic pulmonary inflammation [35]. Regarding cutaneous infections, it was shown that *S. aureus* EVs induce atopic dermatitis (AD) inflammation by enhancing cutaneous production of various cytokines, which promote infiltration of the dermis by mast cells and eosinophils, and consequently the increase in epidermal thickening in mice [30, 37]. In addition to that, *S. aureus* EVs were also shown to exacerbate inflammation in an AD mouse model [38]. Topical application of *S. aureus* EVs resulted in severe eczematous dermatitis, skin thickening, and a massive infiltration by inflammatory and mast cells [38]. These symptoms were not observed when animals were treated with lysed EVs [38]. Finally, an *in vitro* study showed that human dermal microvascular endothelial cells exposed to *S. aureus* EVs produce cell adhesion molecules, such as E-selectin, ICAM1, and VCAM1, which efficiently promote endothelial cell activation and monocyte recruitment, contributing, therefore, to the infiltration of immune cells [36].

Wang et al. demonstrated that EVs derived from the S. aureus JE2 strain could activate TLR2 signaling of NLRP3 inflammasomes in human macrophages through K+ efflux and apoptosis-associated speck-like protein (ASC) recruitment [57]. ASC is a key adaptor complex required for caspase-1 activation, which leads to the release of the mature forms of IL-1β and IL-18 cytokines. They also investigated whether EVs derived from a mutant for the *agr* quorum-sensing system and the SaeRS two-component system could affect inflammasome activation since they control the release of several PFTs, such as hemolysins and leukocidins. Indeed, the Δ*arg*Δ*saeRS* EVs packed a minimum amount of PFTs, leading to the absence of caspase-1 activation and a consequent decrease in the release of IL-1β and IL-18 by human macrophages [57]. Similarly, a mutation in a gene involved in lipidation and maturation of lipoproteins (Δ*lgt*) also decreased the levels of Hla and of the leukocidin LukS-PV present inside EVs, and, consequently, their ability to induce caspase-1 activation and cytokine release [57].

A recent study conducted by Rodriguez et al. demonstrated that nucleic acid associated with *S. aureus* EVs is immunomodulatory [70]. They identified DNA and RNA populations associated with EVs derived from Newman strain and provided evidence that these nucleic acids are delivered into host endosomal compartments [70]. *In vitro* experiments showed that murine macrophages exposed to EVs presented a strong IFN-β mRNA expression after 3 hours of stimulation [70]. Pretreatment of macrophages with inhibitors of endosomal acidification strongly reduced IFN-ß mRNA expression after EV stimulation, suggesting that EVs' processing depends on the acidic endosomal environment to release their immunomodulatory cargo and promote TLR signaling [70]. These results were corroborated when the exposition of TLR3−/−, TLR7−/−, and TLR9−/− mouse macrophages to EVs reflected in a substantial decrease in IFN-ß mRNA expression [70].

As described above, most studies regarding *S. aureus* EVs have focused mainly on clinical human isolates, and to date, there is only one report describing the biological functions of EVs derived from a *S. aureus* animal strain. Tartaglia et al. demonstrated that EVs derived from the bovine mastitis strain Newbould 305 carry several virulence factors and induce cytokine production in a bovine mammary epithelial cell *in vitro* without altering their viability [33]. Additionally, they showed that the intraductal inoculation of EVs in the mouse mammary gland promotes inflammation, tissue deterioration, and cytokine and chemokine production in murine mammary glands [33]. Altogether, these data indicate that staphylococcal EVs can interact with and modulate host cells' immune response, suggesting that EVs can play an important role in staphylococcal pathogenesis.

5. *S. aureus*-EVs delivery to host cells

5.1 *S. aureus*-EVs integrity and cell toxicity

Secretion of molecules and virulence factors is an essential component of *S. aureus* pathogenesis, including toxins, adhesins, and invasins. Molecules such as proteins or nucleic acids released in the surrounding medium may be rapidly degraded by the proteases or nucleases secreted in the extracellular milieu. The bilayered EVs thus appear as protective vehicles for efficient delivery of components in a concentrated manner. Gurung et al. were the first to evidence that Spa delivery via EVs was responsible for host cell death only when EVs were intact, establishing *S. aureus* EVs as effective delivery vehicles to target cells [29].

Other studies confirmed this role of EVs. For instance, disrupted EVs produced by *S. aureus* ATCC 25923 strain were shown to be four times less cytotoxic than intact EVs [65]. Again, whole and lysed EVs derived from strain 03ST17 were both cytotoxic and proinflammatory, however, these properties were more intense when EVs were intact [38, 62]. Nevertheless, in some cases, EV integrity does not influence their cytotoxic properties, as it is the case of *S. aureus* M060 EVs, that in both intact and disrupted states had the same cytotoxicity levels towards HaCaT cells [65]. These results highlight that EVs' integrity is essential and can lead to different outcomes depending on the mode of action of the effector molecules and the mechanism of EV cargo delivery.

5.2 *S. aureus*-EVs internalization into host cells

As important as the transport of cargo by EVs is how they transfer their cargo to recipient cells. They can act extracellularly through ligand-receptor interactions or intracellularly after their internalization into target cells and cargo release [79]. In the latter case, EVs' internalization may occur through several pathways, which all subsequently lead to an intracellular release of their cargo. These pathways include membrane fusion, phagocytosis, macropinocytosis, and lipid-raft-, caveolin- or clathrin-mediated endocytosis [80].

Studies showed that *S. aureus* EVs could interact with host cells via cholesterol-rich membrane microdomain. The cholesterol-sequestering agent Filipin III prevents EV membrane fusion and cargo delivery into host cells [29, 64]. Another study demonstrated that of all pretreatments of human macrophages with different inhibitors for clathrin-, lipid raft-, actin-, and dynamin-dependent endocytosis, only dynasore inhibited the entry of EVs into host cells, suggesting that EV uptake is mediated by dynamin-mediated endocytosis [57]. This finding is supported by a recent report by Rodriguez et al., where macrophages exposed to *S. aureus* Newman EVs had a substantial decrease in IFN-β mRNA expression when cells were also pre-treated with dynasore [70]. They also provided visual evidence through molecule labeling and confocal microscopy that EV-associated RNAs are efficiently delivered into macrophages [70]. Both membrane fusion and endocytosis depend on the integrity of EVs. This may explain why intact EVs usually present higher cytotoxicity since they allow direct delivery of concentrated components into host cells, enhancing, therefore, cell damage and immunomodulation. Although these recent findings highlight the role of cholesterol-rich domains and dynamin in *S. aureus* EV uptake, one cannot exclude that staphylococcal EVs exploit diverse entry routes for their cargo delivery host cells.

6. *S. aureus*-EVs environmental modulation

6.1 Impact of growth conditions in *S. aureus*-EV release

Besides intrinsic bacterial factors, several external factors were also shown to modify EV production. In *S. aureus*, exposure to the antibiotic penicillin significantly increased EV number, size, and protein yield compared to untreated bacterial cultures. In contrast, treatment with the antibiotic erythromycin did not affect EVs release [40]. This can be explained by the nature of each antibiotic action with penicillin affecting cell wall biosynthesis, whereas erythromycin is active on protein translation. Likewise, in another study, *S. aureus* had a significant increase in EVs release after exposure to the β-lactam antibiotics flucloxacillin and ceftaroline due to their ability to weaken the PGN wall [68]. Again, addition of the β-lactam ampicillin increased *S. aureus* EV production in a dose-dependent manner, which corresponded to a 22.4-fold increase at 64 μg/mL concentration [71]. The PGN present in the bacterial cell wall of most bacteria has a rigid structure formed of highly cross-linked polymers composed of polysaccharide chains and short peptides [81]. β-Lactams have been shown to decrease PGN cross-linking by serving as a substrate that irreversible binds and inactivates a transpeptidase involved in cell wall biosynthesis. As a result, it increases cell wall permeability due to the presence of a looser PGN matrix structure, allowing vesicles to cross the cell wall with less resistance, generating, therefore, particles in higher numbers and sizes. The correlation between vesicle release and PGN cross-linking has also been reported for Gram-negative bacteria [10, 82].

6.2 Impact of growth conditions in *S. aureus*-EV cargo composition

Culture conditions also alter EV content since bacteria modulate gene expression and protein secretion to cope with environmental changes. Indeed, comparative proteomic analysis revealed that 131 and 617 proteins were identified in EVs derived from *S. aureus* strain MSSA476 grown in Luria-Bertani (LB) and Brain-Heart Infusion (BHI) broth, respectively, with 109 proteins identified in both conditions [69]. Moreover, EVs derived from LB cultures were two-fold larger than those derived from BHI cultures, even though the latter presented higher protein diversity, which may also explain their significantly higher cytotoxicity towards neutrophils following brief exposure compared to LB-derived EVs [69]. In another study, proteomics identified 156 and 137 proteins in EVs derived from cultures in the presence and absence of a sub-inhibitory concentration of ampicillin, respectively, while only 67 proteins were shared by both conditions [71]. Another example of changes in EVs content was observed in the chemical composition of *S. aureus* EVs following treatment with vancomycin at 1 mg/ml. Compared to EVs produced by untreated bacteria, EVs prepared from vancomycin-treated cultures presented an increase in the ratio of protein relative to carbohydrates [67].

Additionally, EV content can also be impacted by a combination of several factors. For instance, Andreoni et al. evidenced that EVs produced by lysogenic strains had a significantly higher amount of DNA than those of the cured strains when a DNA-damaging SOS antibiotic was used, while the DNA content was unchanged in EVs purified from cultures treated with β-lactam [68]. This can be explained by the prophage-induced cell lysis caused by SOS-response triggering components, leading to an increase of DNA inside EVs, which does not occur with β-lactams since they target bacterial cell wall biosynthesis. These findings evidence that both intrinsic and external factors impact EV release and content, but much research is necessary to better elucidate EV biogenesis and cargo selection in *S. aureus* as well as in other bacteria.

7. *S. aureus*-EVs and host cells specificity

7.1 *S. aureus*-EVs strain specificity

Cytotoxicity and immunomodulation of EVs towards host cells vary according to the *S. aureus* strain and host cell line studied since both can have specific characteristics. As virulence factors vary from an *S. aureus* strain to another, so does the cargo of EVs. This affects cytotoxicity and host cell response to EVs contact. It was demonstrated that the presence of α-hemolysin in EVs is directly related to host cell death, and EVs from α-hemolysin-negative strains have very low or no cytotoxic effect on different cell types [30, 64]. Similarly, EVs from M060 *S. aureus* strain containing exfoliative toxin A (ETA) were highly cytotoxic towards HEp-2 cells, contrary to EVs purified from three other *S. aureus* isolates that lacked the ETA protein [31]. Furthermore, it was also demonstrated that EVs from *S. aureus* ATCC 25923 induces a stronger immune response in HaCaT cells than that of M060 EVs at the same concentrations [65]. These data show that EVs from different *S. aureus* strains indeed have different effects on host cells.

7.2 Host cell lines specificity

On the other hand, the cell lines used *in vitro* also have different responses reflecting differences in host cells-EVs interactions, which result in variable cytotoxicity, and immunomodulation levels. EVs derived from *S. aureus* subsp. *aureus* Rosenbach MSSA476 induced extensive cell death in human neutrophils and THP-1 cells, while it had very low cytotoxicity in HaCaT at the same concentrations [69]. In another study, *S. aureus* JE2 EVs were showed to be less cytotoxic to airway epithelial cells (A549) than to erythrocytes and neutrophil-like HL60 cells [40]. As another example, after exposure to ATCC 14458 *S. aureus* EVs, alveolar macrophages produced TNF-α and IL-6, while A549 cells produced only IL-6 [35]. Together, these findings show that EVs' role in host cell toxicity and immune response is strongly affected by the variations in EV cargo, which itself vary from an *S. aureus* strains to another, and to variations in molecular and physiological characteristics of the host cell types.

8. Applications of bacterial EVs

8.1 Use of EVs as a vaccine platform

As reviewed above, EVs interact with host cells leading to cytotoxicity, immunomodulation, tissue disruption, and other effects that mimic those caused by living bacteria during infection. These characteristics make EVs interesting vectors for delivering antigens and other components, some of which may have adjuvant properties. These features make EVs good candidates for vaccine development. Several studies have shown that EVs can induce adaptive immunity and confer protection against infections caused by both Gram-negative and Gram-positive pathogenic bacteria [83–85]. For instance, mice immunized with 1 μg of *E. coli* derived OMVs resulted in 100% protection against a lethal dose challenge, while the survival rate was only 20% in the untreated group [86]. In another study, intraperitoneal administration of *Streptococcus pneumoniae* BAA-255 EVs protected mice against the EV-producing cells and the pathogenic KCCM-41569 strain, demonstrating EVs' ability in eliciting a cross-protection against different strains [14].

8.2 Use of EVs against *S. aureus* infections

Regarding *S. aureus*, several studies have already reported the use of its derived EVs for immunization, revealing its potential in vaccine design. In 2015, Choi *et al.*

demonstrated that exposition of bone marrow-derived dendritic cells to ATCC 14458 EVs during 24 h enhanced the expression of co-stimulatory molecules CD80 and CD86 and of proinflammatory mediators such as TNF-α, IL-6, and IL-12, suggesting the induction of adaptive immunity [42]. As expected, intramuscular administration with three doses of >5 μg of ATCC 14458 EVs resulted in 100% protection against challenge with a lethal dose of bacteria in a mouse pneumonia model, with a reduction of bacterial colonization, pneumonia, and production of cytokines [42]. They revealed that immunization is mediated mainly by CD4+ T cell response, and transfection of these cells from EVs-immunized mice to naïve mice results in 70% protection after a lethal-dose challenge of *S. aureus*. Finally, they demonstrated that ATCC 14458 EV immunization provides long-term protective immunity and that it is a safe method since the administration of EV doses 10-fold higher were not cytotoxic to mice [42].

In another study, Askarian et al. demonstrated that intraperitoneal vaccination with USA300-derived EVs promoted a high production of antibodies, in addition to the protection of mice against subcutaneous and systemic *S. aureus* infections [69]. Another example of *S. aureus* EVs' application as a vaccine was shown by Wang et al. EVs were purified from the JE2 Δ*agr*Δ*spa* strain containing a plasmid coding for non-toxic Hla and LukE toxins under control of the *spa* promoter, whose activity is enhanced in the absence of the *arg* quorum sensing system [40]. They demonstrated that recombinant non-toxic Hla and LukE are immunogenic, and engineered EVs carrying these detoxified cytolysins protected mice against lethal sepsis infection [40]. Remarkably, reports on OMVs used as vaccine platforms against *S. aureus* infections were also explored. Irene et al. used OMVs derived from *E. coli* to incorporate five *S. aureus* antigens, Hla, SpA, FhuD2, Csa1, and LukE. They were successfully integrated into *E. coli* OMVs, corresponding from 5–20% of the total protein content [87]. The engineered OMVs conferred significant protection against sepsis, kidney, and skin *S. aureus* experimental infections in mice [87].

8.3 Use *S. aureus*-EVs against other infections

Interestingly, Yuan et al. used EVs derived from the *S. aureus* RN4220-Δ*agr* strain to produce particles with a reduced content of virulence factors and a decreased toxicity to generate a safe platform against viral infections [41]. Major components of *S. aureus* EVs were fused to tag sequences able to incorporate viral antigens, generating PdhB-FLAG and Eno-FLAG proteins associated with envelope E domain III, the primary protective domain for prevention of dengue virus (DENV) [41]. These heterologous viral antigens were successfully integrated into EVs, which induced antibodies against four DENV serotypes and protected mice against lethal challenge with DENV-2 [41].

9. Conclusions

As addressed here, EVs transport various types of biomolecules that have been reportedly associated with bacterial survival and host-pathogen interactions. *S. aureus* is, to date, one of the best-documented bacteria in this field. Yet, several research questions remain to be elucidated. First, EVs biogenesis is still poorly understood in Gram-positive bacteria even though recent studies showed *S. aureus*-EVs biogenesis can be affected by a range of intrinsic and external factors, such as PSMs, autolysins, and environmental conditions, such as antibiotics.

DOI: http://dx.doi.org/10.5772/intechopen.96023

Moreover, several studies evidenced that selective cargo sorting exist. Since the EV cargo determines their biological functions, clarifying which components are selected, and how, is of crucial value to understand their role in pathogenesis, and to their use as delivery systems. Second, most studies on *S. aureus* EVs have focused on proteomes. As well as proteins, nucleic acid cargo could play essential roles in *S. aureus* survival and pathogenesis. They could be associated to horizontal gene transfer for antibiotic resistance, and regulation of host cell expression by small regulatory RNAs. Therefore, more research is necessary in this field. Third, the physiological role of *S. aureus* EVs remains elusive. Staphylococcal EV cargo was shown to induce host cell toxicity, and skin and pulmonary inflammations, however, to the best of our knowledge, the exact contribution of EVs during infection remains unclear. The study of EV-free *S. aureus* strains in the infection context could reveal valuable clues to their real contribution to pathogenesis. Nevertheless, to the present, this phenomenon is unknown. Finally, their ability to induce a host immune response has arisen interest in using EVs as vehicles for vaccination. Several studies reported that administration of *S. aureus* EVs induce protection against systemic, pulmonary, and cutaneous infections. Although being a recent field of study, these promising data sheds light onto the possible application of engineered EVs to prevent diseases caused by this important human pathogen.

Acknowledgements

This work was conducted in the frame of BactInflam International Associated Laboratory between INRAE (France) and UFMG (Brazil). This work was part of the CARAVEL project financed by the MICA division from INRAE. BSRL was supported by the International Cooperation Program CAPES/COFECUB at the Federal University of Minas Gerais, funded by CAPES – the Brazilian Federal Agency for the Support and Evaluation of Graduate Education of the Brazilian Ministry of Education (number 88887.179897/2018-00).

Conflict of interest

The authors declare no conflict of interest.

Author details

Brenda Silva Rosa da Luz[1,2], Vasco Azevedo[1*], Yves Le-loir[2] and Eric Guedon[2]

1 Federal University of Minas Gerais, Belo Horizonte, Brazil

2 INRAE, Institut Agro, STLO, Rennes, France

*Address all correspondence to: vasco@icb.ufmg.br

References

[1] Guillaume VN, D'Angelo G, Raposo G. Shedding light on the cell biology of extracellular vesicles. Nat Rev Mol Cell Biol 2018; 19: 213-228. DOI: 10.1038/nrm.2017.125

[2] Stahl PD, Raposo G. Extracellular Vesicles: Exosomes and Microvesicles, Integrators of Homeostasis. Physiology (Bethesda) 2019; 34: 169-177. DOI: 10.1152/physiol.00045.2018

[3] Doyle LM, Wang MZ. Overview of Extracellular Vesicles, Their Origin, Composition, Purpose, and Methods for Exosome Isolation and Analysis. *Cells* 2019; 8, 727. DOI: 110.3390/cells8070727.

[4] Mathieu M, Martin-Jaular L, Lavieu G, et al. Specificities of secretion and uptake of exosomes and other extracellular vesicles for cell-to-cell communication. Nat Cell Biol 2019; 21: 9-17. DOI: 10.1038/s41556-018-0250-9

[5] Gill S, Catchpole R, Forterre P. Extracellular membrane vesicles in the three domains of life and beyond. FEMS Microbiol Rev 2019; 43: 273-303. DOI: 10.1093/femsre/fuy042

[6] Deatheragea BL, Cooksona BT. Membrane vesicle release in bacteria, eukaryotes, and archaea: A conserved yet underappreciated aspect of microbial life. Infect Immun 2012; 80: 1948-1957. DOI: 10.1128/IAI.06014-11

[7] Maas S, Breakefield X, Weaver A. Extracellular vesicles: Unique intercellular delivery vehicles. Trends in Cell Biology. Trends Cell Biol 2017; 27: 172-188. DOI: 10.1016/j.physbeh.2017.03.040

[8] Brown L, Wolf JM, Prados-Rosales R, et al. Through the wall: Extracellular vesicles in Gram-positive bacteria, mycobacteria and fungi. Nature Reviews Microbiology 2015; 13: 620-630. DOI: 10.1038/nrmicro3480

[9] Work E, Knox KW, Vesk M. the Chemistry and Electron Microscopy of an Extracellular Lipopolysaccharide From Escherichia Coli. Ann N Y Acad Sci 1966; 133: 438-449. DOI: 10.1111/j.1749-6632.1966.tb52382.x

[10] Schwechheimer C, Kuehn MJ. Outer-membrane vesicles from Gram-negative bacteria: Biogenesis and functions. Nat Rev Microbiol 2015; 13: 605-619. DOI: 10.1038/nrmicro3525

[11] Lee EY, Choi DY, Kim DK, et al. Gram-positive bacteria produce membrane vesicles: Proteomics-based characterization of *Staphylococcus aureus*-derived membrane vesicles. Proteomics 2009; 9: 5425-5436. DOI: 10.1002/pmic.200900338

[12] Rivera J, Cordero RJB, Nakouzi AS, et al. *Bacillus anthracis* produces membrane-derived vesicles containing biologically active toxins. Proc Natl Acad Sci U S A 2010; 107: 19002-19007. DOI: 10.1073/pnas.1008843107

[13] Brown L, Kessler A, Cabezas-Sanchez P, et al. Extracellular vesicles produced by the Gram-positive bacterium *Bacillus subtilis* are disrupted by the lipopeptide surfactin. Mol Microbiol 2014; 93: 183-198. DOI: 10.1111/mmi.12650

[14] Choi CW, Park EC, Yun SH, et al. Potential Usefulness of *Streptococcus pneumoniae* Extracellular Membrane Vesicles as Antibacterial Vaccines. J Immunol Res; 2017. 2017. DOI: 10.1155/2017/7931982.

[15] López P, González-Rodríguez I, Sánchez B, et al. Treg-inducing membrane vesicles from *Bifidobacterium bifidum* LMG13195 as potential adjuvants in immunotherapy. Vaccine 2012; 30: 825-829. DOI: 10.1016/j.vaccine.2011.11.115

[16] Nishiyama K, Takaki T, Sugiyama M, et al. Extracellular vesicles produced by *Bifidobacterium longum* export mucin-binding proteins. Appl Environ Microbiol 2020; 86. DOI: 10.1128/AEM.01464-20.

[17] Jeon J, Mok HJ, Choi Y, et al. Proteomic analysis of extracellular vesicles derived from *Propionibacterium acnes*. Proteomics - Clin Appl 2017; 11: 2-15. DOI: 10.1002/prca.201600040

[18] Jiang Y, Kong Q, Roland KL, et al. Membrane vesicles of *Clostridium perfringens* type A strains induce innate and adaptive immunity. Int J Med Microbiol 2014; 304: 431-443. DOI: 10.1016/j.ijmm.2014.02.006

[19] Wagner T, Joshi B, Janice J, et al. E*nterococcus faecium* produces membrane vesicles containing virulence factors and antimicrobial resistance related proteins. J Proteomics 2018; 187: 28-38. DOI: 10.1016/j.jprot.2018.05.017

[20] Dean SN, Leary DH, Sullivan CJ, et al. Isolation and characterization of Lactobacillus-derived membrane vesicles. Sci Rep 2019; 9: 1-11. DOI: 10.1038/s41598-018-37120-6

[21] Prados-Rosales R, Baena A, Martinez LR, et al. Mycobacteria release active membrane vesicles that modulate immune responses in a TLR2-dependent manner in mice. MBio 2014; 5. DOI: 10.1128/mBio.01921-14.

[22] Rodovalho VDR, Luz BSRD, Rabah H, et al. Extracellular Vesicles Produced by the Probiotic *Propionibacterium freudenreichii* CIRM-BIA 129 Mitigate Inflammation by Modulating the NF-κB Pathway. Front Microbiol 2020; 11, 1544. DOI: 10.3389/fmicb.2020.01544.

[23] Brown AF, Leech JM, Rogers TR, et al. *Staphylococcus aureus* colonization: Modulation of host immune response and impact on human vaccine design. Front Immunol 2013; 4: 1-20. DOI: 10.3389/fimmu.2013.00507

[24] Solberg CO. Spread of *Staphylococcus aureus* in hospitals: Causes and prevention. Scand J Infect Dis 2000; 32: 587-595. DOI: 10.1080/003655400459478

[25] Salgado-Pabón W, Schlievert PM. Models matter: The search for an effective *Staphylococcus aureus* vaccine. Nat Rev Microbiol 2014; 12: 585-591. DOI: 10.1038/nrmicro3308

[26] Peton V, Le Loir Y. *Staphylococcus aureus* in veterinary medicine. Infect Genet Evol 2014; 21: 602-615. DOI: 10.1016/j.meegid.2013.08.011

[27] Gill SR, McIntyre LM, Nelson CL, et al. Potential associations between severity of infection and the presence of virulence-associated genes in clinical strains of *Staphylococcus aureus*. PLoS One 2011; 6: 1-7. DOI: 10.1371/journal.pone.0018673

[28] Foster TJ. Immune evasion by staphylococci. Nat Rev Microbiol 2005; 3: 948-958. DOI: 10.1038/nrmicro1289

[29] Gurung M, Moon DC, Choi CW, et al. *Staphylococcus aureus* produces membrane-derived vesicles that induce host cell death. PLoS One 2011; 6. DOI: 10.1371/journal.pone.0027958.

[30] Hong SW, Choi EB, Min TK, et al. An important role of α-hemolysin in extracellular vesicles on the development of atopic dermatitis induced by *Staphylococcus aureus*. PLoS One 2014; 9: 1-10. DOI: 10.1371/journal.pone.0100499

[31] Jeon H, Oh MH, Jun SH, et al. Variation among *Staphylococcus aureus* membrane vesicle proteomes affects cytotoxicity of host cells. Microb Pathog 2016; 93: 185-193. DOI: 10.1016/j.micpath.2016.02.014

[32] Lee J, Lee EY, Kim SH, et al. *Staphylococcus aureus* extracellular vesicles carry biologically active β-lactamase. Antimicrob Agents Chemother 2013; 57: 2589-2595. DOI: 10.1128/AAC.00522-12

[33] Tartaglia NR, Breyne K, Meyer E, et al. *Staphylococcus aureus* extracellular vesicles elicit an immunostimulatory response in vivo on the murine mammary gland. Front Cell Infect Microbiol 2018; 8: 1-17. DOI: 10.3389/fcimb.2018.00277

[34] Tartaglia NR, Nicolas A, Rodovalho V de R, et al. Extracellular vesicles produced by human and animal *Staphylococcus aureus* strains share a highly conserved core proteome. *Sci Rep* 2020; 10, 8467. DOI: 10.1038/s41598-020-64952-y.

[35] Kim MR, Hong SW, Choi EB, et al. *Staphylococcus aureus*-derived extracellular vesicles induce neutrophilic pulmonary inflammation via both Th1 and Th17 cell responses. Allergy Eur J Allergy Clin Immunol 2012; 67: 1271-1281. DOI: 10.1111/all.12001

[36] Kim J, Bin BH, Choi EJ, et al. *Staphylococcus aureus*-derived extracellular vesicles induce monocyte recruitment by activating human dermal microvascular endothelial cells in vitro. Clin Exp Allergy 2019; 49: 68-81. DOI: 10.1111/cea.13289

[37] Hong SW, Kim MR, Lee EY, et al. Extracellular vesicles derived from *Staphylococcus aureus* induce atopic dermatitis-like skin inflammation. Allergy Eur J Allergy Clin Immunol 2011; 66: 351-359. DOI: 10.1111/j.1398-9995.2010.02483.x

[38] Jun SH, Lee JH, Kim SI, et al. *Staphylococcus aureus*-derived membrane vesicles exacerbate skin inflammation in atopic dermatitis. Clin Exp Allergy 2017; 47: 85-96. DOI: 10.1111/cea.12851

[39] Davenport V, Groves E, Horton RE, et al. Mucosal immunity in healthy adults after parenteral vaccination with outer-membrane vesicles from *Neisseria meningitidis* serogroup B. J Infect Dis 2008; 198: 731-740. DOI: 10.1086/590669

[40] Wang X, Thompson CD, Weidenmaier C, et al. Release of *Staphylococcus aureus* extracellular vesicles and their application as a vaccine platform. Nat Commun 2018; 9, 1379. DOI: 10.1038/s41467-018-03847-z.

[41] Yuan J, Yang J, Hu Z, et al. Safe Staphylococcal Platform for the Development of Multivalent Nanoscale Vesicles against Viral Infections. Nano Lett 2018; 18: 725-733. DOI: 10.1021/acs.nanolett.7b03893

[42] Choi SJ, Kim MH, Jeon J, et al. Active immunization with extracellular vesicles derived from *Staphylococcus aureus* effectively protects against staphylococcal lung infections, mainly via Th1 cell-mediated immunity. PLoS One 2015; 10: 1-17. DOI: 10.1371/journal.pone.0136021

[43] Haurat MF, Elhenawy W, Feldman MF. Prokaryotic membrane vesicles: New insights on biogenesis and biological roles. Biol Chem 2015; 396: 95-109. DOI: 10.1515/hsz-2014-0183

[44] McBroom AJ, Kuehn MJ. Release of outer membrane vesicles by Gram-negative bacteria is a novel envelope stress response. Mol Microbiol 2007; 63: 545-558. DOI: 10.1111/j.1365-2958.2006.05522.x

[45] Zhou L, Srisatjaluk R, Justus DE, et al. On the origin of membrane vesicles in Gram-negative bacteria. FEMS Microbiol Lett 1998; 163: 223-228. DOI: 10.1111/j.1574-6968.1998.tb13049.x

[46] Elhenawy W, Bording-Jorgensen M, Valguarnera E, et al. LPS remodeling triggers formation of outer membrane

vesicles in salmonella. MBio 2016; 7: 1-12. DOI: 10.1128/mBio.00940-16

[47] Coelho C, Casadevall A. Answers to naysayers regarding microbial extracellular vesicles. Biochem Soc Trans 2019; 47: 1005-1012. DOI: 10.1042/BST20180252

[48] Li S, Huang H, Rao X, et al. Phenol-soluble modulins: Novel virulence-associated peptides of staphylococci. Future Microbiol 2014; 9: 203-216. DOI: 10.2217/fmb.13.153

[49] Andreas Peschel MO. Phenol-soluble modulins and staphylococcal infection. Nat Rev Microbiol 2013; 11, 667-673. DOI: doi:10.1038/nrmicro3110.

[50] Cheung G, Joo H-S, Chatterjee S, et al. Phenol-soluble modulins – critical determinants of staphylococcal virulence. FMES Microbiol 2014; 38: 698-719. DOI: 10.1111/1574-6976.12057

[51] Periasamy S, Joo HS, Duong AC, et al. How *Staphylococcus aureus* biofilms develop their characteristic structure. Proc Natl Acad Sci U S A 2012; 109: 1281-1286. DOI: 10.1073/pnas.1115006109

[52] Laabei M, Jamieson WD, Yang Y, et al. Investigating the lytic activity and structural properties of *Staphylococcus aureus* phenol soluble modulin (PSM) peptide toxins. *Biochim Biophys Acta - Biomembr* 2014; 1838: 3153-3161. DOI: 10.1016/j.bbamem.2014.08.026

[53] Tsompanidou E, Denham EL, Becher D, et al. Distinct roles of phenol-soluble modulins in spreading of *Staphylococcus aureus* on wet surfaces. Appl Environ Microbiol 2013; 79: 886-895. DOI: 10.1128/AEM.03157-12

[54] Björnsdottir H, Rudin AD, Klose FP, et al. Phenol-soluble modulin a peptide toxins from aggressive *Staphylococcus aureus* induce rapid formation of neutrophil extracellular traps through a reactive oxygen species-independent pathway. Front Immunol 2017; 8, 257. DOI: 10.3389/fimmu.2017.00257.

[55] Hanzelmann D, Joo HS, Franz-Wachtel M, et al. Toll-like receptor 2 activation depends on lipopeptide shedding by bacterial surfactants. Nat Commun 2016; 7, 12304. DOI: 10.1038/ncomms12304.

[56] Schlatterer K, Beck C, Hanzelmann D, et al. The Mechanism behind Bacterial Lipoprotein Release : Phenol- Extracellular Vesicle Release from *Staphylococcus aureus*. MBio 2018; 9: 1-13. DOI: 10.1128/mBio.01851-18

[57] Wang X, Eagen WJ, Lee JC. Orchestration of human macrophage NLRP3 inflammasome activation by *Staphylococcus aureus* extracellular vesicles. Proc Natl Acad Sci U S A 2020; 117: 3174-3184. DOI: 10.1073/pnas.1915829117

[58] Łęski TA, Tomasz A. Role of penicillin-binding protein 2 (PBP2) in the antibiotic susceptibility and cell wall cross-linking of *Staphylococcus aureus*: Evidence for the cooperative functioning of PBP2, PBP4, and PBP2A. J Bacteriol 2005; 187: 1815-1824. DOI: 10.1073/pnas.1915829117

[59] Toyofuku M, Cárcamo-Oyarce G, Yamamoto T, et al. Prophage-triggered membrane vesicle formation through peptidoglycan damage in *Bacillus subtilis*. Nat Commun 2017; 8: 1-10. DOI: 10.1038/s41467-017-00492-w

[60] Kim JH, Lee J, Park J, et al. Gram-negative and Gram-positive bacterial extracellular vesicles. Semin Cell Dev Biol 2015; 40: 97-104. DOI: 10.1016/j.semcdb.2015.02.006

[61] Watanabe K. Bacterial membrane vesicles (MVs): novel tools as nature- and nano-carriers for immunogenic antigen, enzyme support, and drug delivery. Appl Microbiol Biotechnol

2016; 100: 9837-9843. DOI: 10.1007/s00253-016-7916-7

[62] Kwon H Il, Jeong NH, Jun SH, et al. Thymol attenuates the worsening of atopic dermatitis induced by *Staphylococcus aureus* membrane vesicles. Int Immunopharmacol 2018; 59: 301-309. DOI: 10.1016/j.intimp.2018.04.027

[63] An Y, Wang Y, Zhan J, et al. Fosfomycin Protects Mice from *Staphylococcus aureus* Pneumonia Caused by α-hemolysin in Extracellular Vesicles via Inhibiting MAPK-regulated NLRP3 Inflammasome. Front Cell Infect Microbiol 2019; 9: 1-18. DOI: 10.3389/fcimb.2019.00253

[64] Thay B, Wai SN, Oscarsson J. *Staphylococcus aureus* α-Toxin-Dependent Induction of Host Cell Death by Membrane-Derived Vesicles. PLoS One 2013; 8: 1-10. DOI: 10.1371/journal.pone.0054661

[65] Kwon H Il, Jeong NH, Kim SY, et al. Inhibitory effects of thymol on the cytotoxicity and inflammatory responses induced by *Staphylococcus aureus* extracellular vesicles in cultured keratinocytes. Microb Pathog 2019; 134: 103603. DOI: 10.1016/j.micpath.2019.103603

[66] Im H, Lee S, Soper SA, et al. *Staphylococcus aureus* extracellular vesicles (EVs): Surface-binding antagonists of biofilm formation. Mol Biosyst 2017; 13: 2704-2714. DOI: 10.1039/c7mb00365j

[67] He X, Yuan F, Lu F, et al. Vancomycin-induced biofilm formation by methicillin-resistant *Staphylococcus aureus* is associated with the secretion of membrane vesicles. Microb Pathog 2017; 110: 225-231. DOI: 10.1016/j.micpath.2017.07.004

[68] Andreoni F, Toyofuku M, Menzi C, et al. Antibiotics stimulate formation of vesicles in *Staphylococcus aureus* in both phage-dependent and -independent fashions and via different routes. Antimicrob Agents Chemother 2019; 63. DOI: 10.1128/AAC.01439-18.

[69] Askarian F, Lapek JD, Dongre M, et al. *Staphylococcus aureus* membrane-derived vesicles promote bacterial virulence and confer protective immunity in murine infection models. Front Microbiol 2018; 9, 262. DOI: 10.3389/fmicb.2018.00262.

[70] Rodriguez B V., Kuehn MJ. *Staphylococcus aureus* secretes immunomodulatory RNA and DNA via membrane vesicles. Sci Rep 2020; 10: 1-22. DOI: 10.1038/s41598-020-75108-3

[71] Kim SW, Seo JS, Park S Bin, et al. Significant increase in the secretion of extracellular vesicles and antibiotics resistance from methicillin-resistant *Staphylococcus aureus* induced by ampicillin stress. Sci Rep 2020; 10: 1-14. DOI: 10.1038/s41598-020-78121-8

[72] Frassinetti S, Falleni A, Del Carratore R. Effect of itraconazole on *Staphylococcus aureus* biofilm and extracellular vesicles formation. Microb Pathog 2020; 147: 104267.

[73] Kim Y, Edwards N, Fenselau C. Extracellular vesicle proteomes reflect developmental phases of *Bacillus subtilis*. Clin Proteomics 2016; 13: 1-8. DOI: 10.1186/s12014-016-9107-z

[74] Bager RJ, Persson G, Nesta B, et al. Outer membrane vesicles reflect environmental cues in *Gallibacterium anatis*. Vet Microbiol 2013; 167: 565-572. DOI: 10.1016/j.vetmic.2013.09.005

[75] Bonnington KE, Kuehn MJ. Protein selection and export via outer membrane vesicles. *Biochim Biophys Acta* 2014; 1843: 1612-1619. DOI: 10.1016/j.bbamcr.2013.12.011

[76] Haurat MF, Aduse-Opoku J, Rangarajan M, et al. Selective sorting of

cargo proteins into bacterial membrane vesicles. *J Biol Chem* 2011; 286: 1269-1276. DOI: 0.1074/jbc.M110.185744

[77] McMahon KJ, Castelli ME, Vescovi EG, et al. Biogenesis of outer membrane vesicles in *Serratia marcescens* is thermoregulated and can be induced by activation of the Rcs phosphorelay system. J Bacteriol 2012; 194: 3241-3249. DOI: 10.1128/JB.00016-12

[78] Veith PD, Chen YY, Gorasia DG, et al. *Porphyromonas gingivalis* outer membrane vesicles exclusively contain outer membrane and periplasmic proteins and carry a cargo enriched with virulence factors. J Proteome Res 2014; 13: 2420-2432. DOI: 10.1021/pr401227e

[79] Caruana JC, Walper SA. Bacterial Membrane Vesicles as Mediators of Microbe – Microbe and Microbe – Host Community Interactions. Front Microbiol 2020; 11: 1-24. DOI: 10.3389/fmicb.2020.00432

[80] Mulcahy LA, Pink RC, Carter DRF. Routes and mechanisms of extracellular vesicle uptake. J Extracell Vesicles 2014; 3: 1-14. DOI: 10.3402/jev.v3.24641

[81] Vollmer W, Blanot D, De Pedro MA. Peptidoglycan structure and architecture. FEMS Microbiol Rev 2008; 32: 149-167. DOI: 10.1111/j.1574-6976.2007.00094.x

[82] Deatherage BL, Lara JC, Bergsbaken T, et al. Biogenesis of bacterial membrane vesicles. Mol Microbiol 2009; 72: 1395-1407. DOI: 10.1111/j.1365-2958.2009.06731.x

[83] Jiang L, Schinkel M, van Essen M, et al. Bacterial membrane vesicles as promising vaccine candidates. Eur J Pharm Biopharm 2019; 145: 1-6. DOI: 10.1016/j.ejpb.2019.09.021

[84] Gerritzen MJH, Martens DE, Wijffels RH, et al. Bioengineering bacterial outer membrane vesicles as vaccine platform. Biotechnol Adv 2017; 35: 565-574. DOI: 10.1016/j.biotechadv.2017.05.003

[85] Peng Y, Yin S, Wang M. Extracellular vesicles of bacteria as potential targets for immune interventions. Hum Vaccines Immunother 2020; 1-7. DOI: 10.1080/21645515.2020.1799667

[86] Kim OY, Hong BS, Park K-S, et al. Immunization with *Escherichia coli* Outer Membrane Vesicles Protects Bacteria - Induced Lethality via Th1 and Th17 Cell Responses . J Immunol 2013; 190: 4092-4102. DOI: 10.4049/jimmunol.1200742

[87] Irene C, Fantappiè L, Caproni E, et al. Bacterial outer membrane vesicles engineered with lipidated antigens as a platform for *Staphylococcus aureus* vaccine. Proc Natl Acad Sci U S A 2019; 116: 21780-21788. DOI: 10.1073/pnas.1905112116

Section 2

Impact on One Health

Chapter 7

Staphylococcus aureus and Dairy Udder

Amjad Islam Aqib, Muhammad Ijaz, Muhammad Shoaib, Iqra Muzammil, Hafiz Iftikhar Hussain, Tean Zaheer, Rais Ahmed, Iqra Sarwar, Yasir Razzaq Khan and Muhammad Aamir Naseer

Abstract

Staphylococcus aureus is a major causative agent of intra-mammary infections in dairy animals with potential virulence of surface components, toxins, and extracellular enzymes. About 74% quarter prevalence of *S. aureus* in bovine udder with overall prevalence exceeding 61% in dairy animals. About 17 different serotypes of dairy originated *S. aureus* have been reported with 24 virulence coding genes for leukocidins (lukED/lukM), pyrogenic toxin super antigen (PTSAg), haemolysins (hla-hlg), toxic-shock syndrome toxin (tst), enterotoxins (sea-seo, seu), exfoliative toxins (eta, etb), and genes for methicillin (mecA) and penicillin (blaZ) resistance. Attainment of refuge inside the macrophages and neutrophils is a major cause of *S. aureus* mastitis persistence. Mammary prebiotics and probiotics are recently being used as alternatives to antibiotic for the prevention of mastitis. Literature showed anti- staphylococcus vaccines with different results depending upon types of immunization, route of administration and adjuvant used. Studies has shown that herd specific as well as commercial *S. aureus* vaccines reduce new infections in dairy animals. Experiments are still in progress for the use of vaccines against *S. aureus* mastitis with optimal efficacy and reliability. Perhaps, there might be bright future because of highly satisfactory trial results of mastitis vaccines in the lab animals.

Keywords: *S. aureus*, dairy udder, transmission, pathogenesis, economic impacts, treatment, prevention

1. Introduction

Staphylococcus aureus is a symbiotic and opportunistic microorganism that can colonize various sites of different animals and humans. This bacteria can cause serious infections in humans and animals [1]. In animals, bovine mastitis, commonly caused by various bacteria, is one of the most devastating disease in dairy farming worldwide. Of these bacteria, *Staphylococcus aureus* is the leading pathogen causing the most dangerous mastitis in cattle and the most difficult dairy product in most countries. *Staphylococcus aureus* has emerged as superbug of dairy udder, compromising animal health and economy [2]. Its virulence is due to its ability of producing wide array of virulence factors that enhances its attachment, colonization, longer persistence and escaping the immune response. Such resistant strains are distinguished by systemic heterogenicity, genetic variety, interactions between complex community and the extracellular matrix of macromolecular substances [3].

Staphylococcus aureus has a variety of strains, most notably multi-drug resistance and biofilm formation. The latter has received a lot of attention due to its ability to minimize the effects of antibiotics, colonize the mucous membrane of the epithelium, last longer, avoid immune reactions, and contribute to etiology [4]. Methicillin resistant *S. aureus* strains have been designated as emerging pathogen in livestock and dairy animals. Hospital acquired MRSA and community associated MRSA are limited to humans only, but livestock occupational personals may have infections with human originated MRSA [5].

The successful mastitis therapy depends on various factors such as accurate diagnosis, elimination of causative agent, stage of disease, severity of the infection, selection of the drugs, route of drugs administration along with other supportive treatments [6, 7] and some other factors regarding mastitis causing organisms. However, irrespective of the appropriate use of antibiotic, the mastitis may not be treated successfully [8]. The treatment failure mainly occurs due to insufficient contact of antimicrobials and disease-causing microorganisms in the udder. Mastitis can incur economic losses in both ways either directly and indirectly [9]. The direct losses include veterinary expenditure, labor costs, reduced production, poor quality milk and discarded milk. Whereas, the indirect losses are not obvious to the producers and are termed as "hidden losses" which include increased risk of other diseases, poor fertility rate, increased culling rate and sometime mortality. So, total cost can be much more than the direct losses [10–12]. This chapter addresses the following aspects such as transmission, pathogenesis, strains spectrum, economic impact, emerging treatment and prevention strategies to control *S. aureus* dairy udder infection.

2. Transmission of *Staphylococcus aureus* in udder infections

The main reservoirs of *Staphylococcus aureus* are infected mammary glands, ducts, and papillary lesions. However, this bacteria also found on the skin, nose and teat passages. The bacteria spread to uninfected areas through the lining of the teat cups, milker's hands, towels and fruit flies. *Staphylococcus aureus* does not persist on healthy teat skin, but tends to colonize damaged skin and teat lesions. The body reproduces the infected lesion, increasing the likelihood of teat colonization and subsequent udder infection. Heifers infected during calf pregnancy are an important reservoir that can be passed on to uninfected *Staphylococcus aureus* herds. There has been much controversy over the route of infection with *Staphylococcus aureus* in early prenatal heifers, but it is possible that the cause is a calf that was fed on a mother infected with *Staphylococcus aureus*. Data is limited, but if you have a problem with *Staphylococcus aureus* on your farm, you should definitely consider choosing scrapes carefully (such as cryo-sterilization). Obviously, a good treatment plan for mastitis will take into account the absence of this disease in heifers [13].

3. Pathogenesis of *S. aureus* in udder infection

Bacterial pathogens can recognize, respond and adapt to the harsh environmental conditions that prevail in mammalian hosts during infection. Despite the host's immune response and antibacterial treatment, it helps to invade, calm, and survive within the host [14]. *Staphylococcus aureus* produces a variety of enzymes, including coagulase, which can coagulate plasma, converting plasma fibrinogen to fibrin, coat bacterial cells, and inhibit nutrition. Hyaluronidase (also called diffusion factor) can break down the hyaluronic acid present in tissues and support the spread of *Staphylococcus aureus* in the host. It also produces DNase (deoxyribonuclease), an enzyme that breaks down DNA. Lipase, which breaks down lipids, and staphylokinase, which breaks down fibrin. It is also known that *Staphylococcus aureus* produces β-lactamase, esterase, elastase and phospholipase for drug resistance, and these enzymes promote colony formation and pathogenicity. Other toxic factors of *Staphylococcus aureus* include leukocidin (which can cause cytolytic destruction of phagocytic cells in some animals) and toxic shock syndrome toxin (TSST). The latter can cause an overproduction of lymphokine, which can lead to tissue damage [15]. Depending on the strain, *Staphylococcus aureus* can release some toxins that are major virulence factors. These toxins act on cell membranes containing superantigens, exfoliating toxins, and some two-component toxins such as alpha toxins, beta toxins, gamma toxins, delta toxins and Panton Valentine's toxins and leukocidin (PVL). It can be divided into three categories, for example toxins [16]. Protein A, which plays an important role in strategies for evading immunity, is immobilized on the staphylococcus-peptide-glycan-pentaglysin bridge using transpeptidase sortase (**Figure 1**). Protein A is able to bind to fragments of the crystal region (Fc) of IgG antibodies (γ-immunoglobulins). This phenomenon is due to the fact that Protein A binds to an IgG antibody produced against the target microorganism and reacts with the corresponding antigen usually present in the patient sample to perform an aggregation test in which a visible aggregation reaction can be observed. The *Staphylococcus aureus* strain is known to produce pigments such as staphyloxanthin and gold carotenoid pigments. These pigment acts primarily as a toxic factor, acting as a bacterial antioxidant and helping microorganisms escape the host's immune system and kill reactive oxygen species used by the pathogen [18]. The toxins produced by *Staphylococcus aureus* destroy the cell membranes and tissues that directly produce milk. White blood cells (leukocytes) are attracted to the area of inflammation and try to fight the infection. First, bacteria damage the tissues lining the teat and mammary gland within 1/4 of a second, eventually leading to scar tissue formation. The bacteria

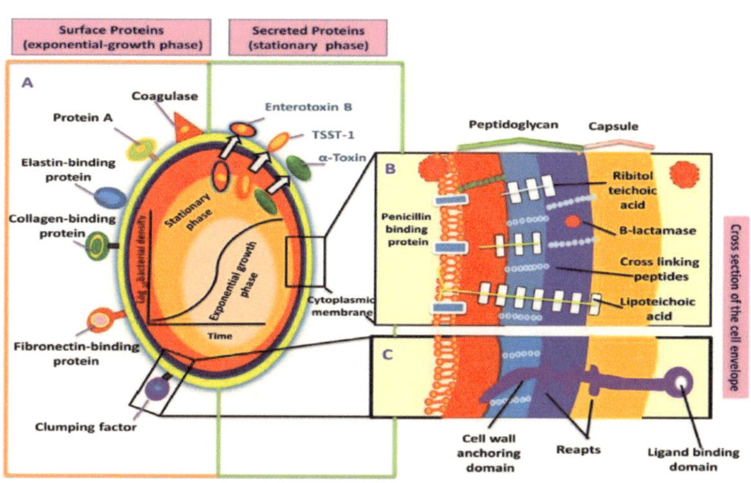

Figure 1.
Various virulence factors of S. aureus [17].

then migrate into the duct system, forming deep-rooted infectious pockets in the lactating (alveolar) cells. The second is the formation of abscesses that prevent their spread, thus avoiding detection by the immune system. Abscesses prevent antibiotics from entering bacteria. This is the main reason for poor response to treatment. However, bacteria can also escape the lethal effects of some antibiotics by hiding in neutrophils (white blood cells) and other host cells preventing exposure to antibiotics. When the white blood cells die (usually within a day or two), the bacteria are released and the infection continues [19].

During infection, the destruction of alveolar and tubular cells reduces the lactation yield. These damaged cells can attach to leukocytes and block the mammary canal that drains the alveolar region, resulting in additional scar tissue, blockage of the canal, and decreased lactation. The teat canal can be opened later, but this usually results in the release of *Staphylococcus aureus* to other areas of the udder. The spread of *Staphylococcus aureus* in the glands leads to the formation of additional abscesses, which can become very large and appear as lumps in the udder (**Figures 2** and **3**). Most cases of *S. aureus* mastitis are asymptomatic, but chronic cows typically have high SCC, abnormal udder tissue, and recurrence of clinical mastitis. Clinically infected areas are usually swollen, milk has visible clots (large clots). Acute infections with *Staphylococcus aureus* usually develops late in lactation. Clinical symptoms such as udder swelling and hardness, milk appearance change) do not appear until the start of the next stage. It is difficult to cure an infection well, because the drug cannot penetrate all foci of infection, and bacteria can avoid contact with antibiotics in the white blood cells. Many strains of *Staphylococcus aureus* have acquired antibiotic resistance (the ability to produce enzymes that

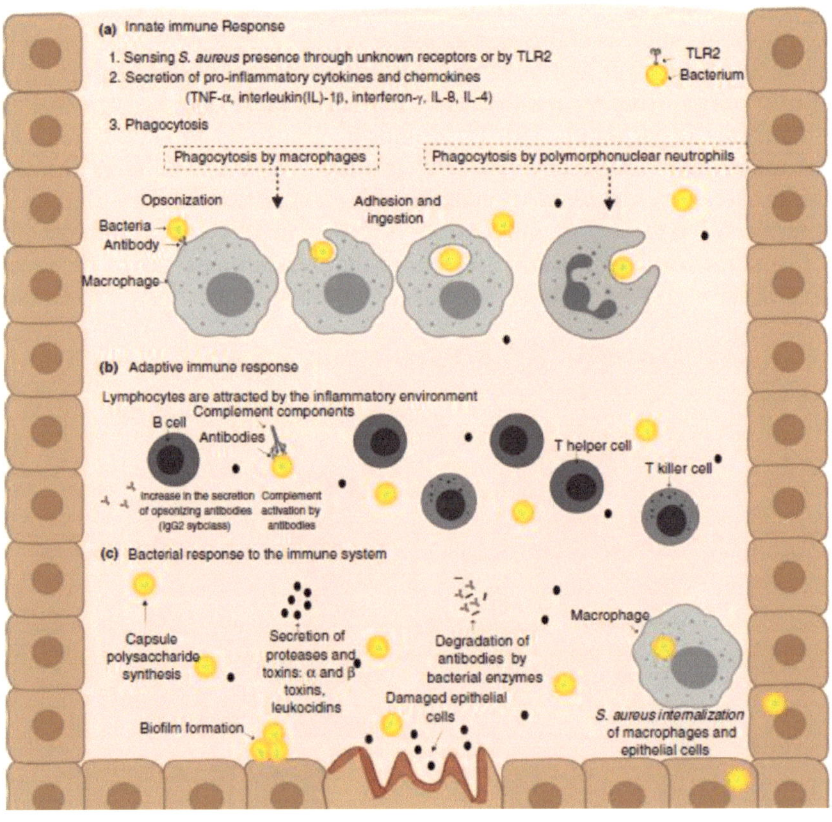

Figure 2.
Immune response to S. aureus *and vice versa inside the mammary gland [20].*

DOI: http://dx.doi.org/10.5772/intechopen.95864

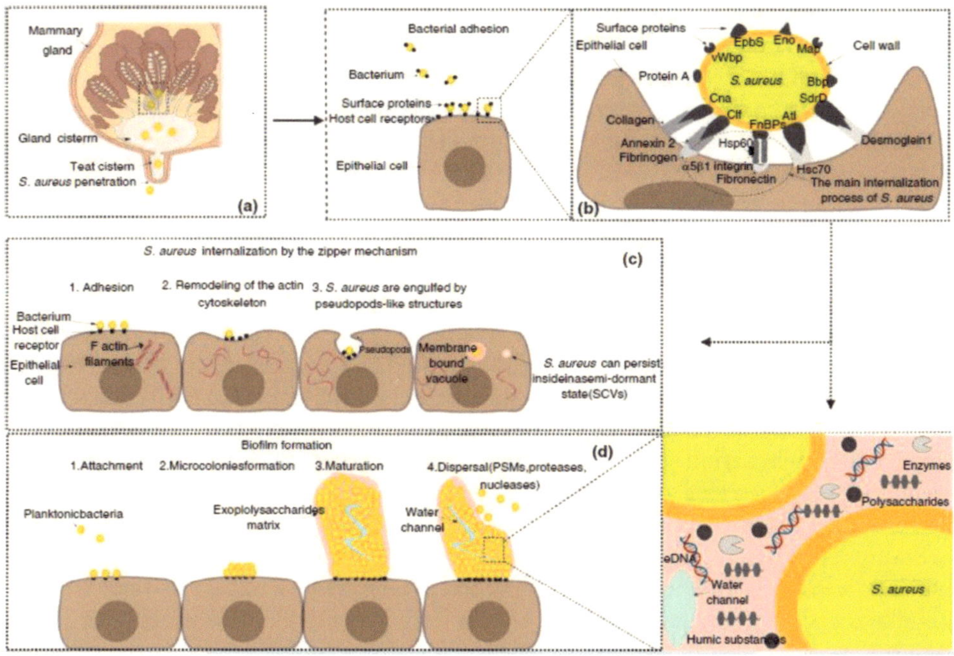

Figure 3.
Intracellular invasion of S. aureus *inside mammary gland [20].*

inactivate penicillin and other antibiotics), making treatment impossible. The development of antibiotic resistance during treatment with certain β-lactam antibiotics (such as penicillin) is another reason for treatment failure [20].

4. *Staphylococcus aureus* strains spectrum

Staphylococcus aureus is a major causative agent of intramammary infections in dairy animals with potential virulence of surface components (adhesins, capsular polysaccharides, protein A), toxins, extracellular enzymes and coagulase [21]. About 74% quarter prevalence of *S. aureus* in bovine udder [22] with overall prevalence exceeding 61% in dairy animals [4]. A wide array of genotypic variations has been observed with great genetic diversity in the isolates of bovine as well as caprine origin. Some of the variants are common throughout the globe as ruminant specific *S. aureus* while others are geographic related in the literature [23]. Inflammatory respondent metabolic pathways (BoLA-DRA, GLYCAM1, FCER1G, B2M, CD74, NFKBIA and SDS), milk constituent associated (CSN2 and CSN3) and immunity related (B2M and CD74) are also specific strains of *S. aureus* of dairy mastitis [24, 25].

Staphylococcus aureus genotyping is mostly done by pulsed field gel electrophoresis(PFGE), multi locus sequence typing (MLST), polymerase chain reaction (PCR), *S. aureus* protein A (spa) typing, agar typing and typing on the basis of virulence and resistance coding genes [23, 26–31]. Thirty-nine electrophoretic types of *S. aureus* with diverse MLST genotyping had been reported, most of them were showed genetic heterogenicity and classified to one of the eight clonal complexes, suggestive of multiclonal nature of the *S. aureus* isolates from single dairy herd [32]. Clonal 8 complex (i.e., USA300), a lineage known for human infections, has also been isolated from bovine mastitis, suggestive of recent host shift and new adoptive genotypic strain of bovine mastitis [27].

PFGE typing of *S. aureus* from dairy origin showed that PFGE type A was significantly related to teat skin while PFGE type Q was more exclusive to milk and exhibit marked biofilm potential [33]. Overall, PFGE clusters of isolates showed same endotoxin coding genes with indistinguishable banding patterns. Phylogenetic studies based on MLST sequencing classified these clusters into clonal complexes with similar staphylococcal endotoxin genetic profiles [23]. Genotyping of dairy originated *S. aureus* showed five clonal types (PFGE A consisting on sequence type 747 [ST747] and spa type t359; PFGE B with spa type ST750 and t1180; PFGE C with spa type t605 and ST126; PFGE D with spa type t127 and ST751; PFGE F with spa type t002 and ST5). About 63% isolates harbor major clone A but negative for Panton-Valentine leukocidin and exfoliative toxin D genes [26]. Another reported PFGE typing of dairy originated *S. aureus* revealed 16 PFGE types (from A – P), with M, I and O as most frequent but not significantly variant strains in the field, respectively. PCR typing based on endotoxin genes presence showed that 11.7, 1.8, 2.7, 0.9 and 7.2% isolates carried seb, seb and sec, sec, see, and tsst-1, respectively with zero prevalence of sea and sej genes. PFGE types M and O showed clustering behavior with β-hemolysin and least prevalence of endotoxin coding genes [34].

Staphylococcal protein A types t084, t304 and t688 from subclinical mastitis showed divergent virulence and heterogenicity traits while a novel spa-type t18546 was also reported from dairy udder ailments [35]. Prevalent clonal types of *S. aureus* from bovine udder exhibited generic alterations of epigenetic modulators to surpass immune response of host. The study reported 35,878 transcripts of these strains which differ 23% from reference genomic cluster. Expressive nature of 20,756 transcripts were observed with more than 1 fragment per kilobase of transcript per million mapped fragments and 25.95% of multi-exonic genes alternatively spliced. Alternative Splicing (AS) events for more than 100 immunogenic genes were noted with 379 alternate AS events coding for transcription and splicing proteins. Spa typing of ovine originated *S. aureus* showed 14 diversified clones, most prominent of which were t1773, t967 and t1534 as 62.32, 5.79 and 5.79% respectively. Three novel spa types were also identified with repeats successions (07–23–12-34-12-12-23-03-12-23), (04–31–17-24-25-17-17) and (04–31–17-24-17-17) [36].

Screening of *S. aureus* for endotoxins (SE) showed that >90% isolates were positive for SE genes while 70.1% with exaggerative response. All isolates were positive for biofilm encoding genes (icaA/D, clf/B, can, fnbA). A total of 7 spa types (1 novel spa type t17182), 5 STs, 14 SmaI-pulso-types and 3agr types (no agrII) were reported. PFGE cluster II-CC1-ST1-t127-agr III was the most prevalent clone (56.3%). Isolates of agr III (PFGE Cluster I/II-CC1-ST1-t127/2279) exhibited higher number of virulence genes than other agr types. The MSSA-ST398-t1456-agr I clone showed higher antibiotic resistance, weak biofilm expression and lower level of virulence genes expression [37]. Another study reported agr-I strain harboring penicillin resistance genes while agr-III strains were devoid of that pattern. Antimicrobial resistance encoding genes (tet (L), tet (K), erm (B) and bla (Z)) were frequent in these strains [36]. Thus, the data narrated agr-I and II as different subspecies of dairy originated *S. aureus* [38]. Disruption of the ica operon in a bap-positive *S. aureus* strain showed no alteration in biofilm expression, indicating Bap gene compensatory mechanism for deficit PIA/PNAG product (a biofilm matrix polysaccharide) [39]. 17 different pulsotypes of dairy originated *S. aureus* have been reported with 24 virulence coding genes for leukocidins (lukED/lukM), pyrogenic toxin superantigen (PTSAg), haemolysins (hla-hlg), toxic-shock syndrome toxin (tst), enterotoxins (sea-seo, seu), exfoliative toxins (eta, etb), and genes for methicillin (mecA) and penicillin (blaZ) resistance. PTSAg-encoding genes and plasmid encoded sei, sed and blaZ genes were frequent in persistent intramammary ailments [40].

Staphylococcus aureus classification based on *mec*A gene is narrated as methicillin susceptible (MSSA) and methicillin resistant (MRSA) strains. Studies reported 84% MSSA prevalence with MRSA isolation rate up to 4%. Spa typing of the isolates showed frequent presence of t034 and t529 in MSSA while t121 was noted in MRSA strains. Both types of isolates were positive for endotoxin B, C, D, and E. MLST and PFGE typing of isolates revealed composite genotype profile of ST 5-PFGE USA100-unknown spa type which is of hospital origin and ST 8-PFGE USA300-spa type t121 genotype, commonly designated as community-associated MRSA clone [28]. Another study reported 77.8% MRSA from goat mastitis as strong biofilm producers. Spa typing revealed 44% t127, 33.3% t2049 and 22.2% t7947 type among total MRSA isolates [41].

5. Economic impacts due to *S. aureus* udder infection

Economic impacts of the mastitis are of great financial importance. Mastitis negatively impacts numerous aspects of cow and herd management. Mastitis can incur economic losses in both ways either directly and indirectly [9]. The direct costs include veterinary expenditure, labor costs, reduced production, poor quality milk and discarded milk. Whereas, the indirect losses are not obvious to the producers and are termed as "hidden costs" which include increased risk of other diseases, poor fertility rate, increased culling rate and sometime mortality. So, total cost can be much more than the direct losses [10–12].

A 15–20% of total cow population of the countries having major share in the milk production is affected by mastitis each year. Production losses per effected quarter are estimated 30% of productivity loss whereas, 15% production is lost during entire lactation/cow. The mastitis rate in the heifer can be up to 97% and *S. aureus* has major significance in imparting the huge economic losses. *Staphylococcus aureus* effects animals of various stage and parity e.g. nulliparous, primiparous, primigravid and multiparous [42, 43].

In Holland, the financial losses resulted due to clinical mastitis by Staphylococci were €293/Cow. Whereas, it was €277/cow in every clinical case of mastitis due to staphylococci in first three months after post calving and €168/cow onward for the rest of the lactation. In USA dairy, the annual losses incurred by the mastitis were estimated around $2billions, while $400 M in Canada and $130 M in Australia excluding the antibiotic residue in human diet, expense to preserve the nutritive quality of milk and to prevent milk degradation [12, 44, 45]. There is variation in cost of each component between the herds, partially due to the performance of herd and partially due to difference in preferences of the farmers when the mastitis is detected. Mastitis can impart economic losses to the farmers in following ways.

5.1 Low milk yield

The loss of yield depends on certain factors of great importance like severity of mastitis, nature of causative agent, stage of lactation at the time of mastitis. Losses are severe in primiparous cows due to clinical mastitis caused by *Staph. aureus*, *E. coli* with *Klebsiella*. However, the maximum loss of production in multiparous is caused by *Streptococcus* spp., *Staphylococcus aureus* and others pathogens [46, 47]. The loss of production is higher in multiparous cows than primiparous. Clinical mastitis occurring before peak production stage/yield causes more extensive loss as compared to rest of the lactation and loss of milk yield is persistent throughout the lactation [12, 48]. According to a study, this yield loss for multiparous could be 300-400 kg (4–6% of lactation) while 200-300 kg in primiparous animals. The magnitude of yield loss in 30% cases of clinical mastitis reached up to 950-1050 kg per lactation. Whereas, in subclinical mastitis the losses incorporated are 80 kg/lactation (1.3%) and 120 kg/lactation (1.7%) in primiparous and multiparous respectively [49, 50].

5.2 Altered milk composition

The mastitis milk is low in fats and casein due to reduction in the synthetic capacity of secretary tissues of the udder parenchyma. The reduction in the fats up to 3-22 kg (1.5–7.5%) and casein protein contents up to 0 to 15 kg (0 to 8.5%) of the milk and higher SCC incurs the penalty to the producers in premium payment [51, 52].

5.3 Veterinary and medicinal cost

The veterinarian cost for treatment fee, travel and labor charges. On an average a handsome expenditure of $444 in clinical mastitis case are charged. This include (128$) directly in term of diagnostic (10$), medicinal expenditure ($36), discarded milk ($25), Veterinary charges ($41), extra labor ($4) while death losses ($32). The indirect costs are ($316) which include ($125) through future production losses and ($182) for culling and replacement and whereas reproductive losses are ($9). Therefore, to take an accurate decision to control the mastitis depends on understanding of economic impact of mastitis [43, 53]. Mastitis is among the main reason in cattle for the use of antibiotics and this exposure of animal to antibiotics is main reason behind the development of antibiotic resistant bacteria and antimicrobial residues in milk which are of a great public health concern [4, 7].

5.4 Discard of milk

Milk of the cow is discarded after mastitis diagnosis or while cow is being treated with antibiotics due to presence of antibiotic residues in milk during withdrawal period. The length of the withdrawal period depends on the drugs used and production system (*i.e.* conventional or organic). This discarded milk cost higher per unit than the milk not produced due to feed costs inclusions [53, 54].

5.5 Extra labor

Clinical mastitis requires extra labor for veterinary visits and medicine administration. Milking order is also changed in the clinical mastitis giving rise to less efficient milking and increasing the labors cost because hours of extra time required to manage the mastitis case [12, 53].

5.6 Subsequent disorders

The probability of subsequent clinical mastitis increases in cows once infected with mastitis. As the affected udder act as reservoir for the pathogen, the affected cows increase the spreading of mastitis in the herd. Cows having experienced one case of clinical mastitis often develop a subsequent case of clinical mastitis later in lactation. Mastitis is associated with increased risk of lameness, ketosis, displaced abomasum (LDA/RDA), and paresis and fertility problems. The economic cost of various disorders and fertility problems arise after mastitis and it is also included in the total cost of mastitis [55–57].

5.7 Culling of animal

The risk of culling and mortality rate is increased with clinical mastitis. Similar to milk loss the increased culling also augments the hidden cost. Involuntary culling is associated with replacement costs and is an important component of total mastitis cost. Economic cost also increases as cows recovered after mastitis do not reach their full production potential [9, 10, 53].

6. Review of emerging treatment options for *S. aureus* of dairy udder

6.1 NSAIDs, plant extracts, and nanoparticles as therapeutic agent

Aqib et al. [58] conducted a study to check the antibacterial of NSAIDs, plant extracts and nanoparticles against mecA positve *S. aureus*. Zinc oxide particles ZnO and Zn (OH) 2 were synthesized by the sorbothermal method and characterized by X-ray diffraction (XRD), calcination and scanning electron microscopy (SEM). Plant extracts were produced by the Soxhlet extraction method. The study showed that 34% (n = 200) of subclinical samples obtained from *Staphylococcus aureus* milk were significantly ($p < 0.05$) associated with suspicious risk factors and pathogens. Antibacterial studies have shown that *Staphylococcus aureus* is 55, 42, 41 and 41% resistant to oxacillin, siroxacin, streptomycin and enoxacin, respectively. Amoxicillin showed higher zone of inhibition increase at 100 mg of *Calotropis procera* extract (31.29%), followed by 1 mg/ml (28.91%) and 10 mg/ml (21.68%) eucalyptus. The combination of amoxicillin with diclofenac, aspirin, ibuprofen and meloxicam up to 500 μg/ml increases the ZOI by 42.85, 37.32, 29.05 and 22.78%, respectively. The Fractional Inhibitory Concentration Index (FICI) shows the synergistic effects of amoxicillin with diclofenac and aspirin, as well as with ibuprofen and meloxicam. Preliminary studies of the combination of micro-particles and amoxicillin in vitro have been found synergistic. In combination with zinc oxide and zinc hydroxide, the ZOI of amoxicillin increases by 26.74% and 14.85%, respectively. NSAIDs, herbal extracts and micro-particles immediately focused on the regulatory resistance of the pathogenic *Staphylococcus aureus* to explore alternative sources of antibacterial agents.

6.2 Lysostaphin as an anti-staphylococcal therapeutic agent

Lysostaphin is a potent staphylococcus-degrading enzyme containing a peptidase that can specifically cleave the polyglycine bridge specific to the cell wall of *Staphylococcus aureus*. Lysostaphin activity is measured by its ability to lyse *Staphylococcus aureus* cells. It is influenced by enzyme concentration, pH, temperature, ion and salt concentration. *Staphylococcus aureus* is enveloped in a thick layer of peptide glycans, and lysostaphin destroys the layer of peptide glycans, causing lysis and cell death. Peptide glycans impart strength and rigidity to the cell walls of gram-positive microorganisms, grow and divide, maintain cell shape, and prevent osmotic lysis of *Staphylococcus aureus*. Recombinant lysostaphin (rLYS) is a zinc metal enzyme that hydrolyzes the glycylglycine bond of a peptide glycan to a pentaglycine bridge on the cell wall of *Staphylococcus aureus*. A rodent model was used for the treatment of mastitis. The first study of rLYS in the sand showed that the rate of reduction of udder infection was over 87%, and the activity of dissolving stones in the body had a detrimental effect on the host. Instead, it reveals that it is a traditional antibacterial agent. Efficacy of rLYS in lactating dairy cows with experimentally induced *Staphylococcus aureus* infection. At least one intra-mammary injection of 100 mg rLYS95 in 60 ml phosphate buffered saline (PBS) cures 95% of udder infection with *Staphylococcus aureus*. The antibacterial activity of rLYS *in vitro* persisted for 72 hours, but *in vivo* most of the infected mammary glands remained in the body for 72 hours after treatment [59].

6.3 Endolysin as therapeutic agent

Staphylococcus aureus is a serious threat to human and animal health, and there is an urgent need to develop new antibacterial agents to combat this pathogen. The aim of this study was to obtain active recombinant hemolysin from a novel bacteriophage (IME-SA1) and to conduct a clinical study of its effectiveness against bovine mastitis. We have isolated phages that are toxic and specific for *Staphylococcus aureus*. The optimal infection multiplier is 0.01. Electro-microscopic examination showed that IME-SA1 belongs to the Myoviridae family with the same head (98 nm) and a long tail (200 nm). Experimental lysis experiments showed a phage incubation time of 20 minutes and a burst size of 80. If the host bacterium is in the early stages of exponential growth, the multiplicity of infection is 0.01, resulting in complete lysis of the bacterium after 9 hours. We cloned the endricin gene (804 bp) into the pET-32a bacterial expression vector and succeeded in obtaining recombinant Trx-SA1 endricin with a molecule size of about 47 kDa. Preliminary results from a milk treatment study indicated that Trx-SA1 can effectively control mild clinical mastitis caused by *Staphylococcus aureus*. Endolicin Trx-SA1 may be another strategy for the treatment of infections (including MRSA) caused by *Staphylococcus aureus* [60].

6.4 Mesenchymal stem cells (MSCs)

Although many methods are effective against bovine mastitis, they do not address the problem of udder tissue regeneration and are associated with increased antibiotic resistance worldwide. Experimentally gold in terms of the safety and efficacy of staphylococcus, given the need for alternative therapies that have a large economic impact on the disease, and reports of mesenchymal stem cell (MSC) regeneration and antibacterial effects. We evaluated this intramammary therapy based on color-induced allogeneic MSCs. In a safety study, heifers received a 2.5 x 10^7 AT-MSCs on day 1 and 10. The animals are clinically examined and blood samples were taken for testing. In efficacy studies, Holstein black-and-white cows were vaccinated with *Staphylococcus aureus*, carrier (NEG; days 4 and 10), antibiotics (ATB; days 4 and 5), or 2.5 x 10^7 AT-. MSC (MSC; 4th and 5th day). Cows are clinically examined daily and somatic cell count (SCC) and colony forming units (CFU) are collected from milk samples. Blood samples are collected to measure serum haptoglobin and amyloid A. Two intra-mammary injections of AT-MSC into healthy dairy animals do not cause changes in clinical or hematological parameters, and pro-inflammatory cytokines. Compared to a quarter of the ATB or NEG infected cows, a quarter of the cows in the MSC group had a similar log/ ml SCC of milk. However, compared to a quarter of NEG cows, a quarter of MSC cows have a lower log CFU/ml. Re-inoculation with 2.5 x 10 allogeneic AT-MSC in the udder does not elicit a clinical or immune response in healthy cows. In addition, anti-inflammatory treatment with MSC reduced the number of bacteria in the milk of cows with clinical *Staphylococcus aureus* mastitis compared with untreated cows. This study provides preliminary evidence for the safety and efficacy of emulsions based on allogeneic intra-mammary MSCs for the treatment of bovine mastitis [61].

6.5 Bacteriophage as therapeutic agent

The lytic effects of bacterial deposition on *Staphylococcus aureus* isolates in milk have been investigated in vitro, and their possible applications in the treatment of udder infections caused by different bacteria have been discussed. The host range of the sequenced lytic phage was determined for 92 strains of *Staphylococcus aureus*. These isolates were taken from a quarter of the forehead samples in cases of clinical and subclinical mastitis. A point test followed by plaque analysis is used to determine the range of phage hosts. Three bacterial products STA1, ST29, EB1, ST11 and EB1, ST27 were selected according to host range, reproductive properties and storage properties to prepare a phage mixture (1: 1: 1) and tested for their lytic activity against *Staphylococcus aureus* in cold sterilized raw milk. It has been found that at least two-thirds of the phage can lyse almost two-thirds of the isolate. The phage mixture can reduce the density of *Staphylococcus aureus* bacteria in cold sterilized milk and retain their regenerative capacity in raw milk. Compared to pasteurized milk, the regenerative capacity is only moderately reduced. The significant decreasing capacity of the mixture of phages in raw milk facilitated further in vivo studies [62].

6.6 *Taraxocum mongolicum* as therapeutic agent

Taraxocum mongolicum is widely used as a traditional Chinese medicine for the treatment of various inflammations and infectious diseases, as well as clinically in the treatment of mastitis. The aim of this study was to investigate the protective effect of *T. mongolicum* against *S. aureus* mastitis and its underlying mechanism. Female ICR mice were given 2.5, 5 and 10 g/kg *T. mongolicum* extract twice daily for 6 consecutive days and infected with *Staphylococcus aureus* via the teat canal to induce mastitis. Anti-inflammatory cytokines such as tumor necrosis factor-α (TNF-α), interleukin-6 (IL-6) and interleukin-1β (IL-1β) levels were measured by ELISA. The activity and distribution of myeloperoxidase (MPO) was measured using a kit and immunohistochemistry. Observe histo-pathological changes in udder tissue with H&E staining. Western blotting was used to demonstrate the expression of talk like receptor 2 (TLR2), phosphorylation of related nuclear factor-κB (NF-κB) proteins, and mitogen-activated protein kinase (MAPK) signaling pathway. *T. mongolicum* reduces TNF- and agr, IL-6- and IL-1. Serum and udder levels of mastitis infected with *Staphylococcus aureus* reduce the activity and spread of MPO. In addition, *T. mongolicum* is effective in reducing histo-pathological damage and cell necrosis in udder tissue infected with *Staphylococcus aureus*. In addition, *T. mongolicum* suppress TLR2 expression and phosphorylation of κBα (IκBα), p65, p38, extracellular signal kinase 1/2 (ERK1/2), and N-terminal c-Jun kinase (JNK). This study showed that *T. mongolicum* prevents mastitis caused by *Staphylococcus aureus* infection by exerting an anti-inflammatory effect by inhibiting the TLR2-NF-κB/MAPK signaling pathway [63].

7. Role of probiotics and prebiotics in prevention of *S. aureus* infection

As mastitis is the most dangerous and costly disease of dairy industry. The use of antibiotics leads to the development of drug resistance due to which it becomes untreatable disease. Also, the presence of antibiotic residues in milk and dairy products render it unused able for consumer. So, there is another approach for prevention and treatment of mastitis [64]. Many successful experiments have been performed in past by using bacteriocin-based products. Nisin has been used as a commercial product for the disinfection of teats. And lacticin is used in the dry cow therapy for sealing teat canal at the time of drying off of cow [54, 65].

7.1 Probiotics

Recently, there is need to use other sources in order to reduce antibiotic administration because antibiotic administration is a major cause of lethal infections in dairy industry. Probiotics are live microorganisms which when administered in sufficient amount provides cure from diseases. The probiotics which prevent diseases are called as probiotic drugs. So, mammary probiotics are recently being used as alternatives to antibiotic for the treatment of mastitis. One of the most useful probiotics are LABs (lactic acid bacteria) which interferes with bacteria associated with mastitis, or interact with mammary epithelial cells. Many experiments were performed and claims the therapeutic and preventive effectiveness of probiotics [66]. Results evaluated by using lactic acid bacteria showed that LABs are pro-inflammatory for the mammary glands and it causes an influx of neutrophils into the milk and at drying off of animals. So, it provides protection against mastitis causing *S. aureus* and their ability to provide cure from mastitis remains to be established [67]. Probiotics interferes with the teat microbiota and prevents adherence and colonization of harmful bacteria with the teat canal. However, oral probiotics provides no cure, but intra mammary preparations can be used with caution to prevent mastitis [66].

Some strains of *Lactobacillus casei* and *weisella* produces some compounds which are active against persistence of *S. aureus* bacteria with the epithelial wall of udder tissues, and thus resisting *S. aureus* bacterial pathogenicity by producing hydrogen peroxide, competing nutritional components, changing of host immune system and its utilization. Prolong use of these probiotics and their metabolites seems to be effective alternatives for the control and prevention of mastitis [66, 68].

There are many mechanisms which explain the mode of action of probiotics.

1. The change of the composition of local bacteria and production of bacteriocins and metabolites helps in the efflux of pathogenic bacteria by competing for nutrients.

2. By increases the barriers of epithelium, either by improvement of epithelial junctions or new formation of epithelial cells and introduction of antimicrobial peptides.

3. Enhancement of general immune response against bacteria. By interacting with many cells like monocytes, macrophages, and dendritic cells and train them for innate immunity.

4. Quick actions of systemic responses, like endocrine modulations or central nervous system via signaling mediators.

Different experiments are going on to unmask the details of action mechanism of probiotics in mastitis alongside boosting up the welfare and production aspects of the animals [67, 69].

7.2 Prebiotics

Antibacterial properties of prebiotics were studied *invitro*. To investigate further efficacy against bacteria studies were conducted in lab animals and their success for treatment and to prevent against bacteria was determined by evaluating liver enzymes (aspartate transaminase and alanine transaminase), bacterial colony count of liver and lungs, and also histological changes. In some studies, raisin was used as prebiotic. But it was less effective than others. So, prebiotics are less effective against *S. aureus* than other things [70]. Synbiotics are also tested against mastitis causing bacteria. Especially, these are more effective against *E. coli* and *listeri*a but less effective against *S. aureus* which is highly resistive to the synergistic effect [66, 70].

8. Vaccination against *S. aureus* udder infection

Mastitis is an important disease of the dairy industry that affects production and has economic losses, losses are due to high medicine cost and unusable milk which goes wasted as a result lowers producers' profit. For control of this disease it is necessary to follow some recommendations like teat sanitization, use of cloth to clean udder before and after milking, antibiotic treatment of clinically ill cases, dry cow therapy and proper management and nutrition of dairy animals [71]. In addition to these, vaccination against many pathogens is recommended for prevention and elimination of disease. One of the most important pathogenic entity in mastitis etiologies is *S. aureus*. In order to improve the general health, welfare, production as well as reproductive efficiency of dairy animals, many therapeutic as well as preventive approaches has been in use with less satisfactory results [72].

Staphylococcus aureus mastitis is found in many herds of dairy cows. Due to the predominant infectivity of this organism, many herds have been able to maintain a low prevalence of IMI caused by this organism. This varies greatly between herds and geographic regions, but it has been shown that calves can be infected with this pathogen during calving [73]. This pathogen usually causes only a small fraction of cases of clinical mastitis, and subclinical infections usually become chronic and refractory to treatment. The ability of this pathogen to establish a long lasting IMI varies from strain to strain. However, many toxic factors increase the viability of microorganisms in the host tissue. For longer periods of infection, fibrin deposits and abscess formation further reduce the effectiveness of the immune response. The ability of phagocytic cells to survive intracellularly affects humoral immunity and drug therapy. In addition, for example, infection with *Staphylococcus aureus*. It rarely elicits a significant innate immune response compared to *E. coli*. This avoids an acute immune response that could compromise the presence of infected tissue [74]. An effective vaccine against this pathogen must overcome some major hurdles. [1] Conservative and universal antigens are required for large variation in strains. [2] Toxic factors of "immunity", especially cell survival and the ability to not be exposed to antibodies. [3] Difficulty in assessing the effect of vaccines on reducing infections and the deleterious clinical effects of actual IMI status. The last point reflects the nature of *Staphylococcus aureus* IMI. It can be regularly excreted by bacteria in milk from infected glands. Due to L-type transformation (no cell wall mutations), *Staphylococcus aureus* can relapse in milk up to 80% of the quarter within 28 days after treatment with careful continuous sampling. IMI One or two samples are less sensitive and can correctly identify negative quarters [75].

Its need of time to control *S. aureus* for profitable business of dairy industry and for comfort of consumers with good quality milk and dairy products. In the past years, much progress was made by the researchers but in spite the use of different strategies to control mastitis, *S. aureus* is still a problem. In the dairy industry, anti-staphylococcus vaccines give different results depending upon types of immunization, route of administration, adjuvant used and involvement of some other factors [76]. Considerable effort, encompassing numerous antigens, virulence factors, and bacterial strains, has been made to develop an efficacious and practical *S. aureus* vaccine.

8.1 Vaccines available in market

Many types of vaccines are in use like commercial and herd specific (autogenous) vaccines. The purpose of vaccines is to protect new infections and to stimulate cows' immune system which may provide protection against clinical mastitis [71, 77]. Vaccination may result in the increased rate of antibodies in blood circulation against *S. aureus* pathogens which decreased bacterial growth rate after entering into the udder. The resulting increased immunity may decrease pathogen damage to milk producing tissues, decreased inflammation, and enhance tissue repair. Commercial preparations of vaccine against mastitis caused by *S. aureus* are available in the market [54]. Currently there are only 2 commercially available vaccines are in use for bovine mastitis control. Lysigin® is available in the United States and Starvac® (hipra) is available in Europe and Canada. Many others are in trials and local practices with no wide range application [6].

8.1.1 Lysigin®

Bacteria containing lysed polyvalent phage-type cultures (including several types of capsular sera) are commercially available in the United States (Lysigin; Boehringer Ingelheim, Ridgefield, CT, USA). This product was derived from a Louisiana study conducted twice every 6 months at 2-week intervals for coagulase-negative staphylococcus (CNS) and *Staphylococcus aureus* calves with decreased IMI. However, the problem that arose was that infection studies showed that this bacteriocin did not prevent IMI, did not increase IMI clearance, and did not affect SCC or post-exposure lactation. The clinical score in heifers treated with Lysigin improved and the clinical course of mastitis was short. Immunization with Lysigin increased the level of bovine serum against *Staphylococcus aureus* IgG1, but did not affect the concentration of IgG1, IgG2 or IgM in milk [75].

Lysigin® is a multivalent vaccine which is prepared by using the mastitis causing strains of *S. aureus*, disintegrated into smaller particles. Early studies showed that this vaccine reduces the risk of new infections, lowers somatic cell count and thus lowers clinical mastitis effects. It is evident from experimental studies that by following a proper vaccination schedule early in life of heifer staphylococcal mastitis can be avoided. Moreover, in some recent studies animals in which this vaccine was administered showed clinical symptoms of mastitis. But these animals recovered earlier than non-vaccinated animals; also, there was no difference in somatic cell count and *anti-S. aureus* antibodies. So, this vaccine failed to provide sufficient antibodies in milk to help leukocytes in the elimination of *S. aureus* bacteria from mammary glands. But Lysigin® vaccinated animals have a higher cure rate as compared to other animals [6, 78].

8.1.2 Starvac®

It's a multivalent vaccine which is mixture of inactivated *E. coli* and inactivated *S. aureus* which shows SAAC (slime associated antigenic complex). This preparation helps reduce clinical mastitis cases to some extent that are caused by *S. aureus* and *E. coli* bacteria. This vaccine increases antibodies but does not provide complete protection from mastitis, but decreases intramammary infections and also decreases rate of transfer of infections [79, 80].

8.1.3 Other formulations/approaches

After experimental infection, it was found that different formulations of bacterial drugs that kill whole cells can reduce the number of infections and a quarter of SCC, but this effect was only reported 13 days after infection. Subsequent field reports of two doses at the same time, lower doses in cattle and additional doses during the subsequent lactation period may produce higher antibodies against *Staphylococcus aureus*. Researchers also report that vaccinated animals consume an average of 0.5 kg of milk per day and have lower SCC levels. In this study, Freund's incomplete adjuvant was used as part of the first biphasic administration. This adjuvant is known to cause significant injection site reactions and is not commonly used in commercial products. More interesting developments from the same research group have identified targets for RNAIII-activated protein (TRAP), a highly conserved membrane protein in many *Staphylococcus* species, including *Staphylococcus aureus*. This antigen can become a specific and universal vaccine against *staphylococcus* [81]. *Staphylococcus aureus* produces adhesin, a pathogenic factor that promotes attachment of host tissues and subsequent attachment between bacterial cells, creating a biofilm that can resist feeding. Surface polysaccharides are an important component of staphylococcal biofilm, and strains expressing high levels of extracellular polysaccharides (surface-associated antigenic complex [SAAC]) have been isolated [82]. A commercial formulation combining SAAC *Staphylococcus aureus* and *E. coli* has been approved by the European Union. Clinical reports have shown that this product can improve udder health by reducing re-infection and SCC in vaccinated animals. The use of vaccines against *Staphylococcus aureus* may be restricted in many dairy farms, especially herds with low IMI prevalence, such as herds with SCC <200,000 cells/ml. Thus, *Staphylococcus aureus* bacteriosin cannot significantly influence the successful control of infectious mastitis through the use of correct milking techniques and milking machine maintenance. Conversely, people who have been vaccinated with the right treatment can experience disappointing results. As previously mentioned, this varies greatly between herds and geographic areas. If the herd has *Staphylococcus aureus*, bacteriosin can also reduce the shedding of bacteria in the milk of infected animals. Researchers have administered *Staphylococcus aureus* bacteriosin to improve antibacterial treatment, but the results are mixed [83].

8.2 Autogenous vaccine against *S. aureus* mastitis

These vaccines are the preparations having specific strains of bacteria obtained from mastitis suffered by animals and used to immunize the herd for protection against further new udder infections with the same strain of bacteria. There are evidences which shows that the use of autogenous *S. aureus* vaccines enhances antibody titer in vaccinated animals as compared to non-vaccinated herd and reduce the risk of both clinical and sub-clinical mastitis [71]. Some studies also show that autogenous vaccines provide almost 70% protection from infection and provide protection from clinically ill mastitis cases challenged with *S. aureus* [80].

Early studies suggest that vaccines for *S. aureus* will increase cure rate and lower SCC but in actuality, it does not work against adult cows. Experimental success was also seen with commercial *S. aureus* vaccine Lysigin® in the young dairy animals. When serum samples from vaccinated animals were checked they showed higher antibody titer as compared to non-vaccinated animals to combat against *S. aureus* infections [71]. So experimental and commercial preparations of *S. aureus* vaccine provide protection against mastitis. Efficacy of these preparations against *S. aureus* ranges between 44%–66% and this strategy for prevention of *S. aureus* in the future, some new antigens and adjuvants are added to the vaccine preparations to enhance their effectiveness [72, 84].

8.3 Vaccine response in vaccinated dairy animals

Staphylococcus aureus is a predominant organism causing mastitis in different species. So, different experiments were conducted in different animal species to determine vaccine efficacy. The production and implementation of *S. aureus* vaccine in milk animals has a great impact towards public health. Inactivated vaccine was prepared and checked by using different adjuvants against *S. aureus* [85].

She camel having sub-clinical mastitis, vaccinal isolates were taken from her having alpha and beta hemolysin toxin, also some were multidrug resistant. Inactivated alum precipitated *S. aureus* vaccine (APSV) and oil adjuvant *S. aureus* vaccine (OASV) were prepared after confirming its antigenicity in rabbits. Experiments showed that APSV and OASV were safe, effective and expressed immunogenic responses in experimental rabbits [86, 87].

S. aureus is a major cause of mastitis in dairy cows causing mild to severe and chronic infections having drastic effects on cow's wellbeing, lifespan and milk production. Irrespective of years of research on mastitis issues still there is no production of an effective vaccine against *S. aureus mastitis.* Experimental studies showed that it's possible to vaccinate *S. aureus* naïve cattle and also this experimental immunization leads to humoral immune response which is different from response that occurs after natural exposure [79, 88].

Experiments are still in progress for the use of vaccine against *S. aureus* mastitis in small ruminants. Still, there is gap in using mastitis vaccine for prevention of *S. aureus* mastitis which is a major issue in dairy industry and causes huge economic losses every year. Perhaps there might be bright future for farmers because trails of mastitis vaccine in lab animals are showing satisfactory results, which is a hope [43, 50].

8.4 Vaccine success rate

Mastitis is one of the most dangerous disease of dairy industry. Vaccination and other managemental practices are the tools to prevent mastitis caused by contagious as well as environmental pathogens. The success rate of immunization depends upon type of vaccine, adjuvant used and route of administration of vaccination regardless of type of vaccine, only vaccine is not enough in the large herds with high mastitis cases. For achieving success, it is necessary to use up to date manage mental practices along with vaccine and culling of chronically ill cases to reduce intra mammary infections [50, 89].

Experiments conducted from last 15 decades show that experimental *S. aureus* vaccines as well as commercial vaccines reduce new infections in dairy heifers. *S. aureus* vaccine was prepared by focusing on two major components of *S. aureus* (pseudo-capsules and alpha toxins). 2 and 4 weeks before calving heifers were given injections in the supra-mammary lymph node of mammary glands. Injections were given subcutaneously. After caving these heifers were challenged with *S. aureus* infections. These heifers showed 46% reduction in *S. aureus* infections as compared with control group of animals. There was almost 70% success rate from infection in vaccinated animals and less than 10% in non-vaccinated animals. Clinical signs of mastitis were also mild in vaccinated herds compared to control group of animals [6, 72].

9. Conclusion

Staphylococcus aureus is a major mastitis causing pathogen which is contagious in nature and persist in the mammary epithelial cell for long period of time and cause further infections. About 74% quarter prevalence of *S. aureus* in bovine udder with overall prevalence exceeding 61% in dairy animals. Cure rate in *S. aureus* mastitis is merely 25–50% during the lactation. A wide array of genotypic variations has been observed with great genetic diversity in the isolates of bovine as well as caprine origin. 17 different pulsotypes of dairy originated *S. aureus* have been reported with 24 virulence coding genes for leukocidins (lukED/lukM), pyrogenic toxin superantigen (PTS Ag), haemolysins (hla-hlg), toxic-shock syndrome toxin (tst), enterotoxins (sea-seo, seu), exfoliative toxins (eta, etb), and genes for methicillin (mecA) and penicillin (blaZ) resistance. The magnitude of yield loss in 30% cases of clinical mastitis reached up to 950-1050 kg per lactation. Attainment of refuge inside the macrophages and neutrophils is a major cause of *S. aureus* mastitis persistence. The antimicrobials cannot penetrate these structures to reach the mastitis causing organisms. This limits the use of antimicrobials to secondary importance in relation to immediate need of supportive treatment. Mammary probiotics are recently being used as alternatives to antibiotic for the treatment of mastitis. One of the most useful probiotics are lactic acid bacteria which interferes with bacteria associated with mastitis, or interact with mammary epithelial cells. Antibacterial properties of prebiotics are also studied *invitro*. Literature showed anti- staphylococcus vaccines with different results depending upon types of immunization, route of administration, adjuvant used and involvement of some other factors. Many types of vaccines are in use like commercial and herd specific vaccines. Commercial vaccines against mastitis caused by *S. aureus* are available in the local markets with variable efficacy around the globe. Studies conducted from last 15 decades show that experimental herd specific *S. aureus* vaccines as well as commercial vaccines reduce new infections in dairy heifers. Experiments are still in progress for the use of vaccine against *S. aureus* mastitis with optimal efficacy and reliability. Still, there is knowledge gap in using vaccines for prevention of *S. aureus* mastitis, needed to be research in focus. Perhaps, there might be bright future for farmers because of highly satisfactory trail results of mastitis vaccines in the lab animals.

Author details

Amjad Islam Aqib[1*], Muhammad Ijaz[2], Muhammad Shoaib[3,4], Iqra Muzammil[2], Hafiz Iftikhar Hussain[1], Tean Zaheer[5], Rais Ahmed[1], Iqra Sarwar[5], Yasir Razzaq Khan[1] and Muhammad Aamir Naseer[5]

1 Cholistan University of Veterinary and Animal Sciences, Bahawalpur, Pakistan

2 University of Veterinary and Animal Sciences, Lahore, Pakistan

3 Institute of Microbiology, University of Agriculture Faisalabad, Pakistan

4 Key Laboratory of New Animal Drug Project, Gansu Province, Key Laboratory of Veterinary Pharmaceutical Development, Ministry of Agriculture, Lanzhou Institute of Husbandry and Pharmaceutical Sciences of CAAS, Lanzhou, China

5 University of Agriculture, Faisalabad, Pakistan

*Address all correspondence to: amjadwaseer@gmail.com

References

[1] Shoaib M, Rahman SU, Aqib AI, Ashfaq K, Naveed A, Kulyar MF-A, et al. Diversified Epidemiological Pattern and Antibiogram of mecA Gene in Staphylococcus aureus Isolates of Pets, Pet Owners and Environment. Pak Vet J. 2020;40(3):331-336.

[2] Aqib A, Nighat S, Ahmed R, Sana S, Jamal M, Kulyar MF, et al. Drug Susceptibility Profile of *Staphylococcus aureus* Isolated from Mastitic Milk of Goats and Risk Factors Associated with Goat Mastitis in Pakistan. Vol. 51. Pakistan J. Zool., Vol. 51, Iss. 1, pp. 307-315 Read more at http://researcherslinks.com/current-issues/Drug-Susceptibility-Profile-of-Staphylococcus/20/1/1880/html#KolwAq8XDDQ2YXZo.99; 2018. 307-315 p.

[3] A Begum H, S Uddin M, J Islam M, Nazir KHMNH, Islam M, Rahman MT. Detection of biofilm producing coagulase positive *Staphylococcus aureus* from bovine mastitis, their pigment production, hemolytic activity and antibiotic sensitivity pattern. 4(1 & 2): J. Bangladesh Soc. Agric. Sci. Technol.4(1 & 2): 97-100; 2007.

[4] Naseer MA, Aqib AI, Ashar A, Saleem MI, Shoaib M, Kulyar MF-A, et al. Detection of Altered Pattern of Antibiogram and Biofilm Character in *Staphylococcus aureus* Isolated From Dairy Milk. Pakistan J Zool. 2020;

[5] Basanisi MG, La Bella G, Nobili G, Franconieri I, La Salandra G. Genotyping of methicillin-resistant Staphylococcus aureus (MRSA) isolated from milk and dairy products in South Italy. Food Microbiol. 2017;62:141-146.

[6] Côté-Gravel J, Malouin F. Symposium review: Features of Staphylococcus aureus mastitis pathogenesis that guide vaccine development strategies*. J Dairy Sci. 2019;102(5):4727-4740.

[7] Hossain SMA. Efficacy of dry cow therapy in mastitis control strategy. MS Thesis. Department of Surgery and Obstetrics, Faculty of Veterinary …; 2004.

[8] Abo-EL-Sooud K. Ethnoveterinary perspectives and promising future. Int J Vet Sci Med. 2018;6(1):1-7.

[9] Radostits OM, Gay CC, Hinchcliff KW, Constable PD. Veterinary Medicine E-Book: A textbook of the diseases of cattle, horses, sheep, pigs and goats. Elsevier Health Sciences; 2006.

[10] van Soest FJS, Mourits MCM, Blanco-Penedo I, Duval J, Fall N, Krieger M, et al. Farm-specific failure costs of production disorders in European organic dairy herds. Prev Vet Med. 2019;168:19-29.

[11] Jingar S, Chhokar MS, Roy A, Sharma R, Lawania P, Kumar A, et al. Economic Loss due to Clinical Mastitis in Crossbred Cows. Int J Livest Res. 2018 Jan;1.

[12] Hagnestam-Nielsen C, Ostergaard S. Economic impact of clinical mastitis in a dairy herd assessed by stochastic simulation using different methods to model yield losses. Animal. 2009 Feb;3(2):315-328.

[13] Petersson-Wolfe CS, Mullarky IK, Jones GM. *Staphylococcus aureus* mastitis: cause, detection, and control. 2010;

[14] Masse E, CHAKRAVARTY S. RNA-dependent regulation of virulence in pathogenic bacteria. Front Cell Infect Microbiol. 2019;9:337.

[15] Quinn PJ, Markey BK, Leonard FC, Hartigan P, Fanning S, Fitzpatrick Es. Veterinary microbiology and microbial disease. John Wiley & Sons; 2011.

[16] Kashif A, McClure J-AM, Lakhundi S, Pham M, Chen S, Conly J, et al. Staphylococcus aureus ST398 Virulence Is Associated with Factors Carried on Prophage $Φ$Sa3. Front Microbiol. 2019;10:2219.

[17] Algharib SA, Dawood A, Xie S. Nanoparticles for treatment of bovine Staphylococcus aureus mastitis. Drug Deliv. 2020;27(1):292-308.

[18] Clauditz A, Resch A, Wieland K-P, Peschel A, Götz F. Staphyloxanthin plays a role in the fitness of Staphylococcus aureus and its ability to cope with oxidative stress. Infect Immun. 2006;74(8):4950-4953.

[19] Zaatout N, Ayachi A, Kecha M. Interaction of primary mammary bovine epithelial cells with biofilm-forming staphylococci associated with subclinical bovine mastitis. Iran J Vet Res. 2019;20(1):27.

[20] Zaatout N, Ayachi A, Kecha M. Staphylococcus aureus persistence properties associated with bovine mastitis and alternative therapeutic modalities. J Appl Microbiol. 2020;

[21] Sutra L, Poutrel B. Virulence factors involved in the pathogenesis of bovine intramammary infections due to Staphylococcus aureus. J Med Microbiol. 1994;40(2):79-89.

[22] Sears PM, Smith BS, English PB, Herer PS, Gonzalez RN. Shedding Pattern of Staphylococcus aureus from Bovine Intramammary Infections. J Dairy Sci. 1990;73(10):2785-2789.

[23] Jørgensen HJ, Mørk T, Caugant DA, Kearns A, Rørvik LM. Genetic variation among Staphylococcus aureus strains from Norwegian bulk milk. Appl Environ Microbiol. 2005;71(12):8352-8361.

[24] Asselstine V, Miglior F, Suárez-Vega A, Fonseca PAS, Mallard B, Karrow N, et al. Genetic mechanisms regulating the host response during mastitis. J Dairy Sci. 2019;102(10):9043-9059.

[25] Filipe J, Bronzo V, Curone G, Castiglioni B, Vigo D, Smith B, et al. Staphylococcus aureus intra-mammary infection affects the expression pattern of IL-R8 in goat. Comp Immunol Microbiol Infect Dis. 2019;66:101339.

[26] Aires-de-Sousa M, Parente CESR, Vieira-da-Motta O, Bonna ICF, Silva DA, de Lencastre H. Characterization of *Staphylococcus aureus* isolates from buffalo, bovine, ovine, and caprine milk samples collected in Rio de Janeiro State, Brazil. Appl Environ Microbiol. 04/20. 2007;73(12):3845-9.

[27] Sakwinska O, Giddey M, Moreillon M, Morisset D, Waldvogel A, Moreillon P. Staphylococcus aureus host range and human-bovine host shift. Appl Environ Microbiol. 2011;77(17):5908-5915.

[28] Haran KP, Godden SM, Boxrud D, Jawahir S, Bender JB, Sreevatsan S. Prevalence and Characterization of *Staphylococcus aureus*, Including Methicillin-Resistant S. *aureus*. J Clin Microbiol. 2012 Mar;50(3):688 LP – 695.

[29] Akpaka PE, Roberts R, Monecke S. Molecular characterization of antimicrobial resistance genes against *Staphylococcus aureus* isolates from Trinidad and Tobago. J Infect Public Heal. 2016/06/23. 2017;10(3):316-23.

[30] Dodémont M, Argudín MA, Willekens J, Vanderhelst E, Pierard D, Miendje Deyi VY, et al. Emergence of livestock-associated MRSA isolated from cystic fibrosis patients: Result of a Belgian national survey. J Cyst Fibros. 2019;18(1):86-93.

[31] Zehra A, Gulzar M, Singh R, Kaur S, Gill JPS. Prevalence, multidrug

resistance and molecular typing of methicillin-resistant Staphylococcus aureus (MRSA) in retail meat from Punjab, India. J Glob Antimicrob Resist. 2019;16:152-158.

[32] Kapur V, Sischo WM, Greer RS, Whittam TS, Musser JM. Molecular population genetic analysis of Staphylococcus aureus recovered from cows. J Clin Microbiol. 1995;33(2):376.

[33] Fox LK, Zadoks RN, Gaskins CT. Biofilm production by Staphylococcus aureus associated with intramammary infection. Vet Microbiol. 2005;107(3):295-299.

[34] Vaughn JM, Abdi RD, Gillespie BE, Kerro Dego O. Genetic diversity and virulence characteristics of Staphylococcus aureus isolates from cases of bovine mastitis. Microb Pathog. 2020;144:104171.

[35] Zayda MG, Masuda Y, Hammad AM, Honjoh K, Elbagory AM, Miyamoto T. Molecular characterisation of methicillin-resistant (MRSA) and methicillin-susceptible (MSSA) Staphylococcus aureus isolated from bovine subclinical mastitis and Egyptian raw milk cheese. Int Dairy J. 2020;104:104646.

[36] Azzi O, Lai F, Tennah S, Menoueri MN, Achek R, Azara E, et al. Spa-typing and antimicrobial susceptibility of Staphylococcus aureus isolated from clinical sheep mastitis in Medea province, Algeria. Small Rumin Res. 2020;106168.

[37] Wang W, Lin X, Jiang T, Peng Z, Xu J, Yi L, et al. Prevalence and Characterization of Staphylococcus aureus Cultured From Raw Milk Taken From Dairy Cows With Mastitis in Beijing, China. Front Microbiol. 2018;9:1123.

[38] Melchior MB, Van Duijkeren E, Mevius DJ, Nielen M, Fink-Gremmels J. Genotyping and biofilm formation of *Staphylococcus aureus* isolates: Evidence for lack of penicillin-resistance in Agr-type II strains. In: Mastitis Control: From Science to Practice. Elsevier; 2008. p. 308.

[39] Cucarella C, Tormo MA, Ubeda C, Trotonda MP, Monzón M, Peris C, et al. Role of biofilm-associated protein bap in the pathogenesis of bovine Staphylococcus aureus. Infect Immun. 2004;72(4):2177-2185.

[40] Haveri M, Roslöf A, Rantala L, Pyörälä S. Virulence genes of bovine Staphylococcus aureus from persistent and nonpersistent intramammary infections with different clinical characteristics. J Appl Microbiol. 2007 Oct;103(4):993-1000.

[41] Angelidis AS, Komodromos D, Giannakou R, Arsenos G, Gelasakis AI, Kyritsi M, et al. Isolation and characterization of Staphylococcus aureus and methicillin-resistant Staphylococcus aureus (MRSA) from milk of dairy goats under low-input farm management in Greece. Vet Microbiol. 2020;247:108749.

[42] Ibrahim N. Review on Mastitis and Its Economic Effect. Can J Sci Res. 2017 Jan;6:13-22.

[43] Rollin E, Dhuyvetter KC, Overton MW. The cost of clinical mastitis in the first 30 days of lactation: An economic modeling tool. Prev Vet Med. 2015 Dec;122(3):257-264.

[44] Dego OK. Current Status of Antimicrobial Resistance and Prospect for New Vaccines against Major Bacterial Bovine Mastitis Pathogens. In: Animal Reproduction in Veterinary Medicine. IntechOpen; 2020.

[45] Klaas IC, Zadoks RN. An update on environmental mastitis: Challenging perceptions. Transbound Emerg Dis. 2018 May;65(S1):166-185.

[46] Mbindyo CM, Gitao GC, Mulei CM. Prevalence, Etiology, and Risk Factors of Mastitis in Dairy Cattle in Embu and Kajiado Counties, Kenya. Vet Med Int. 2020 Aug;2020:8831172.

[47] Tarazona-Manrique LE, Villate-Hernández JR, Andrade-Becerra RJ. Bacterial and fungal infectious etiology causing mastitis in dairy cows in the highlands of Boyacá (Colombia). Vol. 66, Revista de la Facultad de Medicina Veterinaria y de Zootecnia. scieloco; 2019. p. 208-18.

[48] Breen JE, Green MJ, Bradley AJ. Quarter and cow risk factors associated with the occurrence of clinical mastitis in dairy cows in the United Kingdom. J Dairy Sci. 2009;92(6):2551-2561.

[49] Carrillo-Casas EM, Miranda-Morales RE. Bovine mastitis pathogens: prevalence and effects on somatic cell count. In: Milk Production-An Up-to-Date Overview of Animal Nutrition, Management and Health. IntechOpen; 2012.

[50] Contreras Bravo G, Rodríguez J. Mastitis: Comparative Etiology and Epidemiology. J Mammary Gland Biol Neoplasia. 2011 Sep;16:339-356.

[51] Petrovski KR, Buneski G, Trajcev M. A review of the factors affecting the costs of bovine mastitis. J S Afr Vet Assoc. 2006;77(2):52-60.

[52] Janzen JJ. Economic losses resulting from mastitis. A review. J Dairy Sci. 1970;53(9):1151-1160.

[53] Seegers H, Fourichon C, Beaudeau F. Production effects related to mastitis and mastitis economics in dairy cattle herds. Vet Res. 2003 Sep;34:475-491.

[54] Hogeveen H, Huijps K, Lam T, De Vliegher S, Fox LK, Piepers S, et al. Economic aspects of mastitis: New developments. N Z Vet J. 2011;59(1):357-372.

[55] Weller JI, Ezra E, van Straten M. Genetic and environmental analysis of diseases with major economic impact in Israeli Holsteins. J Dairy Sci. 2019;102(11):10030-10038.

[56] Richert RM, Cicconi KM, Gamroth MJ, Schukken YH, Stiglbauer KE, Ruegg PL. Risk factors for clinical mastitis, ketosis, and pneumonia in dairy cattle on organic and small conventional farms in the United States. J Dairy Sci. 2013;96(7):4269-4285.

[57] Esposito G, Irons PC, Webb EC, Chapwanya A. Interactions between negative energy balance, metabolic diseases, uterine health and immune response in transition dairy cows. Anim Reprod Sci. 2014;144(3):60-71.

[58] Aqib AI, Saqib M, Khan SR, Ahmad T, Shah SA, Naseer MA, et al. Non-steroidal anti-inflammatory drugs, plant extracts, and characterized microparticles to modulate antimicrobial resistance of epidemic mecA positive S. aureus of dairy origin. Applied Nanoscience.:1-1

[59] Cardoso CV, Barbosa EV, Liberal MHT, das Chagas EF. Transgenic technology: the strategy for the control and prevention of bovine staphylococcal mastitis? Biotechnol Res Innov. 2019;3(2):291-297.

[60] Fan J, Zeng Z, Mai K, Yang Y, Feng J, Bai Y, et al. Preliminary treatment of bovine mastitis caused by Staphylococcus aureus, with trx-SA1, recombinant endolysin of S. aureus bacteriophage IME-SA1. Vet Microbiol. 2016;191:65-71.

[61] Peralta OA, Carrasco C, Vieytes C, Tamayo MJ, Muñoz I, Sepulveda S, et al. Safety and efficacy of a mesenchymal stem cell intramammary therapy in

dairy cows with experimentally induced Staphylococcus aureus clinical mastitis. Sci Rep. 2020;10(1):1-12.

[62] Titze I, Lehnherr T, Lehnherr H, Krömker V. Efficacy of bacteriophages against Staphylococcus aureus isolates from bovine mastitis. Pharmaceuticals. 2020;13(3):35.

[63] Ge B, Zhao P, Li H, Sang R, Wang M, Zhou H, et al. Taraxacum mongolicum protects against *Staphylococcus aureus*-infected mastitis by exerting anti-inflammatory role via TLR2-NF-κB/MAPKs pathways in mice. J Ethnopharmacol [Internet]. 2020;113595. Available from: http://www.sciencedirect.com/science/article/pii/S0378874120334838

[64] Abdurahman OAS. Udder health and milk quality among camels in the Errer valley of eastern Ethiopia. Livest Res Rural Dev. 2006 Jan;18.

[65] Zadoks RN, Middleton JR, McDougall S, Katholm J, Schukken YH. Molecular epidemiology of mastitis pathogens of dairy cattle and comparative relevance to humans. J Mammary Gland Biol Neoplasia. 2011;

[66] Rainard P, Foucras G. A Critical Appraisal of Probiotics for Mastitis Control . Vol. 5, Frontiers in Veterinary Science . 2018. p. 251.

[67] Soleimani N, Kermanshahi R, Yakhchali B, Sattari T. Antagonistic activity of probiotic lactobacilli against Staphylococcus aureus isolated from bovine mastitis. African J Microbiol Res. 2010 Nov;420:2169-2173.

[68] Rainard P, Riollet C. Innate immunity of the bovine mammary gland. Vet Res. 2006 May;37(3):369-400.

[69] Wilson DJ, Grohn YT, Bennett GJ, González RN, Schukken YH, Spatz J. Comparison of J5 Vaccinates and Controls for Incidence, Etiologic Agent, Clinical Severity, and Survival in the Herd Following Naturally Occurring Cases of Clinical Mastitis. J Dairy Sci. 2007;90(9):4282-4288.

[70] Gadde U, Kim WH, Oh ST, Lillehoj HS. Alternatives to antibiotics for maximizing growth performance and feed efficiency in poultry: A review. Anim Heal Res Rev. 2017;18(1):26-45.

[71] Landin H, Jansson Mörk M, Larsson M, Waller K. Vaccination against Staphylococcus aureus mastitis in two Swedish dairy herds. Acta Vet Scand. 2015 Nov;57:81.

[72] Pereira UP, Oliveira DGS, Mesquita LR, Costa GM, Pereira LJ. Efficacy of Staphylococcus aureus vaccines for bovine mastitis: a systematic review. Vet Microbiol. 2011 Mar;148(2-4):117-124.

[73] Borm AA, Fox LK, Leslie KE, Hogan JS, Andrew SM, Moyes KM, et al. Effects of prepartum intramammary antibiotic therapy on udder health, milk production, and reproductive performance in dairy heifers. J Dairy Sci. 2006;89(6):2090-2098.

[74] Petzl W, Zerbe H, Günther J, Yang W, Seyfert H-M, Nürnberg G, et al. Escherichia coli, but not Staphylococcus aureus triggers an early increased expression of factors contributing to the innate immune defense in the udder of the cow. Vet Res. 2008;39(2):1-23.

[75] Middleton JR, Luby CD, Viera L, Tyler JW, Casteel S. Influence of Staphylococcus aureus intramammary infection on serum copper, zinc, and iron concentrations. J Dairy Sci. 2004;87(4):976-979.

[76] Scali F, Camussone C, Calvinho L, Cipolla M, Zecconi A. Which are important targets in development of S.aureus mastitis vaccine? Res Vet Sci. 2015 Mar;100.

[77] Vasileiou NGC, Cripps PJ, Ioannidi KS, Katsafadou AI, Chatzopoulos DC, Barbagianni MS, et al. Experimental study for evaluation of the efficacy of a biofilm-embedded bacteria-based vaccine against Staphylococcus chromogenes-associated mastitis in sheep. Vet Microbiol. 2019;239:108480.

[78] Middleton JR, Ma J, Rinehart CL, Taylor VN, Luby CD, Steevens BJ. Efficacy of different Lysigin (TM) formulations in the prevention of Staphylococcus aureus intramammary infection in dairy heifers. J Dairy Res. 2006;73(1):10.

[79] Niedziela DA, Murphy MP, Grant J, Keane OM, Leonard FC. Clinical presentation and immune characteristics in first-lactation Holstein-Friesian cows following intramammary infection with genotypically distinct *Staphylococcus aureus* strains. J Dairy Sci. 2020;

[80] Cheng WN. Bovine mastitis: risk factors, therapeutic strategies, and alternative treatments. Asian-Australasian J Anim Sci. 2020 May;

[81] Leitner G, Krifucks O, Kiran MD, Balaban N. Vaccine development for the prevention of staphylococcal mastitis in dairy cows. Vet Immunol Immunopathol. 2011;142(1-2):25-35.

[82] Prenafeta A, March R, Foix A, Casals I, Costa L. Study of the humoral immunological response after vaccination with a Staphylococcus aureus biofilm-embedded bacterin in dairy cows: possible role of the exopolysaccharide specific antibody production in the protection from Staphylococcus aureus induced mastitis. Vet Immunol Immunopathol. 2010;134(3-4):208-217.

[83] Erskine RJ. Vaccination strategies for mastitis. Vet Clin North Am Food Anim Pract. 2012;28(2):257-270.

[84] Reed SG, Bertholet S, Coler RN, Friede M. New horizons in adjuvants for vaccine development. Trends Immunol. 2009 Jan;30(1):23-32.

[85] Tollersrud T, Kenny K, Caugant D, Lund A. Characterisation of isolates of Staphylococcus aureus from acute, chronic and subclinical mastitis in cows in NorwayNote. APMIS. 2000 Oct;108:565-572.

[86] Ali M, Avais M, Ijaz M, Chaudhary M, Hussain R, Aqib A, et al. Epidemiology of Subclinical Mastitis in Dromedary Camels (Camelus dromedarius) of Two Distinct Agro-Ecological Zones of Pakistan. Pak J Zool. 2019 Feb;51.

[87] Aqib AI, Ijaz M, Farooqi SH, Ahmed R, Shoaib M, Ali MM, et al. Emerging discrepancies in conventional and molecular epidemiology of methicillin resistant Staphylococcus aureus isolated from bovine milk. Microb Pathog. 2018;116:38-43.

[88] Shittu A, Abdullahi J, Jibril A, Mohammed AA, Fasina FO. Sub-clinical mastitis and associated risk factors on lactating cows in the Savannah Region of Nigeria. BMC Vet Res. 2012;8(1):134.

[89] Dodd FH. Mastitis--progress on control. J Dairy Sci. 1983 Aug;66(8):1773-1780.

Chapter 8

Progression of β-Lactam Resistance in *Staphylococcus aureus*

Antresh Kumar and Manisha Kaushal

Abstract

Staphylococcus aureus is a notorious human pathogen that causes superficial and invasive infections both in nosocomial and community-acquired settings. The prevalence of staphylococcal infections became more challenging after emerging resistance against topical antibiotics. *S. aureus* evolved resistance to β-lactam antibiotics due to modification and expression of penicillin-binding proteins (PBP), inactivation of drug by β-lactamase synthesis, limiting uptake of drug by biofilm formation, and reducing uptake by expression of efflux pump. The wave of resistance was first observed in penicillin by β-lactamase production and PBPs modification. The second wave of resistance emerged to methicillin by appearing methicillin-resistant *S. aureus* (MRSA) strains. Cephalosporin has long been used as the last resort for preventing MRSA infections, but resistant strains appeared during treatment. In progression to control MRSA or related infections, carbapenems have been used but strains developed resistance. *S. aureus* is among the high-priority resistance organisms that need renewed efforts for the research and development of new antibiotics and innovative preventive approaches. However, a lot of toiling is involved in devising an effective treatment against drug resistant *S. aureus*. This chapter aim is to retrospectively determine the progression of resistance in *S. aureus*, against different β-lactam antibiotics and their challenges of medication.

Keywords: *Staphylococcus aureus*, Drug resistance, β-lactam antibiotics, Penicillin, Methicillin, Cephalosporin

1. Introduction

Infections caused by a variety of bacterial, fungal, viral, and other infectious microorganisms are considered to be the world's most leading problem. Infectious diseases are considered to be the world most leading cause of death, with almost 50,000 deaths per day [1]. Bacterial and fungal infections are the major cause of morbidity and mortality in both developed and developing countries [2]. *Staphylococcus aureus* is a gram-positive, coagulase-positive opportunistic bacterial pathogen, commonly found in the human nasal mucosa in the approximately 20–40% population [3, 4]. It causes a wide range of infections such as skin infections, including abscesses, impetigo, and necrotizing fasciitis; tissue infections, including osteomyelitis and endocarditis; and toxicities, including toxic shock syndrome, pneumonia, sepsis, and surgical site infections [5–7]. The superficial and invasive infections caused by *S. aureus* continue to raise serious health challenges globally as it notoriously exhibits resistance [8, 9].

These infections have rapidly developed resistance against most of the available antimicrobials, which pose serious threats [10–13]. Infections caused by *S. aureus* are associated with significantly higher mortality, because of the limitations of available antimicrobial therapies, difficulties in making a rapid and accurate diagnosis, and the development of multidrug resistance (MDR) [14]. The acute and chronic staphylococcal infections have now become more problematic after emerging multidrug resistance (MDR) against various frontline antibiotics [15, 16]. Antibiotics are small molecules that selectively inhibit the growth of a plethora of bacterial and other infections. These heterogeneous group molecules continue to be save many lives from different bacterial infections. Antibiotics are either naturally synthesized by microorganisms or chemically modified into exciting drugs. β-lactam antibiotics (β-LA) are considered to be the most successful and frequently used antibiotics against a number of bacterial infections. The underlying reason behind this is their wide spectrum activity, oral availability, excellent pharmacokinetics, lack of toxicity, and bactericidal action [17]. Due to the widespread and prolonged practice of β-LA emerged resistance to these resort and became an alarming and emerging problem to the public health. The microbial pathogens tend to adopt different resistance mechanism to skip the cytotoxic effect of β-LA. The progression in β-LA drug resistance to emerge multiple antibiotic-resistant microorganisms has made it difficult to manage many infectious diseases using common anti-infective drugs. In this chapter, we focus on emerging trends of drug resistance in *S. aureus* to the different β-LA.

2. β-Lactam antibiotics (β-LA)

The landmark discovery the beta-lactam penicillin has been developed with the remarkable weapon to control bacterial infections during the Second World War [18]. It was naturally synthesized from *Penicillium chrysogenum* (also known as *Penicillium notatum*). Penicillin G was the first β-lactam antibiotic (β-LA) discovered in 1944, which began the era of antibiotics against a wide range of infectious microorganisms [19]. The development of penicillin led to search its different derivatives (amoxicillin and methicillin) for the betterment of their efficacy, bioavailability, solubility, stability, and other pharmacokinetic properties and to evade steadily emerging problem of multidrug resistance (MDR). Structurally, penicillin is composed of a thiazolidine ring attached to a side chain of a four-membered beta-lactam ring. All penicillins are derivatives of 6-aminopenecillinic acid, which sometimes differ in their side-chain structure. Many β-LA have lactam ring as an integral part of a molecule such as cephalosporins, monobactams, cephamycins, and the carbapenems (imipenem and meropenem). These β-LA antibiotics came into the light to rescue mankind from different Gram –ve and Gram +ve bacterial infections including *S. aureus*. β-LA are the most available and over 34 β-LA approved by the FDA, which together constitute ~50% of all antibiotic prescriptions worldwide. Now, β-LA share the annual consumption of over $15 billion, which contribute almost 65% of the total antibiotics [20].

The β-LA primarily target the cell wall of a bacterial pathogen. Peptidoglycan or murien present in the cell wall provides the mechanical strength to the bacterial cell membrane, which is composed of an alternating unit of *N*-acetylglucosamine (NAG) and *N*-acetylmuramic acid (NAM) residues, joined together by β-1 → 4 linkage. The NAM is further linked with a pentapeptide stem, which is composed of L-Ala-D-Glu- L-Lys-D-Ala-D-Ala. The order and type of amino acids are almost similar in Gram –ve and Gram +ve bacterial with some slight variations. The last D-Ala is lost during maturation and glycan assembly is cross-linked to form a bridge with the carboxyl group of D-Ala at position 4 and the amino group of the amino acid at position 3. Mechanistically, β-LA acts upon a 4-membered "beta-lactam" ring, which shows a resemblance to D-Ala-D-Ala sequence of the cell wall [21]. The primary function of PBP is in the elongation of the cell wall, which is composed of two distinct components termed as PBP1–4. The radioactive analysis revealed that penicillin specifically interacts with PBP protein *via* covalent interactions [22]. The tight binding of β-LA to the transpeptidase domain of PBP (penicillin-binding protein) thereby inhibits the peptidoglycan synthesis by acylating transpeptidase, involved in crosslinking peptide to form peptidoglycan [23].

3. β-Lactam resistance in *S. aureus*

According to the European Centre for Diseases Control (ECDC), antimicrobial resistance is the single biggest threat facing the world in the area of infectious diseases. With the progression of antibiotics discoveries and their prophylactic usages have emerged drug resistance to single or multiple drugs. Antibiotic resistance is a natural selection process when microorganisms are treated with different antibiotics, and microorganisms tend to escape this selection pressure with greater competency to survive and thus show antibiotics resistance. In contrast, bacteria with a susceptible nature are killed with exposed antibiotics. Emerging resistance to β-LA is a serious health concern that causes a major hurdle in the treatment of bacterial infections. The condition of drug resistance is primarily developed by increasing and indiscriminate usage of antibiotics in clinical ailments, unregulated sales of antibiotics, a long course of medication, and poor public health infrastructure. According to a hospital survey, over 80% of clinical samples of *S. aureus* were established resistance to the frontline antibiotics including methicillin [24, 25]. It has been reported that 70% of nosocomial bacterial pathogens have emerged resistance to more than one antibiotic during medication of chronic infections. In contrast, an alarming increase in resistance of community-acquired bacteria has also been observed with significant high rate both in acute and chronic bacterial infections. The emergence of drug-resistant strains of Gram-positive (*Staphylococcus, Enterococcus, Streptococcus sp*) and Gram-negative (*Pseudomonas, Klebsiella, Enterobacter, Acinetobacter, Salmonella sp*) bacteria is the more serious in the present therapeutic scenario. *S. aureus* clearly represents one of the most challenging pathogenic bacteria. Resistance in *S. aureus* strains has been continuously increasing; thus, the ability of these pathogens to spread in both hospital and community settings increased. Bacteria remarkably developed resistant to antimicrobial drugs in several ways. Upon antibiotics treatment, bacteria tend to overcome the selection pressure of the drug by morphological and genetic alterations or drug inactivation. Alterations of membrane integrity and transfer of resistance genes from one strain to another are the common examples of β-LA-mediated resistance in *S. aureus.* β-LA, Penicillin was initially succeeded in the treatment of *S. aureus* infections but widespread and prolonged uses of penicillin were no longer be effective and resistance has been emerged soon after in the 1950s [19]. Antibiotic resistance can be a typical feature of a bacterial species (intrinsic resistance) or acquired by the individual organism that is naturally susceptible (acquired resistance). The acquired resistance is the consequence of chromosomal mutations or acquisition of resistance genes by horizontal gene transfer [26]. Resistance to multiple β-LA can be acquired by individual strains, resulting in multidrug-resistant phenotypes. The high prevalence of drug resistance is primarily adopted by unregulated sales of antibiotics without prescription, a long course of medication, indiscriminate usage of drugs, and poor health infrastructure. The mobility and mortality caused by drug resistance in public health are difficult to evaluate. In 2013, Center for Disease Control and Prevention (CDC) reported more than 11,000 deaths in the USA had a methicillin-resistant *S. aureus* (MRSA)-related infection (CDC 2013). This represents almost 50% of all causalities caused by antibiotic-resistant bacteria. As per WHO report, the MRSA remains among the high-priority multidrug-resistant organisms that need renewed efforts for the research and development of new antibiotics and innovative preventive approaches.

4. Mechanism of β-lactam resistance in *S. aureus*

Different mechanisms of drug resistance in bacterial pathogens are the major hurdle in their treatment. With emerging resistance, it became a serious concern to look into drug resistance mechanism, which can help us to prescribe a specific medication to effectively overcome the problem of resistance.

Several biochemical mechanisms are responsible for β-LA resistance, including enzymatic (β-lactamase) production inactivation of the drug (drug inactivation), modifications of drug target in penicillin-binding protein (PBPs) (target modifications), limiting uptake of drug by biofilm formation (reduced drug uptake), and active efflux of the drug (drug efflux) as shown in **Figure 1** [27, 28]. Bacterial pathogens resist the inhibitory action of antibiotics primarily due to the presence of an enzyme that inactivates the antibiotic or modified antibiotic target by mutation or by the post-translational mechanism, which reduces binding of the antibiotic to the target or bypass of the function dependent on the antibiotic target by an alternative enzyme that is not inhibited by the antibiotic. Moreover, overexpression of drug efflux pumps rendered to reduce uptake of the antibiotic inside the cell, by pumping out the antibiotics from the cell. In contrast, encapsulation of biofilm over the cell boundary reduces the cell permeability to resist antibiotics entry into the cell. The expression of chromosomal β-lactamase can be induced by either producing the plasmid-encoded penicillinase (β-lactamase) enzyme that hydrolyzes β-lactam ring or expression of PBP2a, and a penicillin-binding protein (PBP) encoded by gene *mecA* spread through horizontal gene transfer with low affinity to β-lactam antibiotics is primarily responsible for penicillin resistance [17]. The penicillin-binding cascade induces the blaZ-encoded penicillinase in *S. aureus*, which is transcriptionally regulated by regulatory genes blaI and blaR1 [26, 29].

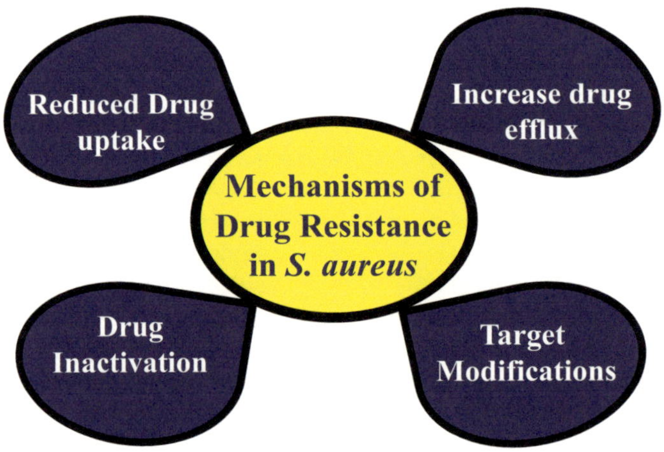

Figure 1.
β-Lactam resistance mechanism of S. aureus.

5. Methicillin resistance in *S. aureus*

Methicillin was introduced in clinical practice for the effective treatment of penicillin-resistant *S. aureus* infections [30]. After 2 years, the second wave of resistance against methicillin came into the light and the first report on methicillin resistance *S. aureus* (MRSA) strain was published by MP Jevons in 1961 [31]. Statistically, incidences of methicillin-sensitive *S. aureus* (MSSA), methicillin-resistant *S. aureus* (MRSA), and vancomycin-resistant *S. aureus* (VRSA) infections have increased up to 54% in both hospital-acquired (HA) and community-acquired (CA) [32]. These antimicrobial-resistant infections cause a significant economic burden on public health. The economic burden of antibiotic resistance in Europe was estimated at almost 1.5 billion euros. However, USA spent more than 55 billion dollars each year on the treatment of antibiotic-resistant infections [9]. It was found that acquisition of methicillin resistance in *S. aureus* was primarily contributed by the integration of a *mecA* gene encoded for low-affinity penicillin-binding protein 2a or 2′ (PBP2a or PBP2′) into the staphylococcal chromosomal cassette (SCC*mec*) element of methicillin-sensitive *S. aureus* (MRSA) [33]. The expression of *mecA* in MRSA is induced by the interaction of methicillin and other antibiotics to the regulatory network. MecIR a regulatory protein, homologous to the BlaIR proteins, controls the expression of *mecA*. It is under the control of MecIR regulatory proteins that are homologous to the BlaIR proteins that regulate BlaZ expression [34, 35]. The SSC*mec* is located specifically with an unknown gene (orfX) of the staphylococcal chromosomal. The function of the unknown gene is mediated by two recombinases termed as *ccrA* and *ccrB* that help in the site-specific integration or excision of DNA elements from the staphylococcal chromosomal [36, 37]. The insertion sequence, transposon (Tn554) or erythromycin- and spectinomycin-encoded resistance genes, and tobramycin and kanamycin resistance-encoded pUB110 plasmid can be additionally jumped in the SSC*mec* region. Typing of SSC*mec* elements is fundamental for the molecular epidemiology of MRSA and categorized majorly into five types, that is, type I-V [38]. The SSC*mec*-type I-III elements are present in hospital-acquired MRSA strains, which are typically resistant to non-β-lactam antibiotics. In contrast, SSC*mec*-type IV-V are only resistance to methicillin, which are primarily present in community-acquired MRSA (CA-MRSA). Different studies revealed that multiple insertions of SCC*mec* elements in the staphylococcal chromosome of MSSA strains yield a MRSA lineage. The *mecC* gene, homolog to *mecA* gene, exhibits 68.7% nucleotide identity is identified in *S. aureus*, *Staphylococcus sciuri*, and *Staphylococcus xylosus* strains [39]. The recent studies revealed that *mecC* carrying *S. aureus* contributes in methicillin resistance in the human population by up to 2.8% of MRSA strains [40–42], while no report was found on mecB-carrying *S. aureus* resistance to methicillin. In many MRSA strains, the expression of *mecA* is also affected either by the synthesis of truncated MecIR regulatory proteins or by repression by *β*-lactamase regulators BlaI and BlaR. The Mec and Bla regulatory proteins can alter the functional behavior and expression of PBP2a-encoded gene in MRSA strains. In a short period, MRSA strains have been identified all around the globe particularly Asia, USA, and Europe [43]. In spite of the rapidly spreading of methicillin resistance, MRSA exhibited broad-spectrum drug resistance against methicillin, penicillins, cephalosporins, and carbapenems. The MRSA cases were increased in hospitals and other healthcare facilities (hospital-acquired), and in communities (community-acquired infections). People with immediate surgeries or stay in healthcare facilities are at MRSA higher risk. Infection also spreads if a medical device has been put in their body or when they come close to contact with MRSA-infected patient. MRSA spreads in communities through uncovered or draining wounds mostly associated with crowded living, sharing personal items, recent stays in healthcare facilities, etc. In 2017, CDC reported that more than a 0.3 million cases and over 10,000 deaths from MRSA-related infections are estimated in-hospital patients with more than 1.7 billion healthcare burdens in the United States. This figure represents mere a 50% of all the mortalities caused by antibiotic-resistant bacteria. The prevalence of MRSA infections in India has been reported to increase from 29% in 2009 to 47% in 2014 [35].

6. Cephalosporin resistance in *S. aureus*

Similar to penicillin or other β-lactams, cephalosporins also target to bind penicillin-binding proteins (PBPs) to inhibit peptidoglycan formation in bacteria. These are effectively used in the treatment of superficial (skin and soft tissue) infections, and nosocomial and community-acquired pneumonia. Different strains of *S. aureus* strains have evolved resistance to cephalosporins, which evolved by reducing the binding affinity of cephalosporins to transpeptidase of PBPs, and also, β-lactamases are produced by bacteria having encoded plasmid for inactivation of therapeutics effect of cephalosporins. The plasmid-mediated β-lactamase resistance is corroborated by the amount and activity of the enzyme produced in bacteria.

Recent studies revealed that the prevalence of cephalosporins resistance in *S. aureus* is comparable to the β-lactamase-resistant penicillin, which accounts for 30–35% [44, 45]. Ceftaroline is the fifth-generation antibiotics, approved by the FDA in 2010, which has a broad-spectrum activity against a plethora of bacterial pathogens. Ceftaroline is active against methicillin-resistant *S. aureus* (MRSA) and has been successfully used for the treatment of different invasive bacterial infections with low adverse effects. This potent third-generation drug was found resistance in MRSA-ST293 strain in different geographical regions. Ceftaroline had the higher affinity to PBP but nonsense or missense mutations in the *mecA* gene alter the amino acid sequence of PBP protein, which causes alteration in the ceftaroline binding to PBPs. In addition, alteration of the promoter sequence of PBP4 by mutation increases PBP4 production that leads to resistance to ceftaroline [46].

7. Carbapenem-resistance

The β-lactam antibiotic carbapenems are the last resort, potent, broad-spectrum antibiotic against Gram +ve and Gram –ve bacterial pathogens. They contain a carbapenem structure linked together with a beta-lactam ring, which primarily targets to bind with PBPs of the cell wall. Due to high potency, low adverse effect appeals to prefer the use of carbapenems. Prolonged and widespread uses of the drug have developed carbapenems resistance, which is contributed by a different mechanism. The resistance that arises to carbapenems is due to β-lactamase gene transfer/production, mutational alteration in PBPs, and expression of efflux pump systems [47, 48]. The carbapenem resistance is mainly contributed by β-lactamase production.

8. Future perspective

Emerging resistance in *S. aureus* is a serious human health problem, which continuously increasing mortality and morbidity rates in both nosocomial and acquired infections. The constant evolution of resistance to topical antibiotics including the continuing appearance of new resistance mechanisms and complexity in multidrug-resistant phenotypes are appealing to find new diagnostic tools and therapeutic strategies to get rid of this problem. However, a lot of toiling has continued to devise a workable treatment against staphylococcal infections particularly for the elimination of MRSA and VRSA pathogens. Emerging MDR in *S. aureus* has evolved major challenges in research and need to expend research to the next level to understand the progression of drug resistance pathways and infections pattern of *S. aureus*. The new search of therapeutics targets and bioactive molecules and their judicious use may be proven significantly to prevent the problem of drug resistance [2, 49]. Reducing the outer membrane permeability of bacterial cells can circumvent the problem of drug resistance. Iron conjugated with the antibiotic method may help to selectively interact to the outer membrane to active transport of antibiotic inside the cell [50]. Another possible approach has been targeted to inhibit quorum sensing that is primarily related to the virulence factors release and associated with the microbial pathogenesis. Chemically, virulence factors are toxic to the host cells that disrupt immune response, along with host cell disruption and cell adhesion. SarA and agr are two main quorum sensing mechanisms of *S. aureus*, which can be targeted to block the quorum sensing for controlling *S. aureus* infections. In addition, bacteriophage therapy is one of the potential methods for controlling the drug resistance in *S. aureus* infection. Phage therapy has many advantages over chemotherapy, for example, very specific, no side effect, environmental friendly, no allergenic effects, and harmless to the eukaryotic host [51]. Phage has been used to eliminate MRSA infections but is still immature in clinical application [51]. The phage-based treatment of resistant *S. aureus* will further be helpful to select the gene responsible for its control. These strategies will pave a way to develop a vaccine in future against the *S. aureus*.

9. Conclusion

It is very clear that bacterium including *Staphylococcus aureus* shows extraordinary adaptability to cope with antibiotic effect and emerge drug resistance against antibiotics. The phenomenon of drug resistance was first observed when β-lactam antibiotics became ineffective after indiscriminative uses and plasmid-responsive β-lactamase (penicillinase) synthesis. The second wave of resistance against methicillin has been primarily contributed by the stable integration of a *mecA* gene-encoded penicillin-binding protein and penicillin-binding protein 2a or 2′ (PBP2a or PBP2′) into the staphylococcal chromosomal cassette (SCC*mec*) element. Cephalosporins have been proven as an effective drug preventing MRSA infections but failed. In progression to antibiotics, carbapenems have been used for preventing *S. aureus* infections, but multidrug resistance (MDR) strains developed. The common cause of bacterial resistance involves horizontal gene transfer, target alteration by point mutations, and expression of efflux pump, which made a variety of antibiotics ineffective and induces persistent infections in both hospital and community settings. Moreover, the prolonged and widespread use of different antibiotics, lack of awareness, and insanitation, primarily contribute in rapidly developing multiple drug resistance (MDR) in developing countries that causes a major financial burden in the treatment of infectious diseases. Though a lot of toiling is involved in devising an effective treatment against staphylococcal infections particularly for the elimination of MRSA and VRSA, the new search of bioactive molecules and their judicious use may be proven significantly to prevent the problem of drug resistance.

Author details

Antresh Kumar[1]* and Manisha Kaushal[2]

1 Department of Biochemistry, Central University of Haryana, Mahendergarh, Haryana, India

2 District Hospital Compound, Amroha, India

*Address all correspondence to: antreshkumar@cuh.ac.in

References

[1] Holmes KK, Bertozzi S, Bloom BR, Prabhat Jha P, Gelband H, DeMaria LM, et al. Major infectious diseases: Key messages from disease control priorities. In: Holmes KK, Bertozzi S, Bloom BR, Jha P, editors. Major Infectious Diseases. 3rd ed. Washington (DC): The International Bank for Reconstruction and Development/The World Bank; 2017

[2] Kumar S, Kumar A, Kaushal M, Kumar P, Mukhopadhyay K, Kumar A. Fungal-derived xenobiotic exhibits antibacterial and antibiofilm activity against *S. aureus*. Drug Discoveries & Therapeutics. 2018;**12**(4):214-223 (IF1.27)

[3] Gorwitz RJ, Kruszon-Moran D, McAllister SK, McQuillan G, McDougal LK, Fosheim GE, et al. Changes in the prevalence of nasal colonization with *Staphylococcus aureus* in the United States, 2001-2004. Journal of Infectious Diseases. 2008;**197**(9): 1226-1234. DOI: 10.1086/533494

[4] Adèle S, Fabienne B, Jean-Louis M, Jean-Marc R, Olivier B. *Staphylococcus aureus* nasal colonization: An update on mechanisms, epidemiology, risk factors, and subsequent infections. Frontier Microbiology. 2018;**9**:2419. DOI: 10.3389/fmicb.2018.02419

[5] Odell CA. Community-associated methicillin-resistant *Staphylococcus aureus* (CA-MRSA) skin infections. Current Opinion in *Pediatrics*. 2010;**22**:273-277

[6] Mohammad H, Thangamani S, Seleem MN. Antimicrobial peptides and peptidomimetics-potent therapeutic allies for staphylococcal infections. Current Pharmaceutical Design. 2015;**21**:2073-2088

[7] Peters PJ, Brooks JT, McAllister SK, Limbago B. Methicillin resistant *Staphylococcus aureus* colonization of the groin and risk for clinical infection among HIV infected adults. Emerging Infectious Diseases. 2013;**19**:623-629

[8] World Health Organization. WHO Antimicrobial Resistance: Global Report on Surveillance. Geneva, Switzerland. Available from: http://www.who.int/drugresistance/documents/surveillancereport/en/: World Health Organization; 2014 [Accessed: 01 January 2019]

[9] Antibiotic resistance threats in the United States. Centers for Disease Control and Prevention. Atlanta, GA. Publisher US Department of Health and Human Services. Available from: https://www.cdc.gov/drugresistance/threat-report-2013/pdf/ar-threats-2013-508.pdf; 2013 [Accessed: 01 January 2019]

[10] Sunagar R, Hegde NR, Archana GJ, Sinha AY. Prevalence and genotype distribution of methicillin-resistant *Staphylococcus aureus* (MRSA) in India. Journal of Global Antimicrobial Resistance. 2016;**7**:46-52

[11] Bouchiat C, El-Zeenni N, Chakrakodi B, Nagaraj S, Arakere G, Etienne J. Epidemiology of Staphylococcus aureus in Bangalore, India: emergence of the ST217 clone and high rate of resistance to erythromycin and ciprofloxacin in the community. New Microbes and New Infections. 2015;**7**:15-20

[12] Thati V, Shivannavar CT, Gaddad SM. Vancomycin resistance among methicillin resistant Staphylococcus aureus isolates from intensive care units of tertiary care hospitals in Hyderabad. The Indian Journal of Medical Research. 2011;**134**:704-708

[13] Uematsu H, Yamashita K, Kunisawa S, Fushimi K, Imanaka Y.

Estimating the disease burden of methicillin-resistant *Staphylococcus aureus* in Japan: Retrospective database study of Japanese hospitals. PLoS One. 2017;**12**:e0179767

[14] Koziel J, Maciag-Gudowska A, Mikolajczyk T, Bzowska M, Sturdevant DE, Whitney AR, et al. Phagocytosis of *Staphylococcus aureus* by macrophages exerts cytoprotective effects manifested by the upregulation of antiapoptotic factors. PLoS One. 2009;**4**:e5210

[15] Duin DV, Paterson D. Multidrug resistant Bacteria in the community: Trends and lessons learned. Infectious Disease Clinics of North America. 2016;**30**:377-390

[16] David MZ, Daum RS. Community-associated methicillin-resistant *Staphylococcus aureus*: Epidemiology and clinical consequences of an emerging epidemic. Clinical Microbiology Reviews. 2010;**23**:616-687

[17] Bush K, Bradford PA. β-Lactams and β-lactamase inhibitors: An overview. Cold Spring Harbor Perspectives in Medicine. 2016;**6**(8):a025247. DOI: 10.1101/cshperspect.a025247

[18] Neushal P. Science, government and the mass production of penicillin. Journal of History of Medicine and Allied Sciences. 1993;**48**(4):371-395

[19] Walsh CT, Wencewicz TA. Antibiotics: Challenges, Mechanisms, Opportunities. Washington, DC: ASM Press; 2016

[20] Thakurla B, Lahon K. The beta lactam antibiotics as an empirical therapy in a developing country: An update on their current status and recommendations to counter the resistance against them. Journal of Clinical and Diagnostic Research. 2013;7:1207-1214

[21] Zango UU, Ibrahim M, Shawai SAA, Shamsuddin IM. A review on β-lactam antibiotic drug resistance. MOJ Drug Design Development & Therapy. 2019;**3**:52-58

[22] Cooper PD, Rowley D. Investigations with radioactive penicillin. Nature. 1949;**163**:480-481

[23] Yocum RR, Rasmussen JR, Strominger JL. The mechanism of action of penicillin: Penicillin acylates the active site of *Bacillus stearothermophilus* d-alanine carboxypeptidase. Journal of Biological Chemistry. 1980;**255**(9): 3977-3986

[24] Turner NA, Sharma-Kuinkel BK, Maskarinec SA, Eichenberger EM, Shah PP, Carugati M, et al. Methicillin-resistant *Staphylococcus aureus*: an overview of basic and clinical research. Nature Reviews Microbiology. 2019;**17**:203-218

[25] Wanda CR. An overview of the antimicrobial resistance mechanisms of bacteria. AIMS Microbiology. 2018;**4**(3):482-501. DOI: 10.3934/microbiol.2018.3.482

[26] Dever LA, Dermody TS. Mechanisms of bacterial resistance to antibiotics. Archives of Internal Medicine. 1991;**151**(5):886-895

[27] Ibrahim ME, Abbas M, Al-Shahrai AM, Elamin BK. Phenotypic characterization and antibiotic resistance patterns of extended-spectrum β-lactamase- and AmpC β-lactamase-producing gram-negative bacteria in a referral hospital, Saudi Arabia. Canadian Journal of Infectious Diseases and Medical Microbiology. 2019;**2019**:6054694. DOI: 10.1155/2019/6054694

[28] Pfeifer Y, Cullik A, Witte W. Resistance to cephalosporins and carbapenems in Gram-negative bacterial pathogens. International Journal of Medical Microbiology. 2010;**300**: 371-379

[29] Guo Y, Song G, Sun M, Wang J, Wang Y. Prevalence and therapies of antibiotic-resistance in *Staphylococcus aureus*. Frontiers in Cellular and Infection Microbiology. 2020;**10**: article107

[30] Jevons M. "Celbenin"-resistant Staphylococci. British Medical Association. 1961;**1**:124-125

[31] Vysakh PR, Jeya M. A comparative analysis of community acquired and hospital acquired methicillin resistant *Staphylococcus aureus*. Journal of Clinical and Diagnostic Research. 2013;**7**(7): 1339-1342

[32] Schulte RH, Munson E. *Staphylococcus aureus* resistance patterns in Wisconsin. 2018 Surveillance of Wisconsin organisms for trends in antimicrobial resistance and epidemiology (SWOTARE) program report. Clinical Medicine & Research. 2019;**17**(3-4):72-81. DOI: 10.3121/cmr.2019.1503

[33] Peacock SJ, Paterson GK. Mechanisms of methicillin resistance in *Staphylococcus aureus*. Annual Review of Biochemistry. 2015;**84**:577-601

[34] Fisher JF, Mobashery S. beta-lactam resistance mechanisms: Gram-positive bacteria and *Mycobacterium tuberculosis*. Cold Spring Harbor Perspectives in Medicine. 2016;**6**:a025221

[35] Hiramatsu K, Ito T, Tsubakishita S, Sasaki T, Takeuchi F, Morimoto Y, et al. Genomic basis for methicillin resistance in *Staphylococcus aureus*. Infection & Chemotherapy. 2013;**45**:117-136

[36] Chambers HF, DeLeo FR. Waves of Resistance: *Staphylococcus aureus* in the Antibiotic Era. Nature Reviews Microbiology. 2009;**7**(9):629-641. DOI: 10.1038/nrmicro2200

[37] Chongtrakool P, Ito T, Ma XX, Kondo Y, Trakulsomboon S, Tiensasitorn C, et al. Staphylococcal cassette chromosome *mec* (SCCmec) typing of methicillin-resistant *Staphylococcus aureus* strains isolated in 11 Asian countries: A proposal for a new nomenclature for SCCmec elements. Antimicrobial Agents and Chemotherapy. 2006 Mar;**50**(3):1001-1012. DOI: 10.1128/AAC.50.3.1001-1012. 2006

[38] Urushibara N, Paul SK, Hossain MA, Kawaguchiya M, Kobayashi N. Analysis of Staphylococcal cassette chromosome *mec* in *Staphylococcus haemolyticus* and *Staphylococcus sciuri*: Identification of a novel *ccr* gene complex with a newly identified *ccrA* allotype (*ccrA7*). Microbial Drug Resistance. 2011;**17**(2):291-297. DOI: 10.1089/mdr.2010.0144

[39] Deplano A, Vandendriessche S, Nonhoff C, Denis O. Genetic diversity among methicillin-resistant *Staphylococcus aureus* isolates carrying the *mecC* gene in Belgium. Journal of Antimicrobial Chemotherapy. 2014;**69**: 1457-1460

[40] Cuny C, Layer F, Strommenger B, Witte W. Rare occurrence of methicillin resistant *Staphylococcus aureus* CC130 with a novel *mecA* homologue in humans in Germany. PLoS One. 2011;**6**:e24360

[41] Paterson GK, Morgan FJ, Harrison EM, Cartwright EJ, Torok ME, Zadoks RN, et al. Prevalence and characterization of human *mecC* methicillin-resistant *Staphylococcus aureus* isolates in England. Journal of Antimicrobial Chemotherapy. 2014;**69**:907-910

[42] Lakhundi S, Zhang K. Methicillin-Resistant *Staphylococcus aureus*: Molecular characterization, evolution, and epidemiology. Clinical Microbiology Reviews.

2018;**31**:e00020-e00018. DOI: 10.1128/CMR.00020-18

[43] Kulkarni AP, Nagvekar VC, Veeraraghavan B, Warrier AR, Deepak TS, Ahdal J, et al. Current perspectives on treatment of gram-positive infections in India: What is the way forward? Interdisciplinary Perspectives on Infectious Diseases. 2019;**2019**:7601847

[44] Deyno S, Fekadu S, Astatkie A. Resistance of Staphylococcus aureus to antimicrobial agents in Ethiopia: A meta-analysis. Antimicrobial Resistance and Infection Control. 2017;**6**:85. DOI: 10.1186/s13756-017-0243-7

[45] Alexander J, Chatterjee SS, Hamilton SM, Eltis LD, Chambers HF, Strynadka N. Structural and kinetic analyses of penicillin-binding protein 4 (PBP4)-mediated antibiotic resistance in *Staphylococcus aureus*. Journal of Biological Chemistry. 2018;**293**: 19854-19865

[46] Meletis G. Carbapenem resistance: Overview of the problem and future perspectives. Therapeutic Advances in Infectious Disease. 2016;**3**:15-21

[47] Meletis G, Exindari M, Vavatsi N, Sofianou D, Diza E. Mechanisms responsible for the emergence of carbapenem resistance in *Pseudomonas aeruginosa*. Hippokratia. 2012;**16**: 303-307

[48] Kumari N, Kumari V, Kumar V, Kumar S, Kumar A. Ouabain potentiates the antimicrobial activity of aminoglycosides against *Staphylococcus aureus*. BMC Complementary and alternative Medicine. 2019;**19**:119-129

[49] Carver PL. The battle for iron between humans and microbes. Current Medicinal Chemistry. 2018;**25**:85-96

[50] Golkar Z, Bagasra O, Pace DG. Bacteriophage therapy: A potential solution for the antibiotic resistance crisis. Journal of Infection in Developing Countries. 2014;**8**:129-136

[51] Dias RS, Eller MR, Duarte VS, Pereira AL, Silva CC, Mantovani HC, et al. Use of phages against antibiotic-resistant *Staphylococcus aureus* isolated from bovine mastitis. Journal of Animal Science. 2013;**91**:3930-3939

Chapter 9

Bacterial Skin Abscess

Mohammed Malih Radhi, Fatima Malik AL-Rubea,
Nada Khazal Kadhim Hindi and Rusull Hamza Kh. AL-Jubori

Abstract

Patients with skin and soft tissue infections may appear with the abscess. Erroneous diagnosis of these entities is common, and should carefully consider the possible alternative diagnoses. Risk for developing skin abscess factors includes disruption of the skin barrier, edema, venous insufficiency, and immune suppression. However, healthy individuals who have no risk factors may also develop these diseases. The most common microbiologic cause of abscess, a commonly group *Streptococcus* or *Streptococcus pyogenes*; *Staphylococcus aureus* (including methicillin-resistant strains) is a notable but less common cause. The most common microbiologic cause of skin abscess is *S. aureus*; a skin abscess can be caused by more than one pathogen. The diagnosis is based on skin abscess usually on the clinical manifestations. It must be subject to patients with disposable abscess incision and drainage, with a test of culture and susceptibility of materials wet. There is no justification for the blood of patients in the cultures of the abovementioned circumstances. It can be a useful radiographic examination to determine whether the skin abscess is present (via ultrasound) to distinguish cellulitis from osteomyelitis (via magnetic resonance imaging). There may be a justification for radiological assessment in patients with immune suppression, diabetes, venous insufficiency, or lymphedema in patients with persistent symptoms of systemic lymphatic obstruction.

Keywords: bacteria, skin, abscess, *S. aureus*

1. Introduction

1.1 Bacterial skin abscess

The most common cause of abscess skin is *Staphylococcus aureus* (either methicillin or midwife to methicillin. *Staphylococcus aureus* aureus), occurring in up to 75% of cases; many patients infected with MRSA do not have risk factors [1–3]. It can be caused by skin abscess more than one pathogens [4]. The isolation of multiple objects (including *S. aureus* CT with Gram-negative bacilli and anaerobes) are more common in patients with skin abscess, which includes the surrounding areas of oral or anal or vaginal [5]. Organisms live by mouth, including anaerobic, you see most often among drug users by intravenous. Include unusual causes of skin abscess such as fungus pneumococcus and *Streptococcus*. Most cysts are caused by infection. However, it can occur in a sterile abscesses put irritants injected. Examples include (especially those drugs Injected that depend on oil), which may not be fully absorbed and remain at the injection site, causing local irritation. Cysts can be transformed into a sterile solid during solid lesions scars [5].

2. Original of abscess

The abscess arise in many tissues and organs of the body, the most important of which are subcutaneous tissue, lymph nodes, soft and adipose tissue around the anus, and breasts in pregnant or lactating women and at the root of the teeth. Cysts can also arise in internal organs such as the liver, lung, brain, kidney and appendix. The abscess has spread significantly in recent years [6]. And the risk factor has been more than 65% including the use of intravenous drugs. In 2005, Dermatology departments received more than 3.2 million people with abscess in the United States [7], while in Australia, about 13,000 patients were hospitalized [8]. Cysts arise in many tissues and organs of the body, the most important of which are subcutaneous tissues (then they are superficially dimple or deep), such as liver, lung, brain abscess, kidney, and appendix. The most important complication is the spread of the abscess (pus) to neighboring tissues by means of treatment tools, which may sometimes cause the death of these tissues (gangrene). Acute inflammation of the abscess originates from the entry of pus bacteria into the affected organ or tissue. Surface cysts are swollen red and painful, accompanied by high fever and pulse [9]. The abscess can also be fatal in rare cases, such as when it is in an area where pressure on vital organs such as the trachea in the case of abscess in the neck area. If the abscess is superficial, it will fluctuate during palpation due to the movement of pus inside. A contributing factor to the formation of an abscess in addition to the use of intravenous drugs [10]. An unconfirmed study suggests that the presence of previous cases of hernia of the vertebrae or any imbalance thereof [11]. While the main cause is pathogenic bacteria, fungi or parasites, the most common cause is methicillin-resistant *Staphylococcus aureus* in the United States and other parts of the world [6]. *Staphylococcus aureus* causes subdural abscesses and parasites to cause abscess, especially in developing countries [12].

3. Epidemiology of skin abscesses

Because of changing the display skin abscess, it was difficult to assess the incidence and prevalence. The incidence of skin abscess is 24.6 per 1000 people per year [13]. Because the majority of the ski abscess tends to melt within 7–10 days, the estimate variable spread significantly. Among patients in hospitals, the rate of prevalence ranges from abscess skiing 7–10% [14, 15]. Among all patients infected in hospitals only infections, skin abscess plays a more important role. Emergency care center, an outlying ski, is the third most common diagnoses after chest pain and asthma [16]. There is an increase in the prevalence rate of men (60–70% of all cases) and patients aged between 45 and 64 years old. It managed approximately 70–75% of all cases in the outpatient setting [13, 16]. With many cases of skin abscess involving the lower leg area (7.9–11). In general, the incidence of benign tumors complex is low (Arasepelas 0.09 per 1000 people per year; inflammation of the lymphatic vessels is 0.16% of all cases of inflammation of cellular tissue and the lymphatic vessels. 16 per 1000 people per year and fasciitis necrotizing 0.04 per 1000 person-years) [13].

The real spread of abscess skin infection is unknown because the light is usually self-occurrence and patients seeking medical care. However, often they face skin abscess in the outpatient and inpatient. According to national statistics for 2011 regarding the cost of health care project and use, skin abscess rate led to 3.4 million visits to the emergency department, or 2.6% of the total emergency department visits, with 13.9% of visits have led to hospitalization [17].

They have caused the infection, skin and soft tissue as well as the case of 500,000 outside the hospital, or 1.4% of total departures, with an average length of stay of 3.7 days and an average cost of $ 18.299 per case. These figures are on the rise due to the prevalence of *Staphylococcus aureus* resistant to methicillin-associated Balmethycelin in the past decade [18–21].

A recent prospective study showed that one out of every 5 patients provide primary care clinic for skin abscess caused by *Staphylococcus aureus* resistant to methicillin (MRSA) require additional interventions at a cost of approximately $ 2000 per patient [22].

4. Risks factors of skin abscesses

The presence of specific risk factors may stimulate the skin abscess, may impose pathogens, disease course and respond to specific treatments. It did not prove the existence of risk factors for the development of skin abscess associated with the seriousness of the disease [23]. It can be organized into two categories of risk factors. First, there are factors associated with the patient, which may provide for the disease or the effects of predictive. Risk factors in this category include serious diseases and the age of the elderly and the situation that suffers from a lack of human immunodeficiency virus and diseases of the liver, kidney and vascular insufficiency (especially the lymphatic or venous) [24]. Since it turns out that the lower part of the leg is more places of infection transmitted through sexual contact common, studies have described risk associated with the patient's infection due to these factors [25]. It was able to determine the likelihood of skin abscess in the lower limbs based on the presence of *Staphylococcus aureus* and/or beta-hemolytic *Streptococcus* in the toe box, erosion or leg ulcers, and/or eradication of the former esophagus. These factors independently associated with the development of skin abscess in the lower leg. In the same population group, if the bacteria found in the toes are absent, the presence of the pedal palm has the ability to moderate predictive secretion of the skin. Moreover, the multiple risk factors associated with the patient may be associated with a poor prognosis of the disease faster, and the development of slow recovery and the causes of the most resistant diseases. Must take into account the specific risk factors (renal failure or chronic kidney, spleen deficiency, immune status, vascular insufficiency or neuropathy) when determining the severity of the disease [26].

Observed factors associated with skin abscess are often among middle-aged adults and older. Erysipelas occurs in young children and the elderly [13].

It includes predisposing factors associated with the risk of skin abscess are:

1. Disable the skin barrier due to trauma (such as corrosion, penetrating wound, pressure ulcers, venous leg ulcers, insect bite, injecting drug use).

2. Inflammation of the skin (such as eczema, psoriasis and radiation therapy).

3. Edema due to poor lymphatic drainage.

4. Edema due to venous insufficiency.

5. Obesity.

6. Immune suppression (such as diabetes or infection with HIV) disease.

7. Skin breaks between these fingers may not be clinically.

8. Dermatitis pre-existing (such as foot frond, herpes, varicella) [27].

Also, acute bacterial skin infections occur when exposure to the risk of loss of skin integrity e.g high bacteria in pregnancy skin or the availability of food bacterial, or excess moisture in the skin, or lack of blood supply, or immune suppression, or a damaged cornea layer. Poor hygiene and the exchange of personal things, physical contact, and crowded living conditions facilitate the spread of infectious diseases. Vascular diseases, peripheral diseases and skin pre-existing increase the risk of acid cellulose. Usually leads to diabetes, a diabetes which is controlled by a bad foot injury. Cause painful events such as wounds, biting and drug abuse by injection injuries increase the risk of skin infections and cysts. The risk of infection on surgical-site support is in the process category, where clean and smaller operations are at the risk of contaminated infections and high-risk operations have a higher risk of injury [28].

Colonization with *Staphylococcus aureus* and *Streptococcus* in the front lines on the skin increases the risk of skin abscess. Considered skin contact to the skin through exercise and attendance in day care or school and live in a place nearby (such as military barracks) risk factors for CAMRSA skin abscess [29].

5. Bacterial invasion of the skin

For as long as microorganisms that colonize the skin of importance to skin diseases and microbiology; I have been collecting our knowledge of these organisms live accurate until recently through the existing studies on the culture. Historically, it is *Staphylococcus aureus* and other *Staphylococcus aureus* negative coagulation as the primary bacterial colonies of the skin. Other microorganisms that are generally regarded as skin colonizers include coryneforms of the phylum Actinobacteria (the genera *Corynebacterium*, *Propionibacterium* and *Brevibacterium*) and the genus *Micrococcus*. Gram-negative bacteria, with the exception of some *Acinetobacter* spp., are generally not isolated from the skin, but are thought to arise in cultures owing to contamination from the gastrointestinal tract [30].

It was isolated from non-bacterial microorganisms from the skin. *Fungal species* are the most common *Malassezia* spp., which is particularly widespread in the fatty areas. Considered mite *Demodex* (such as *Demodex* follicle and *Demodex* brevis), a microscopic arthropods, part of the natural skin flora. They feed on mites *Demodex* sebum and be more prevalent after puberty, preferring to colonize the oily areas of the face. *Demodex* mites may also feed on epithelial cells lining the unit sunscreens space, or even other organisms (such as acne Brobbeoneptariom) that live in the same place. It is not the role of the experimental study of viruses, and is limited research on the molecular and microbiological methods available for the identification and characterization of viruses [31].

Historically, culture-based approach is the standard to describe the microbial diversity. It is now clear that only a minority of bacteria able to thrive in isolation [32]. Choose mainly culture-based laboratory techniques “herbs”: species that thrive under conditions typical nutritional and physiological use of diagnostic microbiology laboratories. This is not necessarily the most abundant organisms in society. This bias is particularly evident when trying to isolate the organisms living in micro skin, which adapted to the nature of cold, dry and acidic environment. Moreover, the hair follicles and sebaceous glands are an oxygen-free environment and are home to the anaerobic microorganisms. Isolate the problem especially anaerobic using routine methods based on culture. These are often slow-growing organisms and require special conditions for growth and during the transfer and processing of samples [33, 34].

The development of molecular techniques to identify and quantify microorganisms has revolutionized our view of the world Microbial. Characterization of genetic diversity of bacterial depends on the sequence of genes for RNA ribosomal 16S, found in all bacteria and analyzes antique, but not in eukaryotes. Genes rRNA contain 16S in highly variable regions of certain types, which allows the classification of classification, and the spaces reserved for the one who, operating Xaah molecular site linking the primers PCR. The emergence of new sequencing technologies (such as pyrosequencing) is to increase productivity significantly while reducing the cost of sequencing. More importantly, the living organism culture does not need to determine the sequence of its kind by 16S rRNA [35].

The skin is the largest organ in the human body, colonized by a variety of tiny, mostly harmless organisms or even beneficial to their hosts. Colonialism is the motivation behind the surface of the skin environment, which is highly variable depending on the site topography, and host factors internal factors, the external environment. The responses can be innate immune and lead to a modified adaptive skin microorganisms in the skin, but microorganisms are also working to educate the immune system. Molecular road development has led to the identification of microorganisms to see the emerging skin bacteria resident are very diverse and variable. The improved understanding of the microbes in the skin is necessary to gain insight into the involvement of microbes in human skin disorders and to enable new methods for therapeutic drugs antimicrobial and antimicrobial therapy [36].

The main barrier against microbial invasion is the skin. It interacts continuously with the external environment, a colonizer with a variety of microbes. The vast majority of plants colony consists of bacteria. To help organize the distribution of plants, one that divides the body into two halves at the waist. The usual things that colonizes the skin above the waist are usually positive types of Gram such as *Staphylococcus epidermidis*, *Corynebacterium species*, *S. aureus* and *Streptococcus pyogenes* [37].

Staphylococcus aureus and *Corynebacterium* spp. It is the most abundant organisms that colonize humid areas, consistent with the data culture that indicate that these organisms prefer high humidity areas. These include navel wet sites (navel), and the basement axillary, and wrinkling inguinal (side thigh) and wrinkling brigades (the upper part of the fold between the buttocks), insole foot, hole popliteal (behind the knee) and the pit antecubital (elbow inner). *Staphylococcus aureus* occupies air position on the skin and may use urea in the race as a source of nitrogen. Insect bacteria are highly sensitive organisms that have slow growth in culture, and such as the role of the skin accurate objects has been appreciated until recently. Treatment of sweat by bacteria and *Staphylococcus* (along with the minute in the basement of underarm living organisms), resulting in a transient characteristic odor associated with sweating in humans [38].

On the other hand, the typical living organisms colonize the skin below the waist Gram-positive and Gram-negative. It is expected that this will be a minor near the anal area difference. Attracted intestinal species, such as the intestinal bacteria, to this region of the skin so-called "Fecal Crust" [36].

Normal distribution pattern consists of the largest population areas in the armpit and groin and thigh, where there is moisture level higher. Microflora tend to fill the upper layer of the cornea and parts of the hair follicles. Specific microbes tend to colonize the anatomical structures based on tropical stimuli and biochemical interactions of the site and the formation of specific tissues of biological membranes. Plants can be significantly by climate group differ, genetics, age, sex, stress, hygiene, nutrition, hospitalization [37].

Skin abscess is the most common manifestations of bacterial infection. Abscess may appear in painful blocks degrade transient without medical intervention, or in severe cases, such as large deep cysts associated with the spread of the blood stream. Although many of the bacteria, causing Gram-positive and Gram-negative cysts, but *Staphylococcus aureus*, especially MRSA associated with the community, it is the causative agent of the most common. Once configured, it can interfere with pus in the lesion Walled significantly with the activity of antibiotics to the extent this makes antibiotic treatment effective to some extent when the abscess exceeds a certain size, with the emergence of the problem of additional scarring. In the case of *EBioMedicine* [39].

Hancock and his colleagues have positive peptide targeted basically describing the formation of cysts. Developed peptides screen anti-biofilm. In the laboratory, which prevent or eliminate biofilms formed by bacteria both Gram-positive and Gram-negative. In non-vertebrate models of infection *P. aeruginosa*, boosted the survival of the host [40].

The main question that arises from the study is the relationship between the strict response and abscess formation. It was responsible for the formation mechanisms kharaj an important topic for research in this field *aureus*. While some defense mechanisms for stress, such as reducing metals and oxidative stress and nitric, appear to have a role in the ability of *S. aureus* to form abscesses, the stringent response in this context has not been clarified yet. It is likely to be the primary contact due to the direct impact of the stringent response CodY regulator. CodY has proven that it affects the severity of the disease in many animal models by changing the expression of the organizers of key, such as agr (RNAIII and RNAII) and saeR, hemolysins (hla), leukocidins (lukSF), the synthesis of the capsule (icaADBC), as well as genes that show it is important to form an abscess. Expression PSMα, which shows that it prevents installed by DJK-5, independently organized through RSH for CodY. Specific factors that regulate the formation of abscess under the strict response remains identified in *Staphylococcus aureus* and other microbes [41].

From a clinical perspective, the siege imposed on the composition of the abscess would be a useful assistant to kill pathogens. Often, infected individuals already infected a large abscess requires Tbarva surgically. For those who provide abscesses smaller or in the early stages which are not viable after discharge surgical, antibiotics are used routinely, but may not be enough to stop the progress of formation of abscess, especially if the pathogen offending is relatively resistant to antibiotics. It can be strict inhibition of the response to the formation of mass abscess useful, and will compare the use of helper inhibitors of protein synthesis inhibition in the treatment of inflammatory toxin mediated by poison. Inhibitors will be particularly useful if they also prevent chronic or recurrent cysts including cases related to chronic bacteria gold that are difficult to treat, such as inflammation of the sweat glands Almqih. Future studies will need to prove that the inhibitors are still effective when used with antibiotics effective or marginal [42].

Other Bacteriologic characteristics. In the monomicrobial form, the pathogens are *S. pyogenes*, *S. aureus*, *V. vulnificus*, *A. hydrophila*, and anaerobic streptococci (i.e., *Peptostreptococcus* species). Can *Staphylococcus aureus* and Streptococcus hemolytic occur simultaneously? Most injuries are obtained from the community and there in the limbs, with nearly two-thirds of cases in the lower limbs. There is often an underlying cause, such as diabetes or vascular disease, atherosclerosis or venous insufficiency with edema. Sometimes, chronic vascular ulcers turn into a more intense process. Fasciitis cases of necrotizing that arise after infection varicella or trivial injuries, such as minor scratches and insect bites, always be the result of bacteria *S. pyogenes*. The mortality rate in this group is high, where close to 50–70% in patients with low blood pressure and organ failure [43].

6. Pathophysiology of abscesses formation

There are other factors, has not yet fully be understood, perhaps play a role. In addition, the large number of organisms found in the abscess, and the presence of an antibiotic inhibitor of enzymes, hostility Anaerobic activity anti-microbial host and defense environment, as well as fibroblasts in the capsule surrounding Boukerg, contributes to the persistence of infection despite antibiotic treatment and the need to exchange. You must remember the contribution of both aerobic and anaerobic organisms in the formation of cysts when one chooses antibiotics to treat such infections [44].

7. Common causes of a skin abscess

When breaking the skin's natural barrier we have, even from simple shock, or small tears, or infections, bacteria can enter the skin. It can be formed where the abscess is trying to kill your body's defenses these germs through the inflammatory response (white blood cells = pus). It can cause blockage of sweat or sebaceous gland or hair follicle or the bag to a pre-existing abscess.

Staphylococcus aureus, *E. coli*, *P. aeruginosa*, and *Streptococcus pyogenes* are the most common types of bacteria that cause skin abscesses in the following areas of the body; the head and neck, parties, armpits, trunk.

There are *Staphylococcus aureus* on the proper surface of the skin. It can cause skin infections, such as skin abscesses and boils, and preferably live in wet areas of the body such as the armpits, groin, and inside the nostrils.

Can some bacteria *S. aureus* produces a toxin called Panton-Valentine leukocidin (PVL), which kills white cells, causing the body to do more white cells to continue to fight infection.

PVL-positive strains of bacteria are therefore more likely to cause skin infections and abscess. They can also cause more serious conditions:

- Septicaemia is blood poisoning caused by bacteria multiplying in the blood.
- Pneumonia is swelling (inflammation) of the lungs caused by an infection. Pus collects in the airways and is coughed up as mucus [45, 46].

8. Types of skin abscesses

- *Impetigo, erysipelas, and cellulitis*. Impetigo may be caused by infection with *S. aureus* and/or *S. pyogenes*. The decision of how to treat impetigo depends on the number of lesions, their location (face, eyelid, or mouth), and the need to limit spread of infection to others.

The tests antibody conjugate *Streptococcus* no value in the diagnosis and treatment of herpes, but they provide a useful supporting evidence of infection *Streptococcus* recent in patients suspected of having inflammation glomerulonephritis after *Streptococcus*. Anti Alstrptullizin O weak response in patients with herpes *Streptococcus* [47], Supposed to be fat in the skin working to suppress Alstrptullizin O response, but the levels consistently high DNase B [48].

Because *S. aureus* currently accounts for most cases of herpes bullosa, as well as for a large part of the non-inflammatory tumor. Complications of herpes retroviruses *Streptococcus* uncommon, for reasons not yet known, rheumatic fever did not occur after herpes *Streptococcus*. On the other hand, are skin infections that affect the strains of the renal group "A" of the main *Streptococcus* previous glomerulonephritis after *Streptococcus* in many regions of the world. There are no conclusive data indicate that the treatment of the skin *Streptococcus* pyoderma prevents nephritis, but this treatment is an important measure of a pandemic in the elimination of strains that infect the college community [49].

9. Abscess, cellulitis, and erysipelas

Cause inflammation of the tissue cell may be many of the original skin living organisms or in specific environmental areas. Inflammation associated with cysts usually caused by *S. aureus*.

9.1 Cellulitis

These terms refer to the spread of skin infections spread, except for infections associated with the well pyogenic inherent, such as skin abscesses and inflammation of the fascia enterocolitis and arthritis Morphological and osteomyelitis. Unfortunately, doctors use the term "cellulitis" and "blush" is inconsistent. For some, it regards the distinction between the two terms deeply inflammation: erysipelas affect the upper dermis, including surface lymphocyte, while the inflammation of the tissue cell includes deep dermis, as well as subcutaneous fat. In practice, it may be difficult to distinguish between inflammation of cellulose and Aloristil clinically, and used some doctors, especially in northern Europe, the term "blush" to describe both infections.

Erysipelas is characterized by clinically from other forms of skin infections following Balmizatan: lesions are raised above the surrounding skin level, and there is a clear line of demarcation between the concerned tissue and tissue is involved [50]. This disorder is more common among infants, young children, and older adults. It is almost always caused by β-hemolytic streptococci (usually group A), but similar lesions can be caused by streptococci from serogroups C or G. Rarely, group B streptococci or *S. aureus* may be involved. In older reports, erysipelas characteristically involved the butterfly area of the face, but at present, the lower extremities are more frequently affected [51].

With early diagnosis and appropriate treatment, the prognosis is excellent. However, the infection rarely extends to the deeper levels of the skin and soft tissue. Is penicillin, which is given either by intravenous or oral according to clinical severity, is the optimal treatment (A-III). In the case of suspected infection *Staphylococcus aureus*, you must choose penicillin-resistant semi-industrial penicillinase or cephalosporin of the first generation. (A-III). In multiple prospective randomized trial, the effectiveness of roxithromycin, anti-Maikaroledat, equivalent to those used in penicillin. Resistance between macrolides streptococci group, however, is increasing in the United States [52].

These infections arise when living organisms enter through breakthroughs in skin. Include predisposing factors for these infection cases that make it more fragile or local host defenses skin is less effective, such as obesity and previous skin damage, edema of venous insufficiency or blockage of the lymphatic or other reasons. The origin of the barrier may be inactivated skin is shock, and skin infections previously existing, such as herpes or eczema, ulceration, and networks toe chapped spots or fungal infections, skin and inflammatory diseases, such as eczema. Often, the commas are in a small skin and is clinically moderate. These infections can occur anywhere, but the most common in the lower legs [53].

Include surgical procedures that increase the risk of inflammation of cellulose, which is assumed to be due to the interruption of lymphatic drainage, eradication of venous bile, and the anatomy of the axillary node breast cancer, surgery for diseases of malignant women involving the lymph node dissection, especially when following radiation therapy node of lymph. The radical hysterectomy [54–56].

Streptococcus responsible in areas of intermittent intra-toe or cracked, underlining the importance of the discovery and treatment of ringworm foot and other causes of toe deformities in these patients. Sometimes, the *Streptococcus* tank is the anal canal or vagina, especially for the group B *Streptococcus*, which causes inflammation of the cellular tissue in patients with cancer, former women treated with surgery and radiation therapy. *S. aureus* less frequent causes inflammation of cellular tissue, and is often associated with penetrating trauma earlier, including the injection sites of drug use illegal [57, 58].

Can many factors other infectious inflammation of the production of cellular tissue, but usually only in special cases. With cat bites or dogs, for example, the administrator would be responsible for the object types Bastorella, especially *P. multocida*, or *Capnocytophaga canimorsus*. This may cause inflammation of the cellulose Alheffilh after immersion in fresh water, while the infection after exposure to salt water can arise from species *Vibrio*, especially *V. vulnificus* in warm climates. In rare cases, *Streptococcus iniae* or *E. rhusiopathiae* may cause infection in persons employed in aquaculture or meatpacking, respectively. Inflammation can occur Salil about the pilgrims caused by *Haemophilus influenzae* in children. It has been reported diagnostic and therapeutic considerations for these infections by the Committee on Infectious Diseases, American Academy of Pediatrics. In anti-neutropenia, infection may be caused by *Pseudomonas aeruginosa* or Gram-negative bacilli, and in patients with HIV, may be in charge of the organism is *Helicobacter sinaada*. From time to time, Alkraatokov neoformans cause inflammation of cellulose in patients with cellular immune deficiency [59, 60].

Due to the low production rate, the blood cultures is not fruitful for the case of typical cases of erysipelas or cellulitis, which were not particularly severe [61]. The aspirations of the needle and skin biopsies also are not necessary in typical cases, which must respond to treatment with antibiotics directed against *Streptococcus* and Staphylococcus. This may be more useful for patients with diabetes procedures, malignant tumors, and factors to prepare non-regular, such as injury immersion, bites and animals, neutropenia, and immune deficiency [62].

Include diseases that are sometimes confused with acute inflammation of the tissue cell, such as resulting from contact with a skin disease, inflammation of the causes of allergies; gout, with skin inflammation significantly extends beyond the affected joint; herpes zoster. Hardening of the skin of acute fatty, which is inflammation of the lip which occurs mostly in obese women with deficient women phlebitis in the lower limb, causing painful areas, erythematous, thin, warm, non-saturated, and sometimes scaly in the medial leg-like inflammation of cellular tissue [63].

The lifting of the affected area, which is an important aspect and is often overlooked in the treatment, the improvement process accelerates by encouraging the discharge of gravity edema and inflammatory substances. Patients should also receive appropriate treatment for any medical condition may be ripe for infection, such as ringworm foot or venous eczema ("stasis dermatitis") or shock.

Each bout of cellulitis cause inflammation and lymphatic perhaps some permanent damage. Acute or recurrent seizures may result from inflammation of the tissue cell to lymph edema, which are in some cases large enough to cause the elephant's disease. Measures to reduce the recurrence of inflammation of the tissue cell treatment maceration between the numbers, maintain skin hydration well emollients to avoid dehydration and cracking, and minimize any essential edema in ways such as raising the upper limb, or compression stockings, or pressure pumps air, and if appropriate, treatment Diuretic. If frequent infections occur despite such measures, prophylactic antibiotics appear reasonable; however, published results demonstrating efficacy have been mixed [64]. Because streptococci cause most recurrent cellulitis, options include monthly intramuscular benzathine penicillin injections of 1.2 MU in adults or oral therapy with twice-daily doses of either 250 mg of erythromycin or 1 g of penicillin V (B-II). An alternative option, but has not been tested, for patients suffering from inflammation of trusted frequent cellulose is an attempt to shorten each episode by providing antibiotics by mouth for them to start treatment as soon as the start of the symptoms of infection. One of the selenium experience by mouth showed a decline in the rate of recurrence of erysipelas in the secondary lymph edema by 80%. This report requires independent confirmation [65].

9.2 Cutaneous abscesses

Skin cysts are collections of pus intradermal skin and deep tissue. Usually red nodules are painful, thin, volatile, often surmounted by a pimple surrounded by the edge of the swelling erythema. Usually multiple microbes skin cysts, and contain bacteria form the regional natural skin flora, and are often combined with living organisms from the adjacent mucous membranes [65]. *S. aureus* is present, usually one nurse, only ~25% of skin cysts in general. Cysts contain up the skin, which often carry the wrong signs as "fat bags," usually on the Flora Leather article in the cornea Aljbnah, even when they are not inflamed. The cultures of the inflamed cysts produce the same living organisms, suggesting that inflammation and vomiting occur in reaction to the rupture of the cyst wall and threw its contents into the dermis, instead of infectious complications [66].

9.3 Furuncles and carbuncles

Strangeness (or "boils") is inflammation of the hair follicles, usually caused by *Staphylococcus aureus*, extending pus through the dermis to the subcutaneous tissue, where a small abscess is formed. It is therefore different from folliculitis, where inflammation is more superficial and there is pus in the skin. Deer can occur anywhere on the skin hairy. Each lesion consists of dogma Inflammatory and upper blister show which hair. When the infection extends to include several contiguous follicles, and produces a homogeneous mass inflammatory with pus distracted from multiple holes porous, called the beauty of the lesion. Muscles tend to develop on the back of the neck is likely to occur particularly in people with diabetes. For small oven, be moist heat, which seems to enhance drainage, satisfactory. Larger Alorfan require larger and all bony rip Tbarva. Systemic antibiotics are usually not necessary, what inflammation Salil or the surrounding fever did not occur on a large scale (E-III). Cases may occur outbreak of inflammation of the thyroid gland caused by MS (MSSA), and as well as MRSA disease in families and other places that involve personal contact and close (such as prisons), especially when the skin are common injury, such as sports teams or Entertainment groups outdoors. The lack of personal hygiene and insufficient exposure to others injured Balfrt predisposing factors important in these circumstances. In some cases, it may harbor fungus organism and facilitate the transmission. Depending on the individual circumstances, it may require control of outbreaks bathing antibacterial soap, such as chlorhexidine; thorough washing of clothes, towels and clothes family; use separate towels and towels. And try to eliminate the transfer of cluster Meningococcal between the colonists [67].

Some individuals have frequent bouts of injury. Have a few of these people, especially children, host responses methodology is not normal, but for most of them, the only Almahb factor that can be determined is the presence of *Staphylococcus aureus* in the front openings or sometimes elsewhere, such as perineum [68].

9.3.1 Soft-tissue infections and the evaluation of MRSA infection

The emerging problem is to increase the spread of the skin and soft tissue infections caused by MRSA acquired by the community. Considered MRSA, which is traditionally considered one of the causes of disease-causing diseases, pathogens that occur in the community, and differ from their counterparts in hospitals in several ways [69]. Cause community strains infections in patients who lack the typical risk factors, such as hospitalization or residence in a long-term care facility; often are susceptible to antibiotics, non-lactam, including doxycycline or clindamycin or trimethoprim—sulfamethoxazole or fluoroquinolone or rifampin; genetically, do not appear to be linked to local hospitals and strains contain a cassette-type SCCmec of the fourth type is unusual in Isolates hospital. Finally, community isolates frequently contain genes for Banoudin Valuksidin, which is associated with mild to severe infections in the skin and soft tissue. It occurred because of an outbreak of MRSA isolates acquired from the community between prison inmates and prisons, injecting drug users and the Native American population and gay men and participants in sports Immobilizer children [70]. Thus, recurrent or persistent furuncles and impetigo, particularly in these high-risk groups, that do not respond to oral β-lactam antibiotic therapy are increasingly likely to be caused by MRSA.

9.3.2 Necrotizing skin and soft-tissue infections

Necrotizing fasciitis may be chronic to bacteria and result from *Cyclococcus*, *Pseudomonas*, or aqueous *Aeromonas*. Recently, necrotizing fasciitis has been prescribed in a patient with MRSA infection. Inflammation of multiple necrotic fasciitis may occur microbes after surgery or in patients with peripheral vascular disease, diabetes, ulcers lie down, tears spontaneous mucous in the digestive tract or the digestive system (i.e., Fournier gangrene). As with renal bone necrosis, unless there is gas in the deep tissue often in these mixed infections [71].

Soft and soft tissue infections skin infections differ from light and surface through clinical presentation and common systemic manifestations and treatment strategies [72]. Are often deep and destructive. It is deep because it may involve fascial compartments and/or muscles; it is devastating because it caused great destruction of tissue and can lead to a fatal outcome. These cases are usually an injury "minor," as it evolves from an initial break in the skin due to trauma or surgery. It can be abnormal (usually containing *Streptococcus* or *Staphylococcus aureus* rarely) or multiple microbes (containing plants from mixed bacterial aerobe-anaerobe). In the initial stages, it may be difficult to distinguish between inflammation of the cellular tissue, which must respond to the treatment of anti-microbial alone necrotizing infection that requires surgical intervention. Many of the clinical characteristics indicate a necrotic infection of the skin and deep structures: (1) severe pain and constant; (2) bubbles, concerning the obstruction of blood vessels deep that traverse the fascia or muscle compartments; (3) the skin or bruises necrosis (bruises) that precedes skin necrosis; (4) gas in the soft tissue, detection palpation or photography; (5) edema extends beyond the margin of erythema; (6) skin anesthesia; (7) of systemic toxicity, manifested in fever, leukocytosis, delirium, and renal failure; and (8) rapid deployment, especially during antibiotic treatment. Bubbles alone is not a diagnosis of deep infections, because they also occur with erysipelas, cellulitis, burned skin syndrome, coagulation diffuse into the blood vessels, Volminac Purpura, some toxins (e.g., those associated with bites of spider brown), skin diseases skin.

10. Necrotizing fasciitis

Fasciitis is an infection necrotizing under the skin are relatively rare tracks on the aircraft along the fascia and extends beyond the surface signs of infection, such as erythema and other skin changes [73]. The term fasciitis sometimes leads to the mistaken impression that the muscle fascia or interruption of urine. The most common fascia is superficial fascia, which consists of all the tissues between the skin and the core muscles (i.e., tissue under the skin).

The clinical characteristic feature is the sense of the wooden tissue under the skin. Inflammation of cellular tissue or blush, can seep tissue under the skin and produces. But in the inflammation of the fascia, the tissue implicit fixed, and cannot distinguish blame and vascular aircraft by palpation. It is often possible to note the course of erythema wide in the skin along the infection during its progress in cattle head. If there is an open wound, the examination of the edges with a sharp tool allows an autopsy on ready-to-aircraft vascular surface that exceed the margins of the wound.

11. Anaerobic streptococcal myositis

Streptococcus anaerobic cause more than other *Streptococcus aureus* infection lazy. Unlike other dead infections, usually associated with muscle injury and aircraft Allvaiah streptococcal anaerobic shock or perform surgery. Incision and drainage necessary. The necrotic tissue and debris eradication but should not remove the inflamed muscles viable, because they can heal and restore function. It must be packed incision with wet bandages. Antibiotic treatment is very effective. All of these organisms susceptible to penicillin or ampicillin, which must be administered in high doses.

12. Pyomyositis

Inflammation of the mouth, which is caused by *Staphylococcus aureus* essentially, is the presence of pus within individual muscle groups. In some cases, the pulmonary S. or Gram-negative intestinal bacillus is responsible. Because of its geographical distribution, often called the case "orbital inflammation of the pus," but it is recognized cases increasingly in temperate climates, especially in patients with HIV or diabetes, lack of. Present the results are local pain in a muscular one, muscle cramps, and fever. This disease occurs mostly, but can share any muscle group, including lumbar muscle or trunk muscles. At first, it may not be possible to contact the separate abscess because localized infection deep within the muscles, but the area has a wooden feeling strong is associated with pain and tenderness. In the early stages, you can perform ultrasound imaging or CT scans to distinguish between this entity and deep venous thrombosis. In the most advanced cases, the abscess is swollen and clinically evident. And appropriate antibiotics in addition to the surgical incision and extensive health and sanitation are required for the proper management [74].

13. Synergistic necrotizing cellulitis

This is simply inflammation of the soft tissue enterocolitis, which includes muscle groups in addition to the surface tissue and fascia. The level of participation depends on the depth and levels of tissue affected by the process of origin or pathological process that precedes infection. Predisposing main causes are cysts circular ischemic. Similar recognition and treatment with inflammation of the fascia grunt, but surgical exploration reveals his innermost.

- *Surgical site infections*. Include infections of soft tissue surgical those that occur after surgery and those severe enough to require surgical intervention for diagnosis and treatment. Clearly provided the algorithm indicates that the infection site surgical rarely occur during the first 48 h after surgery, usually arise fever during that period of non-infectious causes or unknown.

14. Fournier gangrene

Gas gangrene is a rapidly progressive infection caused by *Clostridium perfringens*, *Clostridium septicum*, *Clostridium histolyticum*, or *Clostridium novyi*. Severe penetrating trauma or crush injuries associated with interruption of the blood supply are the usual predisposing factors. *C. perfringens* and *C. novyi* infections have recently been described among heroin abusers following intracutaneous injection of black tar heroin. *C. septicum*, a more aerotolerant *Clostridium* species, may cause spontaneous gas gangrene in patients with colonic lesions (such as those due to diverticular disease), adenocarcinoma, or neutropenia.

This type of inflammation of the soft tissue grunt includes scrotum and penis or vagina and can have a malicious or explosive beginning [75]. The average age of onset is 50 years. Most of the patients suffer from a significant illness, especially diabetes, but 20% of them will not have a clear reason. Most patients initially have an infection around the anus or retroperitoneal spread on aircraft along the fascia to the genitals. Inflammation of the urinary tract, the most common in the event of a narrowing of the urethra, and includes glands around the urethra and extends to the penis and scrotum; or previous trauma to the genital area, allowing the arrival of living organisms to the tissues under the skin.

Infection can start insidious with a separate area of necrosis in the perineum, which is rapidly advancing within 1–2 days with the progress of skin necrosis. In the beginning, it tends to cause surface gangrene, and is limited to the skin and subcutaneous tissue, and extends to the base of the scrotum. Usually save the testicles, glans penis, and the spermatic cord, because they contain a separate blood source. Infection may extend to the perineum and the anterior abdominal wall through the fascia aircraft.

Most of the cases caused by mixed aerobic and anaerobic plants. Often there are types of *Staphylococcus aureus* bacteria *Pseudomonas*, usually in a mixed culture, but in some cases, be *Staphylococcus aureus* is the only pathogen. False is another common object in the mixed culture. As with other infections dead, is the rapid surgical exploration of aggressive and appropriate purification necessary to remove all the dead tissue, while avoiding the deeper structures when possible.

15. Clostridial myonecrosis

Cause gas gangrene *Clostridium* (e.g., muscular muscle necrosis) significantly from *C. perfringens* and *C. novyi* and *C. histolyticum* and *C. septicum*. *C. perfringens* is the most common cause of gas gangrene associated with shocks. Severe pain increasingly begins at the site of infection after 24 h of infection is the first symptom of reliable. The skin may be pale at first, but quickly changed to bronze and then to the red color purple. The area becomes infected tense and smooth, show fluid-filled bubbles blue reddish. There is gas in the tissue, which is detected as crepitus or on the basis of imaging studies, globally present at this late stage. Systemic signs of toxicity, including irregular heartbeats, fever, sweating, develop rapidly, followed by shock and the failure of multiple members.

Both painful gas gangrene and spontaneous are destructive infection requiring accurate intensive care, and support measures, and aggressive surgical revision, and appropriate antibiotics. The role of oxygen therapy high pressure is still unclear. Altemeier and Fullen [76]. It has been reported significant reduction in the mortality rate among patients with gas gangrene using penicillin and tetracycline in addition to aggressive surgery in the absence of high-pressure oxygen. Treatment of experimental gas gangrene proved that tetracycline and clindamycin and chloramphenicol were more effective than penicillin or high-pressure oxygen treatment [77].

16. Clinical manifestations

Abscess clear zones of erythema, edema, and warmth. Evolve as a result of bacteria entering through the breakthroughs in the skin barrier [78]. You can be seen Petechiae and/or bleeding in the skin erythema, and can surface bubbles occur. Fever and other systemic manifestations of infection may also be present. Cysts are always one-sided almost, lower limbs are the most common sites of involvement; bilateral engagement should consider quickly in alternative causes [79].

Cysts deep dermis and subcutaneous fat include; reddish include the upper and lymph dermis surface. Cysts with or without purulent may appear. Erysipelas is grainy [80]. It tends patients with cysts or cellulitis to get more comfortable with the development cycle of topical symptoms over a few days [81].

Patients suffering from erysipelas usually suffer from the emergence of severe symptoms with systemic manifestations, including fever, chills, feeling very upset and headache; these can precede the onset of signs and symptoms of local infections from minutes to hours. In erysipelas, there is a clear demarcation between the involved and associated tissues. There may be raised or erythematous border with central clearing. Classic descriptions of the red leaf notes "butterfly" face involvement. The involvement of the ear (ear tag in Milian) is a distinctive feature of Oryeceblas, because this area does not contain deeper tissues of the skin [82].

Additional features of the abscesses and lymphatic vessels Oristepelas inflammation and enlargement of the regional lymph nodes. Edema surrounding Bbesellat hair may lead to variation in the skin, which creates showing little strength orange peel ("peau d'orange"). This can be seen vesicles bubbles and akimats or Alnchat. Can bleeding skin in the case of a significant inflammation of the skin. Inflammation of the cellular tissue that causes injury and inflammation Alglazi Algrgreeni is an unusual manifestation of inflammation due to cellular Alclaustradia and other anaerobes. It should be the acute manifestations of systemic toxicity with the rapid investigation of additional sources underlying infection [83].

17. Diagnosis of complicated abscess and soft tissues infections

Often begins with a diagnosis of a comprehensive abscesses clinical history and physical examination results, which helps to assess the severity of infection, followed by the study of the living organisms that cause microbearing [84, 85].

Standard procedure is to increase the clinical assessment of laboratory investigations, especially for inpatient. In addition to the patient's history, should be taken into account relevant risk factors such as frequent entry in the hospital factors, diabetes, neutropenia, wounds sting and animal contact, which may indicate a potential junior responsible for the injury of living organisms [86].

Possible complications associated with cysts such as inflammation of the lymph glands and muscle inflammation and inflammation of the intestine and colon, gangrene, osteomyelitis, bacteremia, endocarditis, blood poisoning or poisoning should be taken into account during the diagnosis. It may indicate a significant increase in the number of white blood cells (or leukopenia) syndrome poisoning, while the levels of creatine kinase high may indicate the presence of muscles selflessly caused by inflammation of the fascia or inflammation of the bowel syndrome and colon [87].

Radiological examination and investigations aid imaging of deep tissue infections to assess the location and size of the infection and any involvement of blood vessels that can guide surgical drainage procedures. Tests must be performed culturing microbiological in all cases to distinguish between abscesses and MRSA infections, non-infectious MRSA, and therefore the revision of the final decision on the management of antibiotics to reduce the risk of treatment failure likely [88].

Diagnosis of skin abscess usually depends on the clinical manifestations. Abscess appears Oristepelas in areas of skin erythema, edema, and warmth. It is raised lesions Erysipelas higher than the surrounding skin with a clear delineation of the level of tissue between the concerned and involved. Skin abscess appears as a painful, volatile, erythematous node, with or without a surrounding abscess.

For laboratory tests are not required for patients with uncomplicated infection in the absence of associated diseases or complications. It must be subject to patients with disposable abscess incision and drainage. Routine culture of materials debrided is not necessary in healthy patients who are not receiving antibiotics [89].

There is no justification for the cultures of abandoned materials and cultures of blood (before the addition of antibiotic treatment) in the following cases [90, 91]:

- Severe local infection (e.g., extensive cellulitis).
- Systemic signs of infection (e.g., fever).
- History of recurrent or multiple abscesses.
- Failure of initial antibiotic therapy.
- Extremes of age (young infants or older adults).
- Presence of underlying comorbidities (lymphedema, malignancy, neutropenia, immunodeficiency, splenectomy, diabetes).
- Special exposures (animal bite, water-associated injury).

- Presence of indication for prophylaxis against infective endocarditis.
- Community patterns of *S. aureus* susceptibility are unknown or rapidly changing.

Blood cultures are positive in less than 10% of cellulitis cases [92]. There may be a justification for skin biopsy if the diagnosis is uncertain; cultures from samples of skin biopsy result in pathogens in 20–30% of cases. Cultures of healthy skin wipes are not useful and should not be done [93].

It can be useful radiographic examination to determine whether the skin abscess is present (via ultrasound) and to distinguish between cellulitis and osteomyelitis (via magnetic resonance imaging). There may be a justification for radiological assessment in patients with immune suppression, diabetes, venous insufficiency, or lymphedema in patients with persistent symptoms of systemic. Radiological examination cannot reliably distinguish inflammation from Salil fasciitis or gas gangrene Grunt; if there is clinical doubt for these entities, the imaging should not delay surgical intervention [94].

In patients with recurrent cysts, serological tests for drugs Almnhllh blood beta may be a useful diagnostic tool. Assays include the reaction of an anti Alstrptullizin-O (ASO), or test an anti-desoxyribonuclease b (anti-DNA), or anti Alheialoronidaz test (AHT), or antibody test Alstrepettosem [95].

18. Problems related to the emergence of MDR related abscesses and related clinical management issues

Experimental methods are used to treat a range of cysts surgical treatments and antimicrobial support. However, high resistance of microorganisms to the antibiotics [96]. Resistant organisms medicines in particular, may complicate the treatment of cSSTI. Between the organisms of multi-drug resistance, MRSA, enterococci resistant to vancomycin (VRE), and gentle stretching act-lactamase (ESBL)—producing isolates of *E. coli* and *Klebsiella* spp. It has the highest incidence of [97]. Strains of CA-MRSA differ genetically apparently from HA-MRSA, and thus involve the risk of more severe infections and ease of transmission of resistance [98].

The presence of Pantone assumed—Valentin Okosidin, Botulinum cellular genes coding in MRSA isolated from infection CA—skin to play an important role in this increased virulence strains associated with tissue necrosis, and necrosis of the severity of the largest local and systemic manifestations [99]. Carrying strains of CA-MRSA is also the genes of chromosome mec (SCCmec) *Staphylococcus aureus* (types IV and V), which gives resistance to methicillin and antimicrobial agents β currently available and help in the transfer of resistance easily between living organisms. Although MRSA infection was considered, HA mainly, recent evidence has appeared on the emergence of CA-MRSA rapid even in hospitals [100].

19. Surgical methods and supportive care

The secretions of fluid from the abscess and ulcers are the common features of bacterial abscesses. Therefore, aggressive surgical revision dead tissue/infected by using chemical or mechanical methods of preferred whenever possible to stop the spread of infection and promote wound healing. The delay is known in the final revision of the soft tissue infections is considered one of the most important risk factor for death [101]. Implementation of incision and drainage of inflammatory cysts and purulent [102]. Other roads dressing negative pressure, chronic infection or localized large wounds with excessive secretion [103]. Download closure with the help of the vacuum (as a substitute for wound healing), especially for surgical wounds or subsequent surgery deep infections, infections of the blood clotting involving venous blood clots, and vascular compensation cases involving injuries in the vascular arteries. Supportive care, which includes fluid resuscitation, and members of the support, nutritional, and management to maintain oxygen and tissue perfusion important interventions in the clinical outcomes of these patients are considered [104].

20. Treatment of skin abscess

Some small cysts degrade without treatment, up to the point of disposal. Warm compresses help to speed up the process. It referred to as the incision and drainage when there is a great pain, tenderness and swelling. It is not necessary to wait for volatility. Under sterile conditions, local anesthesia either lidocaine or freezing spray is given [105].

Patients suffering from abscesses intravenous anesthesia large and extremely painful and may benefit pain during the exchange. Often enough having one hole tip stripes to open the abscess. After draining the pus, you must examine the cavity or glove full finger scan sites. Optional normal saline irrigation with gauze used to reduce dead space cavity and prevents the formation of vaccines. Usually the valves are removed after 24–48 h. However, the recent data did not prove the effectiveness of routine irrigation or packing. High local temperature may precipitate inflammation decision [106].

Surgical intervention is the main therapeutic method in cases of fasciitis enterocolitis (A-III). However, many cases of inflammation of the fascia Grunt may begin to Kthab descendant, and if you have been identified fasciitis necrotizing early and treated aggressively, it avoids some patients distort surgical procedures. It must be based on the decision of an aggressive surgery to several considerations. First, there is no response to antibiotics after a reasonable experience is the most common indicator. You must be judged to respond to antibiotics by reducing fever and toxicity and lack of progress. Second, deep toxicity, fever, low blood pressure, or skin and soft tissue provided during antibiotic treatment is an indication for surgical intervention. Third, when the local wound necrosis appears in any skin with easy dissecting along the fascia using a blunt tool, you need to make an incision and a more complete discharge. Fourth, any soft tissue infection accompanied by gas in the injured tissue suggests the presence of tissue necrosis requires Tbarva surgically and/or anesthesia.

Most of the patients must come back with rheumatoid fasciitis Grunt to the operating room over the first 24–36 h after the anesthesia process, and then a day until the surgical team finds no further need debridement. Although separate pus is usually absent, these wounds can discharge abundant amounts of tissue fluid. Aggressive management of fluid is necessary assistant.

You must treat inflammation of the fascia Grunt and/or toxic shock conjugate caused by *Streptococcus* Group A syndrome of streptococci using penicillin and clindamycin (A-II). The rationale for clindamycin in laboratory studies that show both the suppression of toxins and modify the production of cytokines (i.e., TNF), and on animal studies showing the effectiveness of superior versus penicillin, and two studies Rsiditin demonstrating the greater effectiveness of clindamycin for β-antibiotics lactam [107, 108]. You must add penicillin due to increased resistance to Group A *Streptococcus* conjugate of Macroledat, although it is in the United States, only 0.5% of the Group A drug resistance Almacrolad is also resistant to clindamycin.

Cannot be recommended for sure using of beta globulin (B-II) intravenously in the treatment of toxic shock syndrome conjugate *Streptococcus*. Although there is sufficient evidence on the role of toxins *Streptococcus* outside the cellular in shock, organ failure, and the destruction of tissue, containing different sets of IVIG variable amounts of neutralizing antibodies to some of these toxins, and lacked the final clinical data [107]. One of observational studies have shown better results in patients receiving IVIG, but these patients were more likely to undergo surgery and received more than historical control subjects clindamycin [108]. Showed a second study, was a double-blind trial, which placebo-controlled northern Europe, no improvement statistically significant in survival, and specifically for this section, any decrease in due time for the lack of further progress fasciitis necrosis (69 h for IVIG group, compared to 36 h for a placebo) [109]. The results of these studies provide some promise. However, the Committee believes that further studies on the effectiveness of IVIG is necessary before it can make a recommendation on the use of IVIG for the treatment of toxic shock syndrome conjugate *Streptococcus*.

21. Abscess arises from the body parts

21.1 Dental abscess

In the early seventeenth century, death bonds began in London on account of the causes of death with teeth inserted continuously in the list of the main reasons for the fifth or sixth death [110]. By the twentieth century, it has been recognized the possibility of the spread of dental abscesses and cause acute poisoning leading to death. An audit was conducted at the Hull Royal Hospital between 1999 and 2004, an increase in the number of patients who provide services to oral surgery, face and jaws with teeth rot [111]. In the United States, a large prospective study reported that 13% of adult patients sought treatment for dental pain and infection over 24 months of follow-up [112]. The percentage of abscess dentoalveolar occurred 6.4% among children who attended the dental clinic at the outpatient clinics in Nigeria. In India, dental caries affect 60–65% of the general population [113]. Factors involved in the bacteriological cause abscesses teeth consist of a complex mix of strict anaerobic and anaerobic optional. Derived data sets show cultural and molecular studies that have been identified more than 460 unique bacterial species that belong to 100 genus and 9 species in different types of infections pulposus [114]. Signs and symptoms of acute abscess in the teeth are pain, swelling, and erythema are usually localized infected teeth, although suppuration can spread often to nearby tissues, causing fatal complications. Fever, swelling of the mouth and inside the mouth, erythema, tenderness to palpation significantly. Trismus in addition to any changes in the sound, such as hoarseness and a torrent of saliva should pay the doctor to the state of emergency [115].

21.2 Subcutaneous tissue abscess

Respond to simple infections confined to the skin and underlying soft tissues in general to manage outpatient. Among the common symptoms are simple: cellulitis, erysipelas, herpes, folliculitis, fur, shrimp, cysts, infections and injuries. Include complex injuries that extend to the deep underlying tissue, which include deep cysts, ulcers decubitus, fasciitis grunt, Fournier gangrene, infections of human or animal bite. These infections may appear with the inflammatory response syndrome features or systemic sepsis, and sometimes brain necrosis. Inflammation around the anus, and diabetic foot infections, infections in patients with accompanying diseases, and infections of the causes of resistance diseases also represent a complex inflammatory. The diseases of aging, heart disease, or liver, or diabetes, or weakness, or immune poisoning, or obesity, or arterial venous insufficiency or peripheral lymphatic, and psychological trauma among the risk factors of infection of sexually transmitted. The spread of the disease is more common among military personnel during deployment abroad and athletes participating in the nearby sports. Provide with erythema, warmth, edema, and pain on the affected site. Systemic manifestations of infection may follow, reflect the size of the severity of infection. Lower limbs are the most common [116].

21.3 Lymph node abscess

Found swollen lymph node cervical in many different disciplines of general medicine to specialized disciplines such as ear nose and throat surgery or maxillofacial surgery craniofacial. It causes swelling benign or malignant may be. Swellings or even benign cysts as a result of infection due mostly *Staphylococcus aureus* and Group A. Rare disease of animal origin also causes swelling of the lymph node is Altolemia disease. This disease shows all over the northern hemisphere, but the proportion of a 1056 case only registered in the EU in 2016 is very low [117]. Francasla Tolensis, one of the causes of Altolemia disease, is Gram-negative bacteria; been described for the first time in 1911 in the United States of America (USA). Bacteria can be divided into four different strains. Sub-species *F. tularensis* subspecies holarctica spread mostly in Europe, while the sub-species *F. tularensis* subspecies tularensis exist frequently in North America. Although it is the same bacteria can be identified in more than 250 different animal species, but the exact path of transmission to humans is not yet clear [118]. In order to avoid serious illness and complications, it is necessary to appropriate early treatment after identifying pathogens. Active substances of antibiotics are aminoglycosides and fluoroquinolones and tetracycline and chloramphenicol and rifampicin. It should not be used erythromycin as a representative of Macroledat because of natural resistance, especially for the type of mushroom ring [119].

21.4 Perianal abscess

Cysts around the anus are the most common types of cysts anal. These cysts can cause considerable annoyance to patients. It is located at the edge of the anus, and if left untreated can extend into space ischioanal or space intersphincteric because these areas are continuing with the space around the anus. It can also cause systemic infection if left untreated [120]. The prevalence rate of cysts around the anus and anal cysts, in general, is underestimated, since most patients do not seek medical care, or are refusing as the occasional hemorrhoids. It is estimated that there are approximately 100,000 cases of benign anal disease in general. The average age at presentation is 40 years, and that the male mostly of adults twice the rate of infection than females [121]. Abscess around the anus is an indication of the incision and drainage in a timely manner. Antibiotics management alone is inadequate and inappropriate. Once you make an incision and drainage, there is no need to antibiotics unless management require some use of medical problems. Such cases include valvular heart disease, and patients with immune deficiency, diabetes patients, or in the development of sepsis. Antibiotics are also considered in these patients or cases showing signs of infection or systemic inflammation of the cellular tissue surrounding [122].

21.5 Breast abscess

Breast infections are divided into categories of breastfeeding and non-breast-feeding, or postpartum and non-puerperal. It can be associated with the surface of the skin or underlying lesion. The breast abscesses are more common in lactating women, but they also occur when women are breastfeeding. It is important to rule out more serious diseases such as breast cancer when the patient gets unsatisfactory signs and symptoms of breast abscess. The vast majority of these injuries occur in females, but they can also occur in males. Diagnosis and treatment of breast abscess is not difficult, but there is a high percentage of repetition [123]. Abscesses breast disease is often caused by *Staphylococcus aureus* and *Streptococcus* species, it became *Staphylococcus aureus* resistant MRSA increasingly common. Usually breast abscess is a result of a mixed deciduous plants with bacteria *S. aureus* and *Streptococcus* and anaerobic bacteria [124]. Incision and drainage are the standard for the care of breast abscesses. If the patient's back in a primary care centers by the provider is not satisfied with the implementation of these procedures, the patient may start antibiotics and transmit it to a general surgeon for final treatment. You may be trying to suction the needle abscesses smaller than 3 cm or abscesses milk [125].

21.6 Liver abscess

Liver abscess is a pus-filled mass inside the liver [126]. Common causes are cases of abdominal such as appendicitis or diverticulitis because of the spread of blood through the portal vein. Can also develop liver injury complication [127]. The prognosis has improved for liver abscesses. The mortality rate in-hospital is about 2.5–19%. The elderly, ICU admissions, shock, cancer, fungal infections, cirrhosis, chronic kidney disease, acute respiratory failure, severe disease, or disease of biliary origin have a worse prognosis [128]. Antibiotics: metronidazole fourth and third generation cephalosporin/quinolones, antibiotics and β-lactam, and aminoglycosides effective [129].

21.7 Brain abscess

Cysts inside the skull is a common and serious life-threatening. They include brain abscess and subdural empyema or outside the dura and are classified by location anatomic or the causative agent of the disease. The term brain abscess is used in this article to represent all types of cysts within the skull [130]. Abscess formation may occur after nerve surgery or head trauma. In these cases it is often the cause of the bacterial skin infection by, such as *Staphylococcus aureus* and *S. epidermidis*, or negative bacilli Gram. Sinus) it is often caused by *Streptococcus* species 4 but abscesses *Staphylococcus aureus* and microbes (including those resulting from the anaerobic Gram-negative bacilli) also occur [131].

21.8 Renal abscess

Renal cysts and the period surrounding the animal are satisfactory entities that are uncommon due to kidney infections or around it. Moreover, it is a challenge for diagnostic physicians. Delays in diagnosis may lead to higher morbidity and mortality rates [132]. With the availability of computerized tomography (CT) and magnetic resonance imaging (MRI) in the diagnosis of renal cysts, the mortality rate dropped to 12% [133]. The mainstay of the treatment of kidney cysts or perineum is adequate drainage system and antibiotics optimal. Include the classic management of kidney cysts surgical exploration, incision and drainage, or the eradication of the kidney. However, the destructive treatment at the beginning of the 1970s appeared, and the trend towards common conservative treatment due to advances in new imaging techniques and antibiotics. It is noticed several reports that small cysts nephrotic effectively treated through antibiotics intravenously.

Author details

Mohammed Malih Radhi[1], Fatima Malik AL-Rubea[2], Nada Khazal Kadhim Hindi[3]* and Rusull Hamza Kh. AL-Jubori[4]

1 Community Health Nursing, Kut Technical Institute, Middle Technical University, Iraq

2 Microbiology, College of Dentistry, University of Babylon, Iraq

3 Microbiology, Department of Basic and Medical Science, College of Nursing, Babylon University, Babylon Province, Iraq

4 Community Health Nursing, Babylon Health Directorate, Iraq

*Address all correspondence to: nadakhazal@yahoo.com

References

[1] Stevens D, Bisno A, Chambers H. Practice guidelines for the diagnosis and management of skin and soft tissue infections: 2014 update by the infectious diseases society of America. Clinical Infectious Diseases. 2014;**59**(3):147-240

[2] Singer A, Talan D. Management of skin abscesses in the era of methicillin-resistant *Staphylococcus aureus*. The New England Journal of Medicine. 2014;**370**(23):1039-1099

[3] Demos M, McLeod M, Nouri K. Recurrent furunculosis: A review of the literature. The British Journal of Dermatology. 2012;**167**(21):725-780

[4] Summanen P, Talan D, Strong C. Bacteriology of skin and soft-tissue infections: Comparison of infections in intravenous drug users and individuals with no history of intravenous drug use. Clinical Infectious Diseases. 1995;**20**(Suppl 2):279-390

[5] Brook I, Frazier E. Aerobic and anaerobic bacteriology of wounds and cutaneous abscesses. Archives of Surgery. 1990;**125**(37):1445-1499

[6] Talan JA, David A. Management of skin abscesses in the era of methicillin-resistant *Staphylococcus aureus*. England Journal of Medicine. 2014;**370**(11):1039-1047

[7] Singer A, Thode H, Lee C. National epidemiology of cutaneous abscesses: 1996 to 2005. The American Journal of Emergency Medicine. 2009;**27**(3):289-292

[8] Paterson D. Increases in Australian cutaneous abscess hospitalisations: 1999-2008. Microbiology & Infectious Diseases. 2012;**31**(1):93-96

[9] United Kingdom National Health Service. Abscess. 2014;**32**(12):10-30

[10] Kanz G. Diagnostic and treatment options for skin and soft tissue abscesses in injecting drug users with consideration of the natural history and concomitant risk factors. European Journal of Medical Research. 2008;**13**(9):415-424

[11] John K. Spinal subdural abscess following epidural steroid injection. Journal of Neurosurgery. Spine. 2014;**22**(1):90-93

[12] Marx D, John A, Marx M. 8th Chapter 137 Rosen's emergency medicine: Concepts and clinical practice. Skin and Soft Tissue Infections. 2014;**43**(65):4123-4207

[13] Ellis Simonsen S, van Orman E, Hatch B. Cellulitis incidence in a defined population. Epidemiology and Infection. 2006;**134**(21):293-299

[14] Vinh D, Embil J. Rapidly progressive soft tissue infections. Lancet Infectious Diseases. 2005;**5**(31):501-513

[15] Baddour L. Epidemiology, Clinical Features, and Diagnosis of Cellulitis. 2008. Available from: http://www.utdol.com/utd/content/topic.do?topicKey=skin.inf/11185&selectedTitle=1150&source=searc_result2008

[16] Eron L, Lipsky B, Low D, Nathwani D, Tice A, Volturo G. Expert panel on managing skin and soft tissue infections. Managing skin and soft tissue infections: Expert panel recommendations on key decision points. The Journal of Antimicrobial Chemotherapy. 2003;**52**(31):102-202

[17] Dworkin R, Johnson R, Breuer J. Recommendations for the management of herpes zoster. Clinical Infectious Diseases. 2007;**44**(1):1-26

[18] Merritt C, Haran J, Mintzer J. All purulence is local—Epidemiology and

management of skin and soft tissue infections in three urban emergency departments. BMC Emergency Medicine. 2013;**13**(21):26-43

[19] Talan D, Krishnadasan A, Gorwitz R, EMERGEncy ID Net Study Group. Comparison of *Staphylococcus aureus* from skin and soft-tissue infections in US emergency department patients, 2004 and 2008. Clinical Infectious Diseases. 2011;**53**(21):144-149

[20] Edelsberg J, Taneja C, Zervos M. Trends in US hospital admissions for skin and soft tissue infections. Emerging Infectious Diseases. 2009;**15**(31):1516-1518

[21] Gerber J, Coffin S, Smathers S. Trends in the incidence of methicillin-resistant *Staphylococcus aureus* infection in children's hospitals in the United States. Clinical Infectious Diseases. 2009;**49**(20):65-71

[22] Labreche M, Lee G, Attridge R. Treatment failure and costs in patients with methicillin-resistant *Staphylococcus aureus* skin and soft tissue infections: A South Texas Ambulatory Research Network (STARNet) study. Journal of the American Board of Family Medicine. 2013;**26**(98):508-517

[23] Horowitz Y, Sperber A, Almog Y. Gram-negative cellulitis complicating cirrhosis. Mayo Clinic Proceedings. 2004;**79**(21):247-250

[24] Björnsdóttir S, Gottfredsson M, Thórisdóttir A. Risk factors for acute cellulitis of the lower limb: A prospective case-control study. Clinical Infectious Diseases. 2005;**41**(21):1416-1422

[25] Stevens D, Bisno A, Chambers H. Infectious Diseases Society of America. Practice guidelines for the diagnosis and management of skin and soft-tissue infections. Clinical Infectious Diseases. 2005;**41**(32):1373-1406

[26] Quirke M, Ayoub F, McCabe A. Risk factors for nonpurulent leg cellulitis: A systematic review and meta-analysis. The British Journal of Dermatology. 2017;**177**(10):382-609

[27] Cohen J. Clinical practice: Herpes zoster. The New England Journal of Medicine. 2013;**369**(76):255-263

[28] Herman R, Kee V, Moores K. Etiology and treatment of community-associated methicillin-resistant *Staphylococcus aureus*. American Journal of Health-System Pharmacy. 2008;**65**(77):219-225

[29] Mansour S, Pletzer D, De La Fuente-Nunez C, Kim P, Cheung G, Joo H, et al. Bacterial abscess formation is controlled by the stringent stress response and can be targeted therapeutically. eBioMedicine. 2016;**12**(3):219-226

[30] Roth R, James W. Microbial ecology of the skin. Annual Review of Microbiology. 1988;**42**(22):441-464

[31] Dunbar J, Barns S, Ticknor L, Kuske C. Empirical and theoretical bacterial diversity in four Arizona soils. Applied and Environmental Microbiology. 2002;**68**(32):3035-3045

[32] Bowler P, Duerden B, Armstrong D. Wound microbiology and associated approaches to wound management. Clinical Microbiology Reviews. 2001;**14**(76):244-269

[33] Davies C. Use of molecular techniques to study microbial diversity in the skin: Chronic wounds reevaluated. Wound Repair and Regeneration. 2001;**9**(12): 332-340

[34] Hugenholtz P, Pace N. Identifying microbial diversity in the natural environment: A molecular phylogenetic approach. Trends in Biotechnology. 1996;**14**(7):190-197

[35] Vincent Ki M, Coleman Rotstein M. Bacterial skin and soft tissue infections in adults: A review of their epidemiology, pathogenesis, diagnosis, treatment and site of care. Canadian Journal of Infectious Diseases and Medical Microbiology. 2008;**19**(2):173-184

[36] Todar K. The Bacterial Flora of Humans. 2008. Available from: http:// textbookofbacteriology.net/ normalflora.html [Accessed: 12 February]

[37] Iwase T. *Staphylococcus epidermidis* esp inhibits *Staphylococcus aureus* biofilm formation and nasal colonization. Nature. 2010;**465**(89):346-349

[38] De La Fuente-Nunez C, Reffuveille F, Haney E, Straus S, Hancock R. Broad-spectrum anti-biofilm peptide that targets a cellular stress response. PLoS Pathogens. 2014;**32**(55):10-213

[39] Geiger T, Francois P, Liebeke M, Fraunholz M, Goerke C, Krismer B, et al. The stringent response of *Staphylococcus aureus* and its impact on survival after phagocytosis through the induction of intracellular PSMs expression. PLOS Pathogens. 2012;**89212**:43-124

[40] Steer A, Lamagni T, Curtis N, Carapetis J. Invasive group a streptococcal disease: Epidemiology, pathogenesis and management. Drugs. 2012;**72**:1213-1227

[41] Chelsom J, Halstensen A, Haga T, Hoiby E. Necrotising fasciitis due to group A streptococci in western Norway: Incidence and clinical features. Lancet. 1994;**344**(8):1111-1115

[42] Bieluch V, Tally F. Pathophysiology of abscess formation. Clinics in Obstetrics and Gynaecology. 1983;**10**(1):93-103

[43] Hindi NK. Microbiology for Nurses. 1st ed. Alsadiq Printer; 2018 (Chapter 2)

[44] Hirschmann J. Impetigo: Etiology and therapy. Current Clinical Topics in Infectious Diseases. 2002;**22**(3):42-51

[45] Darmstadt G, Lane A. Impetigo: An overview. Pediatric Dermatology. 1994;**11**(12):293-303

[46] Bisno A, Nelson K, Waytz P, Brunt J. Factors influencing serum antibody response in streptococcal pyoderma. Journal of Laboratory and Clinical Medicine. 1973;**81**(22):410-420

[47] Kaplan E, Wannamaker L. Suppression of the anti-streptolysin O response by cholesterol and by lipid extracts of rabbit skin. The Journal of Experimental Medicine. 1976;**144**(66):754-767

[48] Demidovich C, Wittler R, Ruff M, Bass J, Browning W. Im-petigo: Current etiology and comparison of penicillin, erythromycin, and cephalexin therapies. American Journal of Diseases of Children. 1990;**144**(54):1313-1315

[49] Bisno A, Stevens D. Streptococcal infections in skin and soft tissues. New England Journal of Medicine. 1996;**334**:240-245

[50] Chartier C, Grosshans E. Erysipelas: An update. International Journal of Dermatology. 1996;**35**:779-781

[51] Weinstein L, Le Frock J. Does antimicrobial therapy of streptococcal pharyngitis or pyoderma alter the risk of glomerulonephritis? The Journal of Infectious Diseases. 1971;**124**(1):229-231

[52] Dupuy A, Benchikhi H, Roujeau J. Risk factors for erysipelas of the leg (cellulitis): Case-control study. BMJ. 1999;**318**(212):1591-1594

[53] Dan M, Heller K, Shapira I, Vidne B, Shibolet S. Incidence of ery-sipelas following venectomy for coronary artery bypass surgery. Infection. 1987;**15**(6):107-108

[54] Baddour L. Breast cellulitis complicating breast conservation therapy. Journal of Internal Medicine. 1999;**24**(34):5-9

[55] Bouma J, Dankert J. Recurrent acute leg cellulitis in patients after radical vulvectomy. Gynecologic Oncology. 1988;**29**(21):50-57

[56] Semel J, Goldin H. Association of athlete's foot with cellulitis of the lower extremities: Diagnostic value of bacterial cultures of ipsi-lateral interdigital space samples. Clinical Infectious Diseases. 1996;**23**(32):1162-1164

[57] Eriksson B. Anal colonization of group Gb-hemolytic streptococci in relapsing erysipelas of the lower extremity. Clinical Infectious Diseases. 1999;**29**(21):1319-1320

[58] Committee on Infectious Diseases, American Academy of Pediatrics. Antimicrobial agents and related therapy. In: Pickering LK, editor. Red Book 2003 Report of the Committee on Infectious Diseases. Vol. 4(90). 26th ed. Elk Grove Village, IL: American Academy of Pediatrics; 2003. pp. 693-694

[59] Burman W, Cohn D, Reves R, Wilson M. Multifocal cellulitis and monoarticular arthritis as manifestations of *Helicobacter cinaedi* bacteremia. Clinical Infectious Diseases. 1995;**20**(22):564-570

[60] Perl B, Gottehrer N, Raveh D, Schlesinger Y, Rudensky B, Yinnon A. Cost-effectiveness of blood cultures for adult patients with cellulitis. Clinical Infectious Diseases. 1999;**29**(5):1483-1488

[61] Kielhofner M, Brown B, Dall L. Influence of underlying disease process on the utility of cellulitis needle aspirates. Archives of Internal Medicine. 1988;**148**(21):2451-2452

[62] Kirsner R, Pardes J, Eaglstein W, Falanga V. The clinical spectrum of lipodermatosclerosis. Journal of the American Academy of Dermatology. 1993;**28**(11):623-627

[63] Wang J, Liu Y, Cheng D. Role of benzathine penicillin G in prophylaxis for recurrent streptococcal cellulitis of the lower legs. Clinical Infectious Diseases. 1997;**25**(70):685-689

[64] Kasseroller R. Sodium selenite as prophylaxis against erysipelas in secondary lymphedema. Anticancer Research. 1998;**18**(212):2227-2230

[65] Diven D, Dozier S, Meyer D, Smith E. Bacteriology of inflamed and uninflamed epidermal inclusion cysts. Archives of Dermatology. 1998;**134**(217):49-51

[66] Zimakoff J, Rosdahl V, Petersen W, Scheibel J. Recurrent staphylococcal furunculosis in families. Scandinavian Journal of Infectious Disease. 1988;**20**(3):403-405

[67] Hedstrom S. Recurrent staphylococcal furunculosis: Bacteriological findings and epidemiology in 100 cases. Scandinavian Journal of Infectious Diseases. 1981;**13**(9):115-119

[68] Ma X, Ito T, Tiensasitorn C. Novel type of staphylococcal cassette chromosome mec identified in community-acquired methi-cillin-resistant *Staphylococcus aureus* strains. Antimicrobial Agents and Chemotherapy. 2002;**46**(21):1147-1152

[69] Centers for Disease Control and Prevention. Outbreaks of community-associated methicillin-resistant *Staphylococcus aureus* skin infections—Los Angeles County, California, 2002-2003. MMWR. Morbidity and Mortality Weekly Report. 2003;**52**(2):88-121

[70] Miller L, Perdreau-Remington F, Rieg G. Necrotizing fasciitis caused by community-associated methicillin-resistant *Staphylococcus aureusin* Los Angeles. The New England Journal of Medicine. 2005;**352**:1445-1453

[71] Lewis R. Necrotizing soft-tissue infections. Infectious Disease Clinics of North America. 1992;**6**(219):693-703

[72] Giuliano A, Lewis F, Hadley K, Blaisdell F. Bacteriology of necrotizing fasciitis. American Journal of Surgery. 1977;**13**(4):52-57

[73] Sissolak D, Weir W. Tropical pyomyositis. The Journal of Infection. 1994;**29**:121-127

[74] Eke N. Fournier's gangrene: A review of 1726 cases. The British Journal of Surgery. 2000;**87**:718-728

[75] Altemeier W, Fullen W. Prevention and treatment of gas gangrene. JAMA. 1971;**217**:806-813

[76] Stevens D, Bryant A, Adams K, Mader J. Evaluation of hyperbaric oxygen therapy for treatment of experimental *Clostridium perfringens* infection. Clinical Infectious Diseases. 1993;**17**(51):231-237

[77] Raff A, Kroshinsky D. Cellulitis: A review. JAMA. 2011;**316**(337):325-453

[78] Ellis H, Simonsen S, van Orman E, Hatch B. Cellulitis incidence in a defined population. Epidemiology and Infection. 2006;**134**(33):293-321

[79] Liu C, Bayer A, Cosgrove S. Clinical practice guidelines by the infectious diseases society of America for the treatment of methicillin-resistant *Staphylococcus aureus* infections in adults and children. Clinical Infectious Diseases. 2009;**52**(8):18-98

[80] Stevens D, Bisno A, Chambers H. Practice guidelines for the diagnosis and management of skin and soft tissue infections: 2014 update by the infectious diseases society of America. Clinical Infectious Diseases. 2014;**59**(7):147-212

[81] Bisno A, Stevens D. Streptococcal infections of skin and soft tissues. The New England Journal of Medicine. 1996;**334**(99):240-565

[82] Bruun T, Oppegaard O, Hufthammer K. Early response in cellulitis: A prospective study of dynamics and predictors. Clinical Infectious Diseases. 2016;**63**(34):1034-1112

[83] Eron L. Managing skin and soft tissue infections: Expert panel recommendations on key decision points. The Journal of Antimicrobial Chemotherapy. 2003;**98**(90001):3-17

[84] Bassetti M, Baguneid M, Bouza E, Dryden M, Nathwani D, Wilcox M. European perspective and update on the management of complicated skin and soft tissue infections due to methicillin-resistant *Staphylococcus aureus* after more than 10 years of experience with linezolid. Clinical Microbiology and Infection. 2014;**20**(4):3-18

[85] Zilberberg M, Chaudhari P, Nathanson B. Development and validation of a bedside risk score for MRSA among patients hospitalized with complicated skin and skin structure infections. BMC Infectious Diseases. 2012;**12**(1):154

[86] Suaya J, Eisenberg D, Fang C, Miller L. Skin and soft tissue infections and associated complications among commercially insured patients aged 0-64 years with and without diabetes in the U.S. PLoS One. 2013;**8**(4):60057-66809

[87] Fitch M, Manthey D, McGinnis H. Videos in clinical medicine. Abscess incision and drainage. The New England Journal of Medicine. 2007;**357**(11):20-55

[88] Woo P, Lum P, Wong S. Cellulitis complicating lymphoedema. European Journal of Clinical Microbiology & Infectious Diseases. 2000;**19**(31):294-319

[89] Peralta G, Padrón E, Roiz M. Risk factors for bacteremia in patients with limb cellulitis. European Journal of Clinical Microbiology & Infectious Diseases. 2006;**25**(44):619-787

[90] Perl B, Gottehrer N, Raveh D. Cost-effectiveness of blood cultures for adult patients with cellulitis. Clinical Infectious Diseases. 1999;**29**(43):1483-1534

[91] Torres J, Avalos N, Echols L. Low yield of blood and wound cultures in patients with skin and soft-tissue infections. The American Journal of Emergency Medicine. 2017;**350**(7):1159-1212

[92] Stamenkovic I, Lew P. Early recognition of potentially fatal necrotizing fasciitis. The use of frozen-section biopsy. New England Journal of Medicine. 1984;**310**(44):1689-1790

[93] Leppard B, Seal D, Colman G, Hallas G. The value of bacteriology and serology in the diagnosis of cellulitis and erysipelas. The British Journal of Dermatology. 1985;**112**(55):559-643

[94] Dryden M. Complicated skin and soft tissue infection. The Journal of Antimicrobial Chemotherapy. 2010;**65**(3):35-44

[95] Moet G, Jones R, Biedenbach D. Contemporary causes of skin and soft tissue infections in North America, Latin America, and Europe: Report from the SENTRY Antimicrobial Surveillance Program (1998-2004). Diagnostic Microbiology and Infectious Disease. 2007;**57**(1):7-13

[96] Gorwitz R. A review of community-associated methicillin-resistant *Staphylococcus aureus* skin and soft tissue infections. The Pediatric Infectious Disease Journal. 2008;**27**(1):1-7

[97] Loewen K, Schreiber Y, Kirlew M. Community-associated methicillin-resistant *Staphylococcus aureus* infection: Literature review and clinical update. Canadian Family Physician. 2017;**63**(7):512-520

[98] Katayama Y, Ito T, Hiramatsu K. A new class of genetic element, staphylococcus cassette chromosome mec, encodes methicillin resistance in *Staphylococcus aureus*. Antimicrobial Agents and Chemotherapy. 2000;**44**(6):1549-1555

[99] Napolitano L. Severe soft tissue infections. Infectious Disease Clinics of North America. 2009;**23**(3):571-591

[100] Pan A, Cauda R, Concia E. Consensus document on controversial issues in the treatment of complicated skin and skin-structure infections. International Journal of Infectious Diseases. 2010;**14**(4):39-53

[101] Kujath P, Kujath C. Complicated skin structure and soft tissue infections—Are we threatened by multi-resistant pathogens? European Journal of Medical Research. 2010;**15**(12):544-553

[102] Stevens D, Bisno A, Chambers H. Practice guidelines for the diagnosis and management of skin and soft tissue infections: 2014 update by the Infectious Diseases Society of America. Clinical Infectious Diseases. 2014;**59**(2):10-52

[103] Chinnock B, Hendey G. Irrigation of cutaneous abscesses does not improve treatment success. Annals of Emergency Medicine. 2015;**67**(3):379-383

[104] O'Malley G, Dominici P, Giraldo P. Routine packing of simple cutaneous abscesses is painful and probably unnecessary. Academic Emergency Medicine. 2009;**16**(5):470-473

[105] Stevens D. Dilemmas in the treatment of invasive *Streptococcus*

pyogenes infections. Clinical Infectious Diseases. 2003;**37**(21):341-343

[106] Kaul R, McGeer A, Norrby-Teglund A. Intravenous immunoglobulin therapy for streptococcal toxic shock syndrome: A comparative observational study. Clinical Infectious Diseases. 1999;**28**:800-807

[107] Darenberg J, Ihendyane N, Sjolin J. Intravenous immunoglobulin G therapy in streptococcal toxic shock syndrome: A European randomized, double-blind, placebo-controlled trial. Clinical Infectious Diseases. 2003;**37**(95):333-340

[108] Clarke J. Toothaches and death. Journal of the History of Dentistry. 1999;**47**(7):11-13

[109] Carter L, Starr D. Alarming increase in dental sepsis. British Dental Journal. 2006;**200**(4):243-299

[110] Azodo C, Chukwumah N, Ezeja E. Dentoalveolar abscess among children attending a dental clinic in Nigeria. Odonto-stomatologie Tropicale. 2012;**35**(32):41-46

[111] Kaur J. Dental education and oral health problems in India. Indian Journal of Dental Education. 2009;**2**(21):167-171

[112] Siqueira J, Rôças I. Diversity of endodontic microbiota revisited. Journal of Dental Research. 2009;**88**(3):969-981

[113] González-García R, Risco-Rojas R, Román-Romero L, Moreno-García C, López GC. Descending necrotizing mediastinitis following dental extraction. Radiological features and surgical treatment considerations. Journal of Cranio-Maxillofacial Surgery. 2011;**39**(12):335-339

[114] Hersh A. National trends in ambulatory visits and antibiotic prescribing for skin and soft-tissue infections. Archives of Internal Medicine. 2008;**168**(14):1585-1591

[115] EFSA. The European Union summary report on trends and sources of zoonoses. Zoonotic agents and food-borne outbreaks in 2016. EFSA Journal. 2017;**15**(12):5077

[116] Oyston P, Sjostedt A, Titball R. Tularaemia: Bioterrorism defence renews interest in *Francisella tularensis*. Nature Reviews Microbiology. 2004;**2**(12):967-978

[117] Tomaso H, Hotzel H, Otto P, Myrtennas K, Forsman M. Antibiotic susceptibility in vitro of *Francisella tularensis* subsp. *holarctica* isolates from Germany. Journal of Antimicrobial Chemotherapy. 2017;**72**(9):2539-2543

[118] Choi Y, Kim D, Lee D, Lee J, Lee E, Lee S, et al. Clinical characteristics and incidence of perianal diseases in patients with ulcerative colitis. Annals of Coloproctology. 2018;**34**(3):138-143

[119] Amato A, Bottini C, De Nardi P, Giamundo P, Lauretta A, Realis Luc A, et al. Italian society of colorectal surgery. Evaluation and management of perianal abscess and anal fistula: A consensus statement developed by the Italian Society of Colorectal Surgery (SICCR). Techniques in Coloproctology. 2015;**19**(10):595-606

[120] Nguyen V, Jiang D, Hoffman S, Guntaka S, Mays J, Wang A, et al. Impact of diagnostic delay and associated factors on clinical outcomes in a U.S. inflammatory bowel disease cohort. Inflammatory Bowel Disease. 2017;**23**(10):1825-1831

[121] Patani N, MacAskill F, Eshelby S, Omar A, Kaura A, Contractor K, et al. Best-practice care pathway for improving management of mastitis and breast abscess. British Journal of Surgery. 2018;**105**(12):1615-1622

[122] Leung S. Breast pain in lactating mothers. Hong Kong Medical Journal. 2016;**22**(4):341-346

[123] Rao R, Ludwig K, Bailey L, Berry T, Buras R, Degnim A, et al. Select choices in benign breast disease: An initiative of the American Society of Breast Surgeons for the American Board of Internal Medicine Choosing Wisely® campaign. Annals of Surgical Oncology. 2018;**25**(10):2795-2800

[124] Liver Abscess Definition in Medical Conditions Dictionary. 2018. Available from: medconditions.net [Accessed: April 11, 2018]

[125] Medline Plus Encyclopedia Pyogenic liver abscess. Skin abscess. Hong Kong Medical Journal. 2012;**21**(10):323-432

[126] Webb G, Thomas P, Cadman P, Gorard D. Pyogenic liver abscess. Frontline Gastroenterology. 2014;**5**(1):60-67

[127] Akhondi H, Sabih D. Liver Abscess. Vol. 3(12). StatPearls: StatPearls Publishing; 2019. pp. 431-490

[128] Nicolosi A, Hauser W, Musicco M, Kurland L. Incidence and prognosis of brain abscess in a defined population: Olmsted County, Minnesota, 1935-1981. Neuroepidemiology. 1991;**10**(34):122-131

[129] Helweg-Larsen J, Astradsson A, Richhall H, Erdal J, Laursen A, Brennum J. Pyogenic brain abscess, a 15 year survey. BMC Infectious Diseases. 2012;**12**(21):332-400

[130] Yen D, Hu S, Tsai J, Kao W, Chern C, Wang L. Renal abscess: Early diagnosis and treatment. The American Journal of Emergency Medicine. 1999;**17**:192-197

[131] Meng M, Mario L, McAninch J. Current treatment and outcomes of perinephric abscesses. Journal of Urology. 2002;**168**(1):1337-1340

[132] Anderson K, McAninch J. Renal abscesses: Classification and review of 40 cases. Urology. 1980;**16**:333-338

[133] Siegel J, Smith A, Moldwin R. Minimally invasive treatment of renal abscess. Journal of Urology. 1996;**155**(23):52-55

Chapter 10

Bacteriophages as Anti-Methicillin Resistant *Staphylococcus aureus* Agents

Simone Ulrich Picoli, Nicole Mariele Santos Röhnelt and Tiago Sfredo Schenkel

Abstract

Staphylococcus aureus is a colonizing microorganism of the nasal region of both humans and animals and represents an important opportunistic pathogen. The acquisition of the mecA and mecC genes by *S. aureus* led to the emergence of methicillin resistance (MRSA), becoming a public health problem in both human and animal areas. In addition to resistance to β-lactam antibiotics, MRSA strains have multidrug resistance to antimicrobials, significantly limiting therapeutic options, making it crucial to have effective alternatives for treating staphylococcal infections. In this context, the use of lytic bacteriophages, which are viruses that infect and lyse bacteria, as well as the use of their by-products, such as endolysins, has shown potential in the control of *S. aureus*, including MRSA. Due to the specificity of bacteriophages to infect particular prokaryotic hosts, these viruses represent an antibacterial resource for the control of public health relevant microorganisms, especially antibiotic-resistant bacteria.

Keywords: Methicillin resistant *Staphylococcus aureus*, MRSA, phage, phage therapy, phage by-products

1. Introduction

1.1 The role of *S. aureus* in human and animals

Among the different relevant bacterial genus in Veterinary and Human Medicine, *Staphylococcus* is one of the most frequent opportunist pathogens. The species belonging to this genus present themselves as Gram positive cocci and are related to different communitarian and nosocomial infections, in both humans and animals. The members of *Staphylococcus* spp., especially *Staphylococcus aureus*, are constituents of the normal microbiota of the skin, mucous membranes, and upper respiratory tract of humans [1]. Although *S. aureus* is not considered part of the microbiota of dogs, indexes of 5% [2], 10% [3, 4], and even 20% [5] of nasal colonization by the bacterium were described in canines. Similarly, the cats also are included among the pet target-species potentially colonized by *S. aureus* due to their close proximity to humans, as pets [6]. In the context of proximity, the coexistence between man and dogs is still closer in order of canine aptitudes additional to the condition of the pet, as guide dogs, hunting dogs, guard dogs, among others. Thus,

IntechOpen

the pets share daily routines with their owners, establishing affective bonds that emphasizes the importance of the control of transmissible diseases inter-species.

Historically, the first publications related to the human carriage of *S. aureus*, emerged in mid-1940s [7] and showed the relevance of the bacteria in the human infections. On the other side, the approach to this theme in the vet sphere was only evidenced from the year 2000. Regardless, *S. aureus* has zoonotic potential [8], being even more relevant when the bacteria is methicillin-resistant (Methicillin Resistant *S. aureus* or MRSA). The transmission of this emerging zoonotic pathogen among pets and humans [9], including veterinary staff, has been demonstrated [10, 11], implying problems in the public health sphere [12]. In addition, the risk of zoonotic transmission of *S. aureus* may impact directly in the relation between humans and animals, harming the strength of the affective bond. Additionally, the expressive occupational health risk to veterinary professionals must also be considered [13].

1.2 Infections related to *S. aureus* and Methicilli Resistant *S. aureus* (MRSA)

S. aureus is one of the most structured species in order of the high frequency as etiological agent of infections, as well as the growing prevalence of its resistance to antimicrobials [14]. The health complications arising of the infection by *S. aureus* in humans and animals are diversified and depend on intrinsic factors to the bacteria (virulence factors as extracellular enzymes, capsular polysaccharides, surface-associated proteins), as well as the conditions inherent to the host. Clinically, they can limit themselves to localized skin infections, but can cause severe illnesses as septicemia, respiratory tract infections, osteomyelitis, endocarditis, besides food poisoning [9]. Along with the severity of the bacterial infections, the other factor that compromises the recovery of the infected individuals is the bacteria antimicrobial resistance profile. The higher the degree of resistance, the higher will be the restriction to therapeutic alternatives to the treatment of the infection, there may not even be an effective drug. In this regard, the World Health Organization (WHO) suggested in 2017, a list of resistant bacteria considered more relevant in order of antibiotics shortage to treat the diseases. The specialists grouped the pathogens accordingly with the bacterial species and the resistance type shown, resulting in three priority tiers: critical, high, and medium, being Methicillin-Resistant *S. aureus* considered high priority [15].

1.3 Perspectives to MRSA infections treatment

Alternatively, with the development of the new antibiotics to supplant the resistance, there is the possibility of using viral agents to control unwanted bacteria. Viruses termed "bacteriophages" or "phages" are the most abundant agents in the environment and are host-specific, i.e., they infect only prokaryotes that have their own specific receptors for their adsorption. The absence of such receptors makes phage binding to the target cell as well as subsequent infection impossible, characterizing the specificity of these viruses [16, 17]. Phages are easily recovered from soil, sewage, and feces and their numbers are about 3 to 10 times higher than bacterial counts even though variations exist between ecosystems [18, 19]. Like other viruses, bacteriophages are obligate intracellular, and are characterized according to the replication cycle exhibited after infection of the bacterial host. The cycle can be lytic or lysogenic, but only phages that exclusively perform the lytic cycle are of interest for use as therapeutic agents, since they will promote cell lysis at the end of the cycle [18].

2. Methicillin resistant *Staphylococcus aureus* (MRSA)

2.1 What is MRSA?

The *Staphylococcus* genus consists of a variety of opportunistic pathogens of variable relevance in veterinary medicine, being the coagulase-positive *S. aureus* and members of the group *Staphylococcus intermedius*, particularly *Staphylococcus pseudointermedius,* the most important clinically [13]. In human medicine, *S. aureus* can cause clinical manifestations ranging from mild skin and soft tissue infections to severe bloodstream infections. A remarkable skill of this genus is its capacity to acquire antibiotic resistance [20], mainly from the irrational increase in the intensity of its use [21]. Methicillin resistant *S. aureus* (MRSA) are resistant to an important range of antibiotics [20]. The resistance to methicillin, conferred by the presence of the *mec*A or *mec*C gene, is of particular relevance. These genes, located in Staphylococcal Chromosomal Cassette (*SCCmec*) confer the methicillin resistance [22] and codify the production of a penicillin-binding protein (PBP) with low affinity to beta-lactams antibiotics, such penicillin, cephalosporins, and carbapenems [20, 23].

2.2 Laboratory detection of MRSA

Phenotypic tests for laboratory identification of *Staphylococcus* species are relatively simple, with the employment of the catalase and coagulase tests, both positive. However, definitive confirmation requires the employment of additional tests or the Matrix Assisted Laser Desorption Ionization - Time Of Flight Mass Spectrometry (MALDI-TOF) [24], since both *S. aureus* and *S. pseudintermedius* (in addition to other species of staphylococci, such as *S. lugdunensis*) are coagulase positive. The detection of *mec*A and *mec*C genes by polymerase chain reaction (PCR) is also a complementary alternative for the correct identification of methicillin resistant species [25]. Alternatively, phenotypic tests to confirm methicillin resistance are often performed because they have low cost and reliable results. In this context, the behavior of the bacteria is evaluated by disk-diffusion on Mueller Hinton agar with 30 μg Cefoxitin disk for *S. aureus* (MRSA) [24]. The test consists of preparing a bacterial suspension in sterile 0.9% NaCl with density equivalent to 0.5 McFarland standard (1.5 x 10^8 CFU/mL). Next, a cotton swab is soaked in the freshly prepared solution and is seeded on the Mueller Hinton agar surface. After application of the antimicrobial disks and appropriate incubation (35°C/24 hours), the behavior against the antibiotics is verified according to the measurements of the inhibition halos formed around the tested disks [21], and it is interpreted according to the current reference guidelines used in each health service.

2.3 MRSA colonization and MRSA infection

Historically MRSA was described in humans in 1961 [26], while MRSA colonization and infection in animals was first reported in 1972 in asymptomatic dogs in Nigeria and a case of bovine mastitis in Belgium [23]. Around 25–30% of the human population is asymptomatically colonized by *S. aureus* in their nostrils [22, 27]. Humans and animals with nasal colonization by *S. aureus* and MRSA are considered to be at higher risk for developing infections and transmission of bacteria and, since colonization usually precedes infection [26]. In this sense, there is a great public health concern because domestic animals are potential reservoirs of these pathogens, with subsequent transmission to humans. The colonization of people in contact with colonized animals has been described. In addition, it has been shown that transmission can occur from animal to human as well as from human to animal [20]. The epidemiological success of *S. aureus*-related pathogens depends not only on its ability to produce virulence factors but also on its *fitness*, that is, its ability to grow and persist in its hosts, promoting colonization [28].

It is now well established that MRSA isolates are often non-susceptible to different classes of antibiotics and are considered multidrug-resistant (MDR) when resistance is observed for at least three different classes of antimicrobials [25]. The great adaptability of this pathogen is due to its expressive genetic plasticity, in which approximately 25% of the *S. aureus* chromosome consists of mobile genetic elements, such as chromosomal cassettes, transposons, plasmids, and bacteriophages, which can be acquired through horizontal transfer [29].

When human MRSA infections persist, worsen, or recur despite surgical treatment, additional use of systemic antibiotic therapy is required [27]. Different clinical treatment options are available to combat MRSA infections, including vancomycin. Although this drug is the main therapeutic option, there are several limitations in its use, such as the achievement of optimal serum concentration, long-term treatment, renal toxicity, and restricted route of administration (intravenous) [30]. In the veterinary field, there is no effective therapy to treat MRSA infections, so prevention and control measures are critical to contain the further spread of MRSA [21]. While this challenge remains unresolved, successful treatment of infections may require the development of new antibiotics and the use of bacteriophages and phage-derived lytic proteins [29] as alternative therapeutic resources.

2.4 Bacteriophages as anti-MRSA agents

With the emergence of MRSA, staphylococcal infections have become difficult to control. MRSA is typically resistant to beta-lactams and can even present resistance to other antimicrobials [20], thus requiring new therapeutic alternatives. In this sense, phage therapy resurfaces as a promising tool for the control of unwanted bacteria, since it consists of the use of viruses, called bacteriophages, capable of infecting and killing prokaryotes without harming human or animal cells.

2.4.1 What are bacteriophages?

Bacteriophages, also known as phages, are viruses that infect and lyse prokaryotes. They are considered the most numerous infectious entities on the planet, being found in different environmental matrices, such as sewage, water, soil, among others [31]. Phages have been proposed as an alternative resource to the problem of resistant bacteria since they infect bacterial cells and, at the end of their reproduction cycle, promote the lysis of the host bacterium [18, 32]. After their discovery in 1917, phages were successfully used for the treatment of several bacterial infections [31]. However, the advent of antibiotics and their industrial-scale production, coupled with the lack of adequate studies and the poor understanding of phage biology at the time, resulted in the abandonment of studies related to these viruses as therapeutic agents in most institutions. A few places followed up on these studies, such as Eastern Europe, mainly Russia, Georgia, and Poland. Truly, the production and use of phages for prophylaxis and therapy never stopped in the last two countries mentioned [33]. From these countries emerged the main research in the phage therapy field.

Subsequently, the indiscriminate use of antibiotics enabled progressive bacterial resistance, leading to the resumption of studies with phages. Thus, bacteriophages and their products, such as enzymes released at the end of their replication cycle, were once again considered as therapeutic agents [32]. Phage therapy is the use of bacteriophages to eliminate bacterial pathogens, and fortunately, innovative research techniques have made several advances in the field possible. One of the most important discoveries has been the distinction between the replication cycles carried out by phages. The replication of these viruses occurs mainly through two cycles: the lysogenic and the lytic.

2.4.2 Phage replication: Lytic and lysogenic cycles

Frequently, *S. aureus* displays prophages inserted into its DNA and this viral genetic material contributes to bacterial adaptability once it encodes virulence and fitness factors [34]. Although most phages that infect *S. aureus* are temperate, i.e. lysogenic, some of them are strictly lytic and present potential for use as anti-staphylococcal agents. According to the International Committee on Taxonomy of Viruses (ICTV), phages with DNA genetic material belong to the order *Caudovirales* which comprises nine different families: *Siphoviridae, Myoviridae, Podoviridae, Herelleviridae, Drexlerviridae, Demerecviridae, Chaseviridae, Autographiviridae* and *Ackermannviridae* [35]. The phages described so far capable of infecting *S. aureus* belong to the first three families, of which *Myoviridae* and *Podoviridae* involve *S. aureus* phages whose cycle is exclusively lytic [36]. Phages from these families are characterized by having an icosahedral capsid, where the genetic material is located, and are differentiated by the type of tail they have, which can be long and flexible (*Siphoviridae*), long and retractable (*Myoviridae*) or short (*Podoviridae*) [18].

Regardless of the type of cycle (lytic or lysogenic) performed by the bacteriophage, the replication process will begin by the adsorption of the virus to receptors on the surface of the host cell wall. During the infection of Gram-positive bacteria, as is the case of *Staphylococcus* spp., proteins present in the fibers of the viral tail interact with the teichoic acids of the cell wall, and the teichoic acids found in *S. aureus* are distinct from those observed in other *Staphylococcus,* thus allowing the specific binding of the phage [37]. The absence of this receptor in the bacteria renders the phage unable to bind and start its replication cycle, giving the virus the characteristic of being host specific. After the irreversible binding of the phage to the bacterial proteins, the bacterial cell wall undergoes the action of enzymes associated with the phage tail tip complex, forming a pore in the bacterial wall through which the genetic material of the virus is ejected into the cell. In *Staphylococcus* phages of the *Myoviridae* family the ejection of the viral DNA is facilitated by the contraction of the tail sheath [38]; in *S. aureus Siphoviridae* phages occurs the action of enzymes associated with the phage tail tip complex [39] and in *S. aureus Podoviridae* phages are the putative cell wall-degrading enzymes located in the tail spike [40]. Once the viral DNA is inside the host, either the lytic or the lysogenic cycle will be performed according to the characteristics of the phage.

The lysogenic cycle is characterized by phages that are able to infect and integrate their genetic material into the DNA of the bacteria, thus forming a prophage. The ability to integrate its genetic material with the bacteria is due to the presence of genes that encode the integrase protein, an enzyme that mediates the recombination between the phage's DNA and that of the host [41]. Subsequently, proteins are produced that induce viral latency, implying a pause in the transcription of gene products, allowing the prophage to exist with the bacteria for several bacterial generations without major consequences. Furthermore, the prophage induces immunity in the bacteria against infection via new phages. Bacteriophages that exhibit this type of replication cycle are not suitable in the context of phage therapy, since at the end of the viral cycle the death of the bacteria will not necessarily occur. In addition, bacteriophages that perform the lysogenic cycle may be responsible for producing toxic substances and carrying resistance genes [32], implying benefits for the bacteria.

On the other hand, in the lytic cycle there is no integration of the phage genetic material to the prokaryote DNA. At the end of this viral replication cycle, when the new virions are already formed and ready to be released, there is the production of enzymes capable of lysing the bacteria cell wall, inducing bacterial rupture and death for the release of new virions. Therefore, phages whose replication cycle is lytic are the most suitable for use in phage therapy, precisely because they cause bacterial lysis [18]. The schematic representation of the lytic and lysogenic cycles in *S. aureus* is shown below (e.g., **Figure 1**).

2.4.3 History of phage therapy in S. aureus infections

The attempt to use phages for the treatment of infections caused by *S. aureus* began soon after the discovery of phage therapy, and it is likely that the first use was in six patients with skin diseases in 1921. After the discovery of antibiotics, the studies related to phage therapy were abandoned and the few that continued, conducted in Georgia, Russia, and Poland, included efforts to treat staphylococcal infections [31]. Although the main studies target the use of phage therapy in humans, phages have also been proposed for use in veterinary medicine. The first case of application of this therapy in animals was associated with d'Herelle, one of those responsible for the discovery of phages. In 1919, he used the viruses to contain an outbreak of lethal typhoid fever in chickens. After analyzing several dead animals, d'Herelle was able to identify *Salmonella* Gallinarum and after isolated a lytic bacteriophage for the bacterium in question [42]. In another study, *S. aureus* phages were tested in mice, but the results were unsatisfactory because the virus used was not able to protect against a lethal dose of the bacteria [42].

Studies with phages for the control of staphylococcal infections were continued in some regions of the world. In the United States (1952), a laboratory (Delmont Laboratories) licensed, for human use, a bacterial lysate produced from the

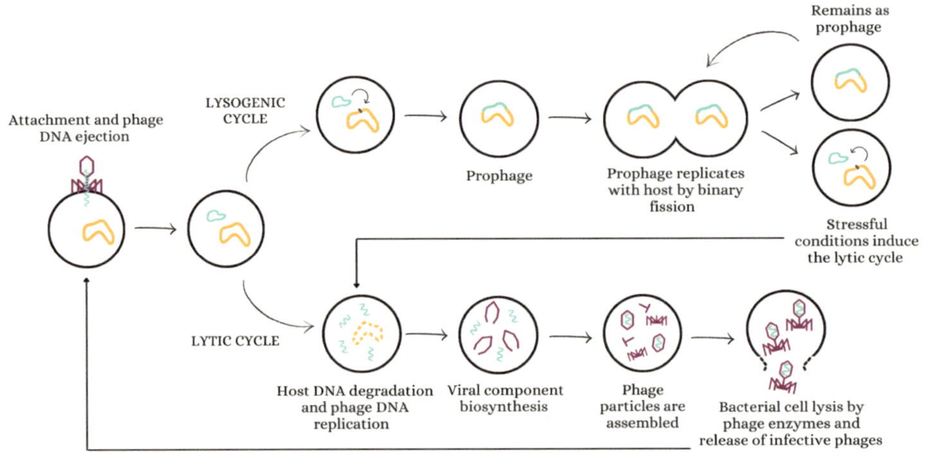

Figure 1.
Lytic and lysogenic cycles.

infection of bacteriophages in two virulent strains of *S. aureus.* Several years later, in 1986, the same product was licensed for veterinary use for the treatment of recurrent canine pyoderma but is no longer marketed for human use. This lysate, whose commercial name is "Staphage Lysate SPL", consists of bacterial cell wall fragments, intracellular components released during bacterial lysis, culture media ingredients, and viable bacteriophages. In 1981, it was demonstrated to be able to protect 80–100% of infected mice compared to the group not treated with SPL [43]. In dogs, SPL has been used effectively to treat chronic staphylococcal blepharitis as well, where weekly injections were administered to control the disease without adverse effects on the animals [44].

Because of the resistance of *S. aureus* to antimicrobials, some studies have sought to evaluate the activity of phages and their products against MRSA isolates. In 2008, one study evaluated the potential use of phages to eliminate or reduce nasal colonization by *S. aureus*, concluding that decolonization may be beneficial for certain patient groups, and phages were able to effectively combat induced infections in animal experiments [45]. A recent review concluded that phages are effective as topical antimicrobials against *S. aureus*, being able to combat MRSA in skin infections regardless of whether they are used with or without combination to topical antibiotics [46]. In addition to the phage itself being used as an antimicrobial agent, its products, such as lytic enzymes (endolysins), are also the subject of investigation. Phages and their products can be administered orally, inhaled, intravenously, subcutaneously, and topically, as suspensions for ocular use or application to bacteria-infected burns. The use of bacteriophages in therapeutics has advantages, mainly the high viral specificity that allows them to bind only to bacterial cells with the specific receptors, not affecting human or animal cells, thus avoiding significant side effects. Furthermore, phages can be used in the control of bacteria that show resistance to antibiotics [32]. Additionally, these viruses can adapt to the resistance mechanisms developed by bacteria, evolving in parallel to their host.

2.4.4 Commercial phage products anti-staphylococcal

Commercial products containing phages or enzymes produced by them are manufactured and available in some countries, mainly in Russia and Georgia, but also in Canada, the Netherlands and the Czech Republic. The following table (e.g., **Table 1**) gathers different commercial phage products, the target bacteria of each product, their main uses and the manufacturer [47–50].

In recent years, different studies involving commercial phage products with anti-staphylococcal activity have been undertaken. Most of them were related to *S. aureus Myoviridae* phages and demonstrated very promising results. Among them, it was shown that 100% (10/10) of multidrug resistant *S. aureus* isolates were lysed by Fersisi phage cocktail; 90% (9/10) were lysed by Instesti bacteriophage and 80% (8/10) by Pyo phage cocktail, showcasing the high lytic activity of commercial phage cocktails of Eliava BioPreparations, Georgia [51]. Similarly, 95% of clinical isolates of staphylococci, including 3 MRSA and 17 Methicillin susceptible *S. aureus* (MSSA) were sensitive to the action of Pyofag® polyvalent bacteriophage (Pharmex Group LLC, Ukraine for NeoProbioCare Inc.) Moreover, the same commercial phage cocktail was able to control furuncles in a patient with skin lesions by topical application of Pyofag®, as well as orally and nasally, for 14 days [52].

Some commercial products with the same name, but produced by different manufacturers, are proposed for the control of *S. aureus* in skin and wound infections, including Pyophage (polyvalent purified) cocktails from Microgen (Russia) and Pyophage from Eliava BioPreparations (Georgia). One study evaluated the performance of both cocktails against 20 MSSA and 31 MRSA clinical isolates

Product name	Active against	Informations/use	Manufacturer
Complex Pyo bacteriophage	*Staphylococcus, Streptococcus, Enterococcus, P. mirabilis, P. vulgaris, K. pneumoniae, K. oxytoca, P. aeruginosa,* enteropathogenic *E. coli*	Mix of sterile lysate phages. Used for the treatment of diseases of the eyes/ear/ nose, throat, infections of respiratory tract, lungs, surgical sites, urogenital, enteric, septic diseases. operational and newly infected wounds, for the prevention of hospital-acquired infections.	Microgen (Russia)
Fersisi bacteriophage	*S. aureus, S. epidermidis, S. pyogenes, S. sanguis, S. salivarius, S. agalactiae*	Sterile filtrate of phage lysates. Used for the treatment of otolaryngological diseases; infections of skin, urogenital, gynecologic, enteric, pyo-inflammatory disease in children (including newborns).	Eliava BioPreparations (Georgia)
Gladskin Acne, Gladskin Eczema, Gladskin Rosacea, Gladskin Shaving Irritation	*S. aureus,* Metichillin Resistant *S. aureus* (MRSA)	Endolysin XZ.700. Used for the treatment of skin disorders (acne, eczema, rosacea, psoriasis).	Micreos (Netherlands)
Intesti bacteriophage	*S. flexneri* serotypes 1,2,3,4, *S.* Paratyphi A and B, *E. coli, S.* Typhimurium, *S. enteritidis, P. vulgaris, S.* Cholerasuis, *S. sonnei, S.* Oranienburg, *P. mirabilis*	Mix of sterile filtrates of phage lysates. Used for the treatment of enteric infections.	Eliava BioPreparations (Georgia)
Intesti-bacteriophage	*S. flexneri* serotypes 1,2,3,4,6, *S. sonnei, S.* Paratyphi A and B, *S.* Typhymurium, *S.* Cholerasuis, *E. coli, S.* Oranienburg, *S. enteritidis, P. vulgaris, P. mirabilis, Enterococcus, Staphylococcus, P. aeruginosa*	Mixture of sterile filtrates of phage lysates. Used for the treatment of bacterial dysentery, dyspepsia, disbacteriosis, enterocolitis, colitis, salmonellosis.	Microgen (Russia)
Pyophage	*S. aureus, S. pyogenes, S. sanguis, S. salivarius, S. agalactiae, E. coli, P. aeruginosa, P. mirabilis, P. vulgaris*	Mix of sterile lysate phages. Used for the treatment of infections of upper respiratory tract, dermatological, surgical site, ocular urogenital, gastrointestinal, purulent septic infections in children, for prevention of post- operational complications and hospital infections.	Eliava BioPreparations (Georgia)

Product name	Active against	Informations/use	Manufacturer
Pyofag® polyvalent bacteriophage	*S. pyogenes, S. aureus, E. coli, P. aeruginosa, P. vulgaris, P. mirabilis*	Solution in vial with bacteriophages. Used for the treatment of pyoinflammatory diseases of ears, throat, nose, oral cavity, eyes, surgical infections, burn wounds; urogenital, gynecologic, and enteric infections.	Pharmex Group LLC (Ukraine) for NeoProbioCare Inc. (Canada)
Stafal ®	*S. aureus*, MRSA, including biofilms	Polyvalent bacteriophages of the family *Myoviridae* and genus *Kayvirus*.	Bohemia Pharmaceuticals (Czech Republic)
Staphefekt ™	*S. aureus* and MRSA	Endolysin XZ.700. Used for treatment of inflammatory skin conditions such as eczema, acne, rosacea, psoriasis.	Micreos (Netherlands)

Table 1.
Commercially available anti-S. aureus phage products.

and concluded that both products had greater than 75% coverage, but Microgen's Pyophage was extremely effective against MRSA, killing 97% of the bacterial isolates. Genomic analyses of the *S. aureus* phages contained in these commercial products revealed great similarities (*Myoviridae, Kyavirus* genus), however Microgen's cocktail additionally featured a *S. aureus Podoviridae* component that possibly contributed to the higher coverage observed against MRSA [53].

In a recent study, the action of Stafal® (a preparation with polyvalent bacteriophages active *on S. aureus)* on planktonic cells as well as on biofilms produced by MSSA and MRSA was demonstrated. Bacterial cells immersed in the biofilm required high phage concentrations and longer exposure time to be destroyed compared to planktonic forms [54]. It is likely that this occurred because of the difficulty of the phage to access the host cell surface within the biofilm matrix. Still, the phages were active on the biofilms, whereas antimicrobials are known to be ineffective due to the limitation of their diffusion through the extracellular polymeric substances matrix. Similarly, enzymes encoded by bacteriophages called endolysins have shown promising advances against bacterial biofilm formation. Such enzymes are responsible for lysis of the host bacterial cell wall promoting the release of viral progeny at the end of the replication cycle of lytic phages [55]. Experimental assays showed that the phage-derived lysine named "LysH5" was able to remove *S. aureus* biofilm, even eliminating persistent cells (subpopulation of cells that showed high resistance to antibiotics). During treatment of staphylococcal biofilm with LysH5 (0.15 μM), complete inhibition in biofilm formation was also seen in certain *S. aureus* isolates [56].

Commercially, the recombinant endolysins Staphefekt SA.100 and Staphefekt XDR.300 (Micreos Human Health BV, Netherlands) which act on *S. aureus* (including MRSA) are available for use. A few clinical studies have been conducted with Staphefekt SA.100 and all have demonstrated remission and/or improvement of chronic *S. aureus* skin infections (folliculitis, rosacea, and eczema) [57, 58], reinforcing the utility of this therapeutic resource. Moreover, it is believed that endolysins may be better therapeutic alternatives than bacteriophages themselves since bacteria have the possibility to develop resistance to the phage. On the other hand, it is necessary to consider that endolysins present limitations, such as: i) induction of inflammatory response of cytokines and neutralizing antibodies that imply the reduction of the half-life time (*in vivo*); ii) their systematic use *in vivo* will provoke an immune response that will promote the loss of the lytic activity of the enzyme [59]; iii) lower activity on Gram-negative bacteria due to the presence of the external membrane in the cell wall [60].

Other commercially available products are: Bronchophage, Otophage, Phagodent, Phagoderm, Phagogyn, Phagovet, Vetagyn (Micromir, Russia); ENKO bacteriophage, SES Bacteriophage, Staphylococcal bacteriophage (Eliava BioPreparations, Georgia); Dysentery bacteriophage, *E. coli* bacteriophage, *E. coli-Proteus* bacteriophage, *Klebsiella* purified polyvalent bacteriophage, Sextaphag® polyvalent pyo bacteriophage, *Streptococcus* bacteriophage (Microgen, Russia); Phagestaph, Phagyo, Septaphage (Biochimpharm, Georgia); and Intestifag® polyvalent bacteriophage (Pharmex Group LLC, Ukraine for NeoProbioCare Inc., Canada). Detailed information can be found in related sources [47–50].

2.4.5 Non-commercial anti-S. aureus bacteriophages

Fortunately, since the year 2000, different studies have contributed to a better understanding of phages as anti-*S. aureus* therapeutic agents. For example, the efficacy of the bacteriophage named ØMR11 against a lethal infection caused by *S. aureus* in mice was evaluated. Initially, the phage was isolated, had its bacteriolytic activity determined, and finally, *in vivo* infection experiments were performed by introducing *S. aureus* intraperitoneally, including MRSA strains, causing bacteremia and eventual death of the mice. After peritoneal administration of the isolated phage in infected animals, suppression of *S. aureus*-induced lethality occurred [61]. Similarly, the use of cloned lysins encoded by the phage ØMR11 was efficient in cell lysis, including MRSA. These lysins are enzymes produced at the end of the replication cycle of bacteriophages and are responsible for degrading the bacterial wall and releasing virions. After sequencing the phage ØMR11 the possible genes related to lysins were identified, these were cloned, and their protein products were purified on a large scale. The results showed high activity of lysins against MRSA isolates both in mice contaminated intranasally and subsequently treated with the intranasal lysins, as well in animals infected intraperitoneally, showing that the enzyme can be used for the control of *S. aureus* in humans and domestic animals [62].

A cocktail containing two bacteriophages, designated K and 44AHJD, was tested against clinical isolates of *S. aureus*, showing 85% of lytic action on the bacteria. The *in vivo* efficacy of the cocktail was evaluated through the murine nasal colonization model. Efficient decolonization was verified after eight days of intranasal administration in animals treated with the phage cocktail, while the control group (received only the bacteria) and the group treated with placebo remained colonized [63]. Although different studies have already demonstrated the efficiency of phages on *S. aureus*, few clinical trials have been conducted to validate their efficacy and safety. According to the records of clinical trials involving *S. aureus* and bacteriophages, in progress or already concluded [64] it appears that they are scarce and that few countries, mainly the U.S., have invested in clinical trials that corroborate the use of phages in clinical practice (e.g., **Figure 2**). The lack of large clinical studies that can effectively consolidate the use of phages *in vivo* is an obstacle to be overcome.

The Clinical Trials platform, a database of clinical studies conducted worldwide, reports the existence of eight studies related to the use of bacteriophages against *S. aureus* [64]. These are intended for the use of viruses for the treatment of ulcers infected by *S. aureus* in diabetic patients, prevention, and treatment of infection by *S. aureus* and other bacteria in burn patients, use for patients with covid-19

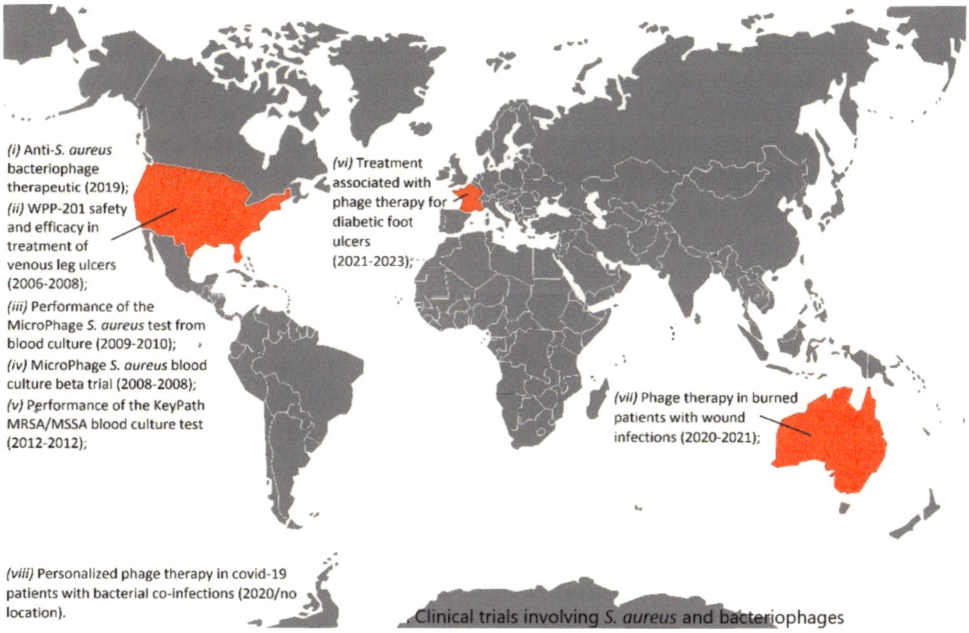

Figure 2.
Clinical trials involving S. aureus *and bacteriophages. Available at: www.pngwing.com*

affected with pneumonia or bacteremia/septicemia due *S. aureus* infection, use in patients with serious or immediate risk of life, and patients with venous leg ulcers. In addition, three studies that use phages as a diagnostic method. When considering regulatory measures for the application of phages as therapeutic agents, it is likely that, initially, such viruses are more easily used prophylactically in order to reduce the frequency of infections. In contrast, phage therapy aimed to eradicate systemic bacterial infections will inevitably be more complex [65].

2.4.6 Advantages and challenges of phage therapy

Among the principal attractive aspects of phage therapy, the main ones are: i) high specificity of the virus for the bacteria providing freedom from side effects on cells that are not targeted by the therapy; ii) activity against different bacteria, including multidrug resistant bacteria; iii) reduced treatment costs compared to antibiotic therapy; iv) prevention to the growth of secondary pathogens; v) ability to degrade bacterial biofilm by lysing bacteria; vi) high body distribution and vii) high efficacy compared to antimicrobials [32]. On the other hand, there are some limitations to the use of phages in therapy, among them: i) the possibility of antibody production by the immune system; ii) the difficulty of measuring the application dose; iii) the possibility of gene transfer among pathogens through phages, which may be responsible for passing pathogenic determinants and virulence factors, resulting in a possible resistance of bacteria; iv) the ability of bacteria to develop resistance against bacteriophages; v) elucidation of the correct route of administration and treatment time and vi) accurate and rapid diagnosis of the microorganism that is provoking the illness [32].

Fortunately, for all the limitations previously indicated, there are already studies that aim to circumvent these problems. For example, viral genome sequencing avoids the use of phages that are lysogenic or contain toxic and resistant genes. Along with this is the progressive search for new phages to be used if antibodies are produced by the immune system, or to replace phages for which the bacteria have become resistant. In addition, it is already known that viruses can mutate and adapt to resistance mechanisms created by bacteria. In other words, after the creation of barriers that make it impossible for the phage to replicate in the bacteria, changes occur in the viruses that allow their replication cycle to continue, even with the presence of the bacterial adaptations [32]. Further in this context, the use of new diagnostic resources allows the rapid differentiation of the disease-causing bacteria, in addition to the use of cocktails with different phages for the same bacterium, enhancing even more the specificity and avoiding the manifestation of resistance [32, 66].

3. Conclusions

MRSA represents a global threat due to its progressive resistance to antimicrobials, as well as the future prospect of no effective antibiotics. The use of lytic bacteriophages and their by-products are promising alternatives for bacterial control, since they infect and lyse the pathogen without the inconvenience of side effects, as well as contributing to lower consumption of antimicrobials, reflecting in the reduction of antibiotic resistance rates. The study of phages has always occurred in countries such as Georgia and Russia, where phage-based commercial products are relevant antibacterial alternatives. Although different *in vivo* studies have already evidenced the efficacy of phage therapy in prophylaxis and treatment of staphylococcal infections, including those caused by MRSA, some aspects should be considered before its clinical use. Among them, the restriction and scarcity of clinical trials along with the lack of robust randomized clinical trials evaluating the safety and efficacy of phage therapy are important limitations for the therapeutic use of these viruses. We highlight the need to foster studies in the area of phage therapy, especially given the scenario of increasing multi-resistant bacteria worldwide and the scarcity of new antimicrobial drugs.

Acknowledgements

The authors would like to thank Ana Carolina Klein for the graphic art.

Author details

Simone Ulrich Picoli*, Nicole Mariele Santos Röhnelt and Tiago Sfredo Schenkel
Feevale University, Novo Hamburgo, Brazil

*Address all correspondence to: simonepi@feevale.br

References

[1] Wertheim HF, Melles DC, Vos MC, van Leeuwen W, van Belkum A, Verbrugh HA, Nouwen JL. The role of nasal carriage in *Staphylococcus aureus* infections. Lancet Infectious Diseases. 2005;5(12):751-762. DOI: 10.1016/S1473-3099(05)70295-4

[2] Daley P, Bajgai J, Penney C, Williams K, Whitney H, Golding GR, Weese S. A cross sectional study of animal and human colonization with methicillin-resistant *Staphylococcus aureus* (MRSA) in an aboriginal community. BMC Public Health. 2016;16:595. DOI: 10.1186/s12889-016-3220-9

[3] Boost MV, O'Donoghue MM, James A. Prevalence of *Staphylococcus aureus* carriage among dogs and their owners. Epidemiology and infection. 2008;136(7):953-964. DOI: 10.1017/S0950268807009326

[4] Yunita MN, Effendi MH, Rahmaniar RP, Arifah S, Yanestria SM. Identification of spa gene for strain typing of methicillin resistant *Staphylococcus aureus* (MRSA) isolated from nasal swab of dogs. Biochemical Archives. 2020;2999-3004. DOI: 10.35124/bca.2020.20.S1.2999

[5] Gómez-Sanz E, Torres C, Ceballos S, Lozano C, Zarazaga M. Clonal dynamics of nasal *Staphylococcus aureus* and *Staphylococcus pseudintermedius* in dog-owning household members. Detection of MSSA ST^{398}. PLoS One. 2013;8(12):10.1371/annotation/8f8893cc-1367-410d-a450-d72a19a56643. DOI: 10.1371/journal.pone.0069337

[6] Deurenberg RH, Stobberingh EE. The evolution of *Staphylococcus aureus*. Infect Genet Evol. 2008;8(6):747-763. DOI: 10.1016/j.meegid.2008.07.007

[7] Gillespie EH, Devenish EA, Cowan ST. Pathogenic staphylococci: Their incidence in the nose and on the skin. Lancet, 1939; 870-873. DOI: 10.1016/S0140-6736(00)62957-4

[8] Tyasningsih W, Effendi MH, Budiarto B, Syahputra IR. Antibiotic resistance to *Staphylococcus aureus* and methicillin resistant *Staphylococcus aureus* (MRSA) isolated from dairy farms in Surabaya, Indonesia. The Indian Veterinary Journal. 2019;96(11):27-31. ISSN 0019-6479, E ISSN 0974-9365

[9] Algammal AM, Hetta HF, Elkelish A, Alkhalifah DHH, Hozzein WN, Batiha GE, El Nahhas N, Mabrok MA. Methicillin-resistant *Staphylococcus aureus* (MRSA): One health perspective approach to the bacterium epidemiology, virulence factors, antibiotic-resistance, and zoonotic impact. Infection and Drug Resistance. 2020;13:3255-3265. DOI: 10.2147/IDR.S272733

[10] Loeffler A, Pfeiffer DU, Lloyd DH, Smith H, Soares-Magalhaes R, Lindsay JA. Meticillin-resistant *Staphylococcus aureus* carriage in UK veterinary staff and owners of infected pets: New risk groups. The Journal of Hospital Infection. 2010;74(3):282-288. DOI: 10.1016/j.jhin.2009.09.020

[11] Feßler AT, Schuenemann R, Kadlec K, Hensel V, Brombach J, Murugaiyan J, Schwarz, S. Methicillin-resistant *Staphylococcus aureus* (MRSA) and methicillin-resistant *Staphylococcus pseudintermedius* (MRSP) among employees and in the environment of a small animal hospital. Veterinary Microbiology. 2018;221:153-158. DOI: 10.1016/j.vetmic.2018.06.001

[12] Reddy BS, Kumari KN, Sivajothi S. Methicillin-resistant *Staphylococcus aureus* (MRSA) isolated from dogs with recurrent pyoderma. Journal of Dairy, Veterinary & Animal Research.

2016;3(2):62-65. DOI: 10.15406/jdvar.2016.03.00073

[13] Weese JS, van Duijkeren E. Methicillin-resistant *Staphylococcus aureus* and *Staphylococcus pseudintermedius* in veterinary medicine. Veterinary Microbiology. 2010;140(3-4):418-429. DOI: 10.1016/j.vetmic.2009.01.039

[14] Rahmaniar RP, Yunita MN, Effendi MH, Yanestria SM. Encoding gene for methicillin resistant *Staphylococcus aureus* (MRSA) isolated from nasal swab of dogs. The Indian Veterinary Journal. 2020;97(2):37-40. ISSN 0019 - 6479, E - ISSN 0974 – 9365

[15] WHO. WHO publishes list of bacteria for which new antibiotics are urgently needed [Internet]. 2017. Available from: https://www.who.int/en/news-room/detail/27-02-2017-who-publishes-list-of-bacteria-for-which-new-antibiotics-are-urgently-needed [Accessed: 2021-01-17]

[16] Dowah ASA, Clokie MRJ. Review of the nature, diversity and structure of bacteriophage receptor binding proteins that target gram-positive bacteria. Biophysical Reviews. 2018;10(2):535-542. DOI: 10.1007/s12551-017-0382-3

[17] Silva JB, Storms Z, Sauvageau D. Host receptors for bacteriophage adsorption. FEMS Microbiology Letters. 2016;363(4):fnw002. DOI: 10.1093/femsle/fnw002

[18] Orlova E. Bacteriophages and their structural organisation. In: Kurtboke, I. editors. Bacteriophages. 1nd ed. Rijeka, Croatia: InTec; 2012; 3-30. DOI: 10.5772/1065

[19] Withey S, Cartmell E, Avery LM, Stephenson T. Bacteriophages: Potential for application in wastewater treatment processes. Science of The Total Environment. 2005;339(1-3):1-18. DOI: 10.1016/j.scitotenv.2004.09.021

[20] McGuinness WA, Malachowa N, DeLeo FR. Vancomycin resistance in *Staphylococcus aureus*. The Yale Journal of Biology and Medicine. 2017;90(2):269-281. PMID: 28656013 PMCID: PMC5482303

[21] Decline V, Effendi MH, Rahmaniar RP, Yanestria SM, Harijani N. Profile of antibiotic-resistant and presence of methicillin-resistant *Staphylococcus aureus* from nasal swab of dogs from several animal clinics in Surabaya, Indonesia. International Journal of One Health. 2020;6(1): 90-94. DOI: 10.14202/IJOH.2020.90-94

[22] Lindsay JA. Hospital-associated MRSA and antibiotic resistance-what have we learned from genomics? International Journal of Medical Microbiology. 2013;303(6-7):318-323. DOI: 10.1016/j.ijmm.2013.02.005

[23] Schmitt S, Stephan R, Huebschke E, Schaefle D, Merz A, Johler S. DNA microarray-based characterization and antimicrobial resistance phenotypes of clinical MRSA strains from animal hosts. Journal of Veterinary Science. 2020;21(4):e54. DOI: 10.4142/jvs.2020.21.e54

[24] Ma GC, Worthing KA, Gottlieb T, Ward MP, Norris JM. Molecular characterization of community-associated methicillin-resistant *Staphylococcus aureus* from pet dogs. Zoonoses Public Health. 2020;67(3): 222-230. DOI: 10.1111/zph.12677

[25] Horváth A, Dobay O, Sahin-Tóth J, Juhász E, Pongrácz J, Iván M, Fazakas E, Kristóf K. Characterisation of antibiotic resistance, virulence, clonality and mortality in MRSA and MSSA bloodstream infections at a tertiary-level hospital in Hungary: A 6-year retrospective study. Annals of Clinical Microbiology and Antimicrobials. 2020;19(1):17. DOI: 10.1186/s12941-020-00357-z

[26] Marshall C, Wesselingh S, McDonald M, Spelman D. Control of endemic MRSA-what is the evidence? A personal view. The Journal of Hospital Infection. 2004;56(4):253-268. DOI: 10.1016/j.jhin.2004.02.001

[27] Witte W. Community-acquired methicillin-resistant *Staphylococcus aureus*: What do we need to know? Clin Microbiol Infect. 2009;Suppl 7:17-25. DOI: 10.1111/j.1469-0691.2009.03097.x

[28] Otto M. Community-associated MRSA: what makes them special? International Journal of Medical Microbiology. 2013;303(6-7):324-330. DOI: 10.1016/j.ijmm.2013.02.007

[29] Salas M, Wernecki M, Fernández L, Iglesias B, Gutiérrez D, Álvarez A, García L, Prieto E, García P, Rodríguez A. Characterization of clinical MRSA isolates from northern Spain and assessment of their susceptibility to phage-derived antimicrobials. Antibiotics (Basel). 2020;9(8):447. DOI: 10.3390/antibiotics9080447

[30] Vanamala K, Tatiparti K, Bhise K, Sau S, Scheetz MH, Rybak MJ, Andes D, Iyer AK. Novel approaches for the treatment of methicillin-resistant *Staphylococcus aureus*: Using nanoparticles to overcome multidrug resistance. Drug Discovery Today. 2021;26(1):31-43. DOI: 10.1016/j.drudis.2020.10.011

[31] Guttman B, Raya R, Kutter E. Basic phage biology. In: Kutter E, Sulakvelidze A, editors. Bacteriophages: Biology and Applications. 4nd ed. 2005;42-79. DOI: 10.1201/9780203491751.ch3

[32] Wittebole X, De Roock S, Opal SM. A historical overview of bacteriophage therapy as an alternative to antibiotics for the treatment of bacterial pathogens. Virulence. 2014;5(1):226-235. DOI: 10.4161/viru.25991

[33] Klem J, Dömötör D, Schneider G, Kovács T, Tóth A, Rákhely G. Bacteriophage therapy against staphylococci. Acta Microbiologica et Immunologica Hungarica. 2013;60(4):411-422. DOI: 10.1556/AMicr.60.2013.4.3

[34] Lindsay, JA. Genomic variation and evolution of *Staphylococcus aureus*. International Journal of Medical Microbiology. 2010;300:98-103. DOI: 10.1016/j.ijmm.2009.08.013

[35] ICTV International Committee on Taxonomy of Viruses [Internet]. 2019. Available from: https://talk.ictvonline.org/ [Accessed: 2021-01-10]

[36] Azam AH, Tanji Y. Peculiarities of *Staphylococcus aureus* phages and their possible application in phage therapy. Applied Microbiology and Biotechnology. 2019;103(11):4279-4289. DOI: 10.1007/s00253-019-09810-2

[37] Winstel V, Liang C, Sanchez-Carballo P, Steglich M, Munar M, Broker BM, Penades JR, Nubel U, Holst O, Dandekar T, Peschel A, Xia G. Wall teichoic acid structure governs horizontal gene transfer between major bacterial pathogens. Nature Communications. 2013;4:2345. DOI: 10.1038/ncomms3345

[38] Leiman PG, Shneider MM. Contractile tail machines of bacteriophages. Advances in Experimental Medicine and Biology. 2012;726:93-114. DOI: 10.1007/978-1-4614-0980-9_5

[39] Davidson AR, Cardarelli L, Pell LG, Radford DR, Maxwell KL. Long noncontractile tail machines of bacteriophages. Advances in Experimental Medicine and Biology. 2012;726:115-142. DOI: 10.1007/978-1-4614-0980-9_5

[40] Hrebík D, Štveráková D, Škubník K, Füzik T, Pantůček R, Plevka P. Structure

and genome ejection mechanism of Podoviridae phage P68 infecting *Staphylococcus aureus*. bioRxiv. 2019; 447052. DOI: 10.1101/447052

[41] Groth AC, Calos MP. Phage integrases: Biology and applications. Journal of Molecular Biology. 2004;335(3):667-678. DOI: 10.1016/j.jmb.2003.09.082. PMID: 14687564

[42] Sulakvelidze A, Barrow P. Phage therapy in animals and agribusiness. In: Kutter E, Sulakvelidze A, editors. Bacteriophages: Biology and Applications. 4nd ed. 2005;326-371. DOI: 10.1201/9780203491751.ch13

[43] Esber HJ, DeCourcy SJ Jr, Bogden AE. Specific and nonspecific immune resistance enhancing activity of staphage lysate. Journal of Immunopharmacology. 1981;3(1):79-92. DOI: 10.3109/08923978109026420

[44] Chambers ED, Severin GA. Staphylococcal bacterin for treatment of chronic staphylococcal blepharitis in the dog. Journal of the American Veterinary Medical Association. 1984;185(4):422-425. PMID: 6469840

[45] Mann NH. The potential of phages to prevent MRSA infections. Research in Microbiology. 2008;159(5):400-405. DOI: 10.1016/j.resmic.2008.04.003

[46] Moghadam MT, Khoshbayan A, Chegini Z, Farahani I, Shariati A. Bacteriophages, a new therapeutic solution for inhibiting multidrug-resistant bacteria causing wound infection: Lesson from animal models and clinical trials. Drug Design, Development and Therapy. 2020;14:1867-1883. DOI: 10.2147/DDDT.S251171

[47] Bacteriophages[Internet]. 2021. Available from: https://bacteriophages.info/en/bacteriophage/ [Accessed: 2021-02-20]

[48] Biochimpharm [Internet]. 2021. Available from: http://biochimpharm.ge; [Accessed: 2021-02-20]

[49] Eliava Biopreparations [Internet]. 2021. Available from: http://phage.ge; [Accessed: 2021-02-20]

[50] Bacteriophage products [Internet]. 2021. Available from: https://www.bacteriophage.news/phage-products [Accessed: 2021-02-20]

[51] Ozkan I, Akturk E, Yeshenkulov N, Atmaca S, Rahmanov N, Atabay HI. Lytic activity of various phage cocktails on multidrug-resistant bacteria. Clinical and Investigative Medicine. 2016;39(6):S66-S70. PMID: 27917795

[52] Poniatovskyi V, Bondarchuk O, Prystupiuk M, Smikodub O, Shyrobokov V. Bacteriophages against methicillin resistant *Staphylococcus aureus* strains. Medical Perspectives. 2020;25(4):73-80. DOI: 10.26641/2307-0404.2020.4.221232

[53] McCallin S, Sarker SA, Sultana S, Oechslin F, Brüssow H. Metagenome analysis of Russian and Georgian Pyophage cocktails and a placebo-controlled safety trial of single phage versus phage cocktail in healthy *Staphylococcus aureus* carriers. Environmental Microbiology. 2018;20(9):3278-3293. doi: 10.1111/1462-2920.14310

[54] Dvořáčková M, Růžička F, Dvořáková Heroldová M, Vacek L, Bezděková D, Benešík M, Petráš P, Pantůček R. Therapeutic potential of bacteriophages for staphylococcal infections and selected methods for in vitro susceptibility testing of staphylococci. Epidemiol Mikrobiol Imunol. 2020;69(1):10-18. PMID: 32326711

[55] Abdelrahman F, Easwaran M, Daramola OI, Ragab S, Lynch S, Oduselu TJ, Khan FM, Ayobami A,

Adnan F, Torrents E, Sanmukh S, El-Shibiny A. Phage-encoded Endolysins. Antibiotics. 2021;10(2):124. DOI:10.3390/antibiotics10020124

[56] Gutiérrez D, Ruas-Madiedo P, Martínez B, Rodríguez A, García P. Effective removal of staphylococcal biofilms by the Endolysin LysH5. PLoS One. 2014;9(9): e107307. DOI: 10.1371/journal.pone.0107307

[57] Totté JEE, van Doorn MB, Pasmans SGMA. Successful treatment of chronic *Staphylococcus aureus*-related dermatoses with the topical Endolysin Staphefekt SA.100: A report of 3 cases. Case Reports in Dermatoly. 2017;9(2): 19-25. DOI:10.1159/000473872

[58] de Wit J, Totté JEE, van Mierlo MMF, van Veldhuizen J, van Doorn MBA, Schuren FHJ, Willemsen SP, Pardo LM, Pasmans SGMA. Endolysin treatment against *Staphylococcus aureus* in adults with atopic dermatitis: A randomized controlled trial. Journal of Allergy and Clinical Immunology. 2019;144(3):860-863 DOI: 10.1016/j.jaci.2019.05.020

[59] Fischetti VA. Bacteriophage lysins as effective antibacterials. Current Opinion in Microbiology. 2008;11(5):393-400. DOI: 10.1016/j.mib.2008.09.012

[60] Gajdács M. The concept of an ideal antibiotic: Implications for drug design. Molecules. 2019;24(5):892. DOI: 10.3390/molecules24050892

[61] Matsuzaki S, Yasuda M, Nishikawa H, Kuroda M, Ujihara T, Shuin T, Shen Y, Jin Z, Fujimoto S, Nasimuzzaman MD, Wakiguchi H, Sugihara S, Sugiura T, Koda S, Muraoka A, Imai S. Experimental protection of mice against lethal *Staphylococcus aureus* infection by novel bacteriophage phi MR11. The Journal of Infectious Diseases. 2003;187(4):613-624. DOI: 10.1086/374001

[62] Rashel M, Uchiyama J, Ujihara T, Uehara Y, Kuramoto S, Sugihara S, Yagyu K, Muraoka A, Sugai M, Hiramatsu K, Honke K, Matsuzaki S. Efficient elimination of multidrug-resistant *Staphylococcus aureus* by cloned lysin derived from bacteriophage phi MR11. The Journal of Infectious Diseases. 2007;196(8):1237-1247. DOI: 10.1086/521305

[63] Narasimhaiah MH, Asrani JY, Palaniswamy SM, Bhat J, George SE, Srinivasan R, Vipra A, Desai SN. Therapeutic potential of staphylococcal bacteriophages for nasal decolonization of *Staphylococcus aureus* in mice. Advances in Microbiology. 2013;3(1):52-60. DOI: 10.4236/aim.2013.31008

[64] Clinical Trials [internet] 2021. Available from: www.clinicaltrials.gov [Accessed: 2021-12-20]

[65] Jassim SA, Limoges RG. Natural solution to antibiotic resistance: Bacteriophages 'The living drugs'. World Journal of Microbiology & Biotechnology. 2014;30(8):2153-2170. DOI: 10.1007/s11274-014-1655-7

[66] Sulakvelidze A, Alavidze Z, Morris Jr JG. Bacteriophage therapy. Antimicrobial Agents and Chemotherapy. 2001;45(3):649-659. DOI: 10.1128/AAC.45.3.649-659.2001

Chapter 11

Antimicrobial Resistance Leading to Develop Livestock-Associated Methicillin-Resistant *S. aureus*, and Its Impact on Human, Animal, and Environment

Muhammad Farooq, Ifra Siddique and Zia Ullah

Abstract

The most important microbe in humans is *Staphylococcus aureus*, which has caused worldwide dispersion in both nosocomial and community settings. The impact of Gram-positive *Staphylococcus Aureus* on the host is extremely detrimental to illness development. The life form is noteworthy for its ability to receive anti-toxin protection from a variety of anti-toxin classes. The development and distribution of methicillin-resistant *Staphylococcus Aureus* (MRSA) strains, which are generally multi-drug resistant in clinics and, as a result, in the population, cause severe mortality and bleakness. The research of MRSA illness transmission has advanced since its underlying event, which necessitates a complete clinical approach to dealing with take on this microorganism. For long term use drug of choice is vancomycine nevertheless its efficacy has been put to the test by rise in opposition. More modern anti-MRSA anti-infection medicines have been approved for clinical usage in the last 10 years or so. The aim of this chapter is to offer related data on the genus Staphylococcus and the evolution of antibiotic resistance in addition a discussion of the most important antibiotic resistance mechanisms. Although they are notorious for causing anti-infection blockage, there is a constant need for exploring innovative MRSA antagonists from various sources, including plants, and assessing non-anti-toxin draws close.

Keywords: antibiotics, staphylococci, MRSA, environment, livestock infection

1. Introduction

Staphylococci are most seen in humans and other animals. They were usually separated into two groups based on their size to collect blood plasma. The most pathogenic species, *S. aureus*, is established by coagulase-positive staphylococci. There are currently over 30 distinct types of coagulase-negative staphylococci (CNS). CNS constant skin commensals, even though a few animal species can produce adulterations. It is now evident that the separation of staphylococci into positive and negative strains is unnatural and, at times, misleading. Coagulation is a marker for *S. aureus*; however, there is no immediate confirmation that it is a virulence factor [1]. Similarly, several of *S. aureus*'s distinctive secludes are defective in it. In any event, the span is still widely used by clinical microbiologists. Some of it binds to protein and polysaccharides, which are linked to virulence. The combined effect of various factors transmitted during illness causes harm [2]. Antibodies for staphylococcal toxins and compounds neutralize them; however, vaccines are not available. Antimicrobial therapy and clinical drainage are commonly required to treat blisters, massive bubbles, and looping illnesses. These are difficult to treat with anti-toxins alone and frequently necessitate the removal of the device. A rare strain in which hospitalized patients are resistant to the maximal usage of antibiotics for contaminations, vancomycin is the final medicine to which opposition has not been produced [3].

2. Strains of *S. aureus*

Although *S. aureus* is normally a commensal part of the human microbiota, its role sometime as opportunistic pathogen, which causes several diseases in skin as abscesses, sinusitis as respiratory diseases, and food poisoning. Pathogenic strains regularly promote infections by causing virulence causes including strong protein toxins and the creation of a cell-surface protein that attaches to and deactivates antibodies. The enhancement of antibiotic-resistant types of *Staphylococcus aureus*, such as methicillin-resistant *Staphylococcus aureus* (MRSA), is a worldwide scientific problem. Even though there are wide investigation and expansion, no *S. aureus* vaccine has been approved. There are now 32 species and the genus Staphylococcus has eight subspecies, numerous of which specially inhabit the human body, although *Staphylococcus aureus* and *Staphylococcus epidermidis* are the two most explained and examined strains.

3. Staphylococcal infections in humans

S. aureus disease are normally pyogenic and severe, and if not treated, they can disperse to neighboring tissue or metastatic sites via bacteremia [2]. Several common diseases caused by *S. aureus* include furuncles or boils, cellulitis, impetigo, and post-operative wound diseases in several sites. *S. aureus* causes several skin and soft tissue disorders, including mastitis. Staphylococcal mastitis has received less attention than *S. aureus* suppurations in humans. According to estimates, 1–3% of nursing mothers suffer with mastitis. Infection usually appears two to three days after birth, with symptoms ranging from abscess formation to cellulitis development [4]. In extreme cases, general signs such as a common cold and fever may arise.

Toxic shock syndrome (TSS), and staphylococcal food poisoning are examples of staphylococcal diseases produced exclusively by the production of staphylococcal toxins. Enterotoxins are resistant to heat and may live circumstances that would normally destroy bacteria [5]. Furthermore, enterotoxins are resistant to the action of proteolytic enzymes and can remain active in the digestive tract after consumption [6, 7]. After consuming toxic food, nausea and vomiting ensue, and the incubation period is brief. Possible adverse effects include diarrhea, hypotension, and dehydration. Enterotoxin production has been found in *S. xylos*, *S. chromogenes*, *S. cohnii*, *S. pseudintermedius*, *epidermidis*, *S. lentus*, *S. lugdunensis*, *S. sciuri*, *S. saprophyticus*, *S. warneri*, and *S. hyicus*, among others [3, 6]. Approximately partial of the CNS species found to be involved for human diseases, particularly *S. epidermidis*, are often accountable for nosocomial and suppurative infections linked with prosthetic devices [8, 9]. The increased suppuration rate is related to the bacterium's ability to produce an extracellular polysaccharide. The development of the protective advantages and biofilms on bacteria is discussed in further detail below.

Joint infections, septicemia, urinary tract infections, peritonitis, infections, wound infections, and endocarditis are the second most common CNS conditions associated with human suppuration. Staphylococcus saprophyticus, another opportunistic bacterium, causes urinary tract infections in humans [2, 10].

As novel zoonotic pathogens, *S. lugdunensis* and *S. schleferi* identified. *Staphylococcus lugdunensis*, another human pathogen, has lately emerged as animal pathogen involved in respirational and skin diseases. It has previously been linked to skin infections as well as invasive diseases including osteomyelitis, endocarditis, and sepsis. *Staphylococcus schleiferi*, formerly related to skin infections in dogs, has recently been linked to human metastatic infection, endocarditis, and endophthalmitis [11, 12].

4. Staphylococcal infections in animals

The only bacteria that cause significant disease in animals are *Staphylococcus aureus*, *Staphylococcus epidermidis*, *Staphylococcus hyicus*, and *Staphylococcus pseudintermedius*. Other Staphylococcus species exist primarily correlated with devious animal infections. *S. aureus* produces septic arthritis in hens, as well as subcutaneous abscesses. *S. aureus* is a common cause of dermatitis in goats and sheep, and it can cause botryomycosis in horses and pigs, a persistent, suppurative granulomatous illness. *S. aureus*, like *S. pseudintermedius*, causes suppurative illnesses in companion animals. *Staphylococcus hyicus* causes exudative epidermitis, called as greasy pig sickness. In several countries, methicillin-resistant *S. pseudintermedius* is becoming a significant clinical issue in veterinary medicine [13].

Intramammary infection causes in different animals: Even though bovine IMIs are the most economically significant, staphylococci IMIs can generate substantial losses in locations where sheep and goats are raised for milk. Similarly, substantial financial losses have been reported in places where buffalo or camel milk is generated because of mastitis. Due to IMI problem, financial loss occurs in different ways—rejection of milk because of its poor quality or milk withdrawal after or before medication, high treatment fees, high labor cost all these include [12, 14]. Aside from the apparent economic losses caused by IMIs, there are sum of indirect expenditures that are difficult to measure. Subclinical diseases in a herd usually go undiagnosed, causing in a steady drop in milk supply and a reduction in total milk value. This results in a consistent loss of income surplus, even when found, can take a considerable amount money and time to cure [9].

This species *S. aureus* is possibly the most well-known mastitis pathogen because once infection occurs due to this species, its unable to treat and become persistent [15].

5. Structure

5.1 Taxonomy

RNA hybridization, ribosomal DNA (r-RNA), and approximately 16 oligonucleotide r-RNA analyses also reveal that Staphylococci compile family level infidelity. This social problem occurred in a wide group of Bacillus-Lactobacillus-Streptococcus, which described Gram-positive bacteria with low G + C DNA components. In any event, Biochemica discovered 30 different kinds of staphylococci [3, 16].

Eleven of these may be secured with individuals such as guests. *S. aureus* (nares) and *S. epidermidis* (nares, skin) are fundamental visitors with the highest pathogenic potential. *S. saprophyticus* (skin, occasionally) is another common cause of urine plot contamination. *S. hemolyticus, S. simulans, S. cohnii*, and *S. warter* are all bacteria. Furthermore, *S. lugdunensis* can cause illness in people [6].

5.2 Morphology

Gram-positive cells are found in *S. aureus* cells and appear to be in good health. When seen *via* a light magnifying device, they are frequently in bunches that resemble grapes after staining. The Greek name for these bacteria is 'Staphylococcus,' which means "in the shape of (staphyle) grapes packed with berry (kokkos)" [17]. Filtering electron small perception reveals primarily circular shaped cells with smooth surfaces [18]. The width of the cells ranges from 0.5 to 1.0 M [19]. On electron microscopy, a thick cell divider may be seen, as well as an obvious and shapeless cytoplasmic layer and shapeless cytoplasm [20].

5.3 Isolation and identification

The existence of staphylococci in a real-world problem can be linked from the start following testing with a second Gram stain. In any event, little amounts of microorganisms in blood obstruct minute examination and must be improved from the outset. Striking raw material from the clinical model into strong medium, such as different agar including blood, tryptic soy, or heart implantation, separates living things. Models that are at risk of being harmed by different bacteria can grow on mannitol salt agar containing 7.5% sodium chloride, which allows crown indulgent staphylococci to grow [21]. In an ideal world, a Gram stain of the solution would be done, as well as tests for catalase and coagulase production, allowing the coagulase-positive *S. aureus* to be identified quickly. The creation of thermostable deoxyribonuclease is another enormous test for *S. aureus*. Testing conditions might need *S. aureus* to agglutinate with latex particles, coated with immunoglobulin G and fibrinogen, which bind protein and the batching factor autonomously on the bacterial cell surface [5, 22–24]. These are available from business sources (e.g., Staphaurex). The most recent latex test (Pastaurex) uses monoclonal antibodies against serotype 5 and 8 capsular polysaccharides to reduce the number of false negatives. (Some novel clinical isolates of *S. aureus* necessitate the production of coagulase in the same way that packaging factors do, which can make checking tedious.) The association of *S. epidermidis* (and, to a lesser extent, other coagulase-negative staphylococci) with no so-called comial illnesses associated with possessing gadgets suggests that partition of these microorganisms from blood will undoubtedly be significant, especially if reformist blood social orders are positive. Nowadays, *S. epidermidis* and other types of Staphylococci are identified using commercial biotype ID units such as as API Staph Ident, API Staph-Trac, Vitek GPI Card, and Micro breadth Pos Combo. Preformed strips containing test substrates are among them [20, 25].

5.4 *S. aureus* infection pathogenesis

S. aureus communicates several cell surface-related and extracellular proteins that are potentially toxic. Pathogenesis is complex for most diseases caused by this living creature. Along these lines, it is difficult to properly determine the role of some random element. This also reflects the shortcomings of many animal models for staphylococcal diseases. In any event, linkages between strains unrelated to specific illnesses and articulation of specific variables suggest their importance in pathogenesis. In the case of some toxins, symptoms of human illness may be replicated in animals with pure proteins [26]. The use of atomic physics has resulted in late progress in the understanding of the pathophysiology of staphylococcal diseases. Potentially hazardous components have been cloned and sequenced, and proteins have been screened. This has sparked atomic-level research into their modes of action, both *in vitro* and in model frameworks. Furthermore, characteristics encoding potential harmfulness factors have been deactivated, and the destructiveness of the mutants in creature models has been compared to the wild-type strain. Any reduction in harmfulness traps the missing component. If destructiveness is reinstated when the quality is returned to the freak, then "Sub-atomic Koch's Postulates" have been satisfied. This approach has confirmed a couple of *S. aureus's* damaging components [23, 27].

6. Infection in the general population

S. aureus is responsible for a wide range of contaminations in humans. Clinical illnesses caused by *S. aureus,* square measure divided into native space and health facility categories based on the onset of illness. These two strains square measure apparent in clinical indicators of contamination, anti-infection quality, and therefore the genetic basis of the contaminating *S. aureus* strains [21]. For a long period, *S. aureus* has been primarily a health care organism, and it may be a major source of mortality and dullness in medical clinics. Regardless, the native space *S. aureus* illnesses are increasing in square measure. Many clinical bacteriemia, infective carditis, skin and sensitive tissue contaminations, osteoarticular disorders, and pleuropulmonary contaminations are all caused by *S. aureus*. Other clinical contaminations include epidural sore, meningitis, dangerous shock situation, and urinary plot infections. According to European research, the prevalence of osteoarticular infections in children ranges from 7 to 22 per 100,000 person-years. In males, its ratio is more as compared to female as result of children in France are 24 per 100,000 for boys and for girls its ratio is 19 per 100,000 per year. Some ethnic groups may be more vulnerable, with Maori and Pacific Islander people overrepresented in a New Zealand study of 813 instances of acute OM. Since 2000, CA-MRSA has become a far more common cause of acute osteoarticular infections in the United States. In a study of 158 cases in Tennessee, the proportion of osteoarticular infections caused by CA-MRSA increased from 4 to 40% between 2000 and 2004. Similarly, in Dallas, TX, the proportion of cases of acute OM caused by CA-MRSA was 6% from 1999 to 2001 and 31% from 2001 to 2003. Between 2001 and 2010, 195 of 376 (52%) cases of *S. aureus* OM in Houston, TX, were caused by MRSA. *S. aureus* produces a wide range of SSTIs, from the benign (e.g., impetigo and simple cellulitis) to the potentially fatal. It is the most often isolated pathogen from surgical site infections (SSIs), cutaneous abscesses, and purulent cellulitis. We discuss the epidemiology, pathogenesis, clinical characteristics, and the management of *S. aureus* SSTIs, with a focus on the recent community-associated MRSA pandemic (CA-MRSA) [28].

7. Factors that cause harm

S. aureus has complete control over the harmfulness variables. Components enable live beings to function as microorganisms, which cause a wide range of animal contaminations, including human contamination. Destructive factors aid in the connection of cells, the separation of the host's resistant shield, tissue infiltration, the cause of sepsis, and the inspiration of poison interceded circumstances. This is the cause of persistent staphylococcal infections in the absence of a strong host immune response [8].

8. The study of disease transmission

8.1 Nasal carriage

S. aureus is a commensal bacterium that acts as a leader. The natural claim to fame of the head is the front nares, where the animal colonizes in individuals. *S. aureus* nasal carriage increases the risk of infection, particularly in health care settings [29]. *S. aureus* nasal carriage may affect up to 30% of humans [30]. Because nasal carriage enhances the chance of the advancement of cautious site, lower respiratory, and flow framework diseases in health care facilities, attempts are being performed to eliminate the carriage utilizing diverse methodologies [11, 12].

8.2 Rise and advancement of MRSA

S. aureus is a commensal bacterium that is also a pioneer. Front Nares is a particular head of the environment in which animals invade people. Nasal *S. aureus* heightens the disease's risk, particularly in clinical settings [29]. *S. aureus* can reach 30% of the human population by normal nasal transportation [30]. Because nostrils enhance the danger of careful location, decreasing illness, and circulation of respiratory systems in medical clinics, attempts are being made to publish it.

Sarman is a strain of *S. aureus* that transmits the MECA quality, which encodes penicillin proteins that restrict extras, PBP2A. Anti-microbial beta-lactams work by inactivating penicillin-limiting proteins (PBP), which is a critical accelerator for the conjunction of bacterial cell dividers. In all situations, this anti-infective drug has only a modest affinity for PBP2A; nonetheless, this chemistry escapes inactivation and is part of the essential PBP involving the integration of cell dividers and bacteria, even in the presence of beta-lactam anti-microbes. Sarman is resistant to most beta-lactam anti-infection drugs because of the presence of MECA [15]. Penicillin was discovered in 1928 as an anti-toxin primary beta-lactam and was found to captivate weapons against *S. aureus* infection. There were instances of *S. aureus* tension that resisted penicillin in the 1940s, which was faster following the presentation in the institution [7]. This stress caused Beta-lactamase plasmid beta-lactamase (penicillinase) to be produced, which breaks beta-lactam penicillin rings, resulting in non-active anti-microbes [31, 32]. In the 1950s, penicillin resistance was restricted to the closure of the *S. aureus* emergency clinic. In the late 1960s, due to the mobility of plasmid quality penicillin (Blaz) and diffusion of clones from safe strains, more than 80% of *S. aureus* was captivated, independent of area and the establishment of an emergency clinic, was extremely resistant to penicillin [9, 33]. The researchers then examined methicillin, a semi-designed penicillin that was resistant to enzymatic corruption from penisination, in *S. aureus* with opposition penicillinase intervention. Methicillin was introduced to the center in 1961; however, after one year, *S. aureus* blockage restricts the use of methicillin (MRSA) [34]. For the next 10 years and beyond, the MRSA outbreak is projected in many regions of the world, particularly in European nations [35, 36]. The Sarman appears in the form of a supported microbiological clinic, and the major components of these reports are from an emergency clinic. In 1981, the Battle-Lactam anti-infection protection system in the Sarjor separator was described [4]. As previously stated,

MRSA Supegate provided a high-quality MEC code for PBP2A. Quality is a variable genetic component ranging from 21 to 60 KB known as a Meca ribbon (SCMCECA) from the chromosome (SCMCECA). Two ideas describe the origins of MRSA. The specific clone idea proposes that the adaptable hereditary components join the *S. aureus* popula at an event and bring a specific MRSA clone framework, which disseminated all over the globe. Other most common theory is that MRSA is created by how many times the process of exchanging portable hereditary components becomes phylogenetic, including *S. aureus* (MSSA) strains (MSSA) [MSSA] [9, 32–35]. Related Medical Care and Local Sarma Area

8.3 Medical care related to MRSA (HA-MARM)

SRSA in medical therapy (HA-MRASA) is *S. aureus* collected from patients at least two days after in hospital or with the danger of Sarma (history of hospital today, medical procedures, dialysis, or homes at the Advisory Office are drawn in one year earlier). The existence of a catheter that is directly eternal clinic or percutaneous gadgets (such as tracheotomy tubes, gastrostomy cylinders, or Foley catheters) with Cultural Clock. Alternatively, on the other side of MRSA termination [4, 36], MRSA for local regions (Ca-Mrasa) occurs when *S. aureus* discharges patients after 2 days in hospital and without the previously described MRSA danger concerns. MRSA was previously and resistant to non-beta lactam anti-infection agent until the 1990s.

8.4 Health care-associated MRSA

MRSA has traditionally been thought of as a clinic- or health care-related pathogen (HA-MRSA), affecting those patients by doing surgery or some medical devices implants and as well as those who are immunocompromised. Health care-related MRSA strains are often multidrug resistant and contain SCCmec types I, II, and III [37]. Most HA-MRSA types worldwide are CC5, CC8, CC22, CC30, and CC45 [28, 37].

9. Resistance of staphylococci to antimicrobial drugs

Clinic strains of *S. aureus* often impervious to various anti-infection agents. Without a doubt, strains are impervious to all clinical medications, paying little attention to vancomycin and teicoplanin glycopeptides, it has been clarified [38]. The term MRSA reference methicillin obstruction and most of the methicillin strains likewise increase. Plasmid-aniseed vancomycin opposition has been distinguished in a few Enterococci and the obstruction determinant has been moved from Enterococci to *S. aureus* in the lab and can happen normally [23]. *S. epidermidis* nosocomial secludes sturdy to a few anti-toxins including methicillin. Notwithstanding, *S. aureus* expresses protection from disinfectant and affection, for example, the quartier ammonium compound, which can help its endurance in the medical clinic climate. Since the start of the anti-microbial time, *S. aureus* has reacted to the presentation of new medications by securing quickly with an assortment of hereditary instruments including (1) plasmid extraction some procurement or extra data in chromosomes through transposon or DNA inclusion type and (2) with a chromosomal quality change [5].

Many determinants-encoded plasmids are recently put into chromosomes on sites related to the determinant of the methicillin resistance. There may be benefits for organisms that have a determinant of resistance in the genetic material due to more stability. The four basic mechanism of resistance to bacteria are as follows: (1) enzymatic deactivation of drugs, (2) changes to target area of the drug to prevent binding, (3) enhanced drug efflux to avoid toxic absorptions collects in cells, and (4) permit mechanisms in which an analytical resistant type is stated [10, 11, 38].

9.1 Antimicrobial drugs

Penicillin first time in *S. aureus* showed exceptional adaptability. The impediment has resulted in tone prescriptions in a short period of time. A few strains are now resistant to the most used anti-microbials. He is concerned that no new anti-infection drugs are on the horizon. Every new advancement may be traced back to an existing medication [5, 34].

The initial approach used by the pharmacological production to identify antimicrobial medicines is to channel organic products and designed synthetic compounds for antibacterial activity. After that, the activity instrument is considered. Another technique for determining the antimicrobial age has been obtained. The likely aims, for example, chemicals, are up to the major capacities (e.g. in cell division) are recognized based on microbial and metabolic physiology information. The identification approach is then refined to differentiate some objective atomic inhibitors. Similarly, given specific atomic knowledge on the target particles, precise inhibitors may be devised [22].

9.1.1 Mechanism of methicillin resistance in staphylococci

Methicillin resistance develops because of the mecA gene being acquired, which determines a complementary penicillin-binding protein, with a poor attraction for -lactam antibiotics [37], Despite of inactivation of cells' natural penicillin-binding protein, the production of PBP2a allows bacterial cell wall production to continue in the existence of lactam antibiotics. Cephalosporins and cefamycins have resistant to lactam antibiotics, which are conferred *via* the mecA gene.

The mecA gene is part of the Staphylococcal Cassette Chromosome mec (SCCmec), a large mobile genetic element [19, 39].

International classification of Staphylococcal types of chromosome elements now contains 11 kinds of different SCCmec elements. Mec gene is protected by this Staphylococcal chromosomal which has been found in CPS and CNS [10]. In CNS, the structure of SCCmec elements is polymorphous with abundant amount of CCRmec sequences found, but not used for MRSA [40]. For the development of novel MRSA, clones' greater frequency and diversity of SCCmec elements required that play a vital role in CNS and CNS is reservoir of mec elements. Horizontal transfer of SCCmec elements to *S. aureus* from CNS is still not found [38]. For many years, scientists have speculated about the origin of the mecA gene. mecA gene homologous have been discovered in *S. sciuri* and *S. vitulinus*, neither instance is the mecA gene present in a mecA complex like SCCmec [22]. Two scientists named as Tsubakishita and colleagues discovered a mecA gene similar in *S. fleuretti* that had almost 100% sequence with MRSA strain N315 and resided on a structure that was nearly matching to the mecA complex. *Staphylococcus fleuretti* is a commensal bacterium that belongs to the *S. sciuri* group of staphylococci [18]. Direct detection of methicillin resistance gene in staphylo which lives in animals serves as reservoir for making new SCCmec elements [20].

Molecular research on a S. A new mecA homolog was discovered after a methicillin-resistant *S. aureus* strain was reported to be phenotypically resistant to methicillin but on other hand when tested with polymerase chain reaction (PCR) assay it was negative [1]. The bacterial strain in which the gene was originally sequenced, *S. aureus*

LGA251, shares 70% nucleotide similarity with the conventional mecA gene [23]. The investigation of Garca-lvarez and colleagues revealed that mecALGA251 was discovered in *S. aureus* lineages commonly linked with cattle, such as clonal complex (CC)130, CC1943, and sequence type (ST)425, implying the presence of a zoonotic MRSA reservoir. Furthermore, evidence of mecALGA251-carrying MRSA strains being transmitted from animal to human has been observed [30]. The IWCC renamed the mecA variant mecC [41] in 2012. The mecC gene is located on a new SCCmec element known as SCCmec XI [14]. S. methicillin-resistant *S. aureus* strains with the mecC gene have been proven to cause a variety of illnesses in people, and they appear to be mostly community associated.

9.2 One health and antibiotic resistance

One well-being concept reveals that human well-being is inextricably linked to the environment and its inhabitants. Because the well-being of animals, people, and the environment are all intertwined, interdisciplinary approaches to advancing the strength of each of these areas are required. As the human population grows, more people come into touch with animals, increasing the risk of disease transmission between humans and larger animals. The concept of one's well-being is quite related to the idea of environmental change and global travel risks. The achievements of Robert Koch, Rodolph Virchow, and William Osler in the development of vaccinations and their impact on human health, the management of zoonosis, and germ theory formed the framework of one health [25] (**Figure 1**).

9.3 New resistance variants continue to emerge

With a Gram-positive entrance to multi-fiditive Gram-negative microscopic organisms, which is a limited or completely less handling option, large variations in the degree of opposing predominance occur. Some attention has been drawn to the quality that encodes the novel metallo-lactamase 1 (NDM-1) (NDM-1) (NDM-1) which renders Gram-negative enterobacteria resistant to the line's most recent anti-toxins, such as Carpenem [10]. Indeed, this is an AMR concern since there has been

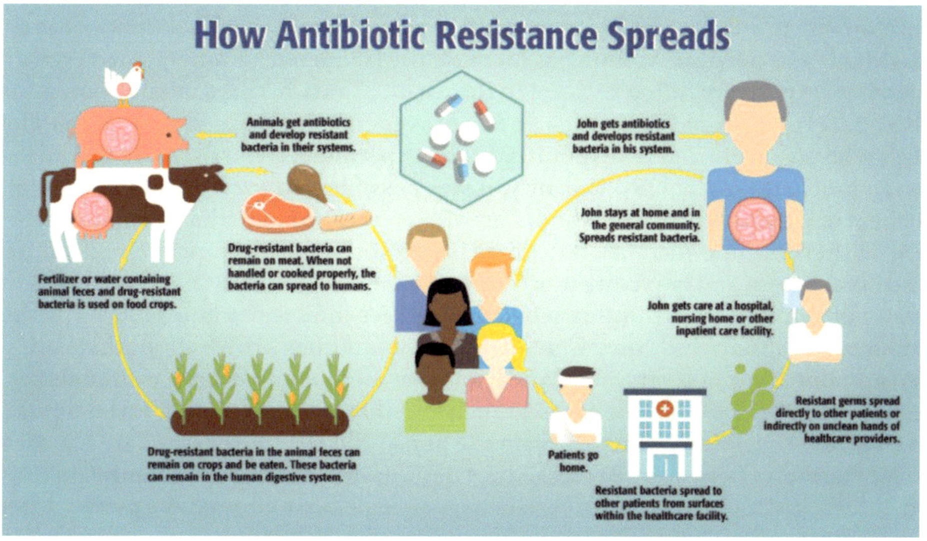

Figure 1.
How antibiotics spreads.

an overall increase in the risk of delivering enterobacteria in Europe and throughout the world as to most carpenemase characteristics. Another issue that has emerged in the last decade is multi- or enlarged TB, Neisseria (microorganisms causing gonorrhea) that is resistant to the most current cephalosporins, and problematic clostridium that causes a severe moxifloxacin safe flat mate. Regardless, progress has been made in comprehending the unpredictable nature of opposing reversibility [40]. The investigation discovered that there was a minimal or no risk of AMR reversals after being defined in Community and non-Community situations [37, 38].

9.3.1 Antibiotic-resistant bacteria transmission

The emergence of multi-obstruction detonates, particularly among Gram-negative bacteria, has drawn attention to the growing relevance of genetic component coding transfer for multi-resistance, as well as the potential zoonotic transmission (creature based). The term "resistome" represents new information regarding the transmission of AMR bacteria [22]. Resistments are a group of characteristics that were first discovered in terrestrial microscopic organisms. It is necessary to be accountable for the development of various defense mechanisms that allow soil microorganisms to survive in the face of anti-microbials found naturally in the environment. It is considered that attributes from blockage might perhaps be transferred to non-land microscopic creatures, therefore exacerbating opposition difficulties. Regardless of whether it is debated, research reveals that some safe microorganisms have been more successful in sustaining extensively and enduringly owing to the resistome [23]. Antimicrobial misuses outside of human medicine is an additional aggravating element in AMR, notably the development of AMR in animals and humans [14, 24, 41]. The use of antimicrobials in agriculture can provide a large source of antimicrobial safe microscopic organisms that can spread to people through food supply when critters are eaten. This includes non-therapeutic applications, such as development progression. This also includes using it as a prophylactic to try to prevent illnesses from developing in food species and as a useful specialist to cure debilitated creatures. See the previous section. Farming serves as a reservoir for AMR microorganism transfer to and from humans [13]. However, it remains difficult to correlate the anti-microbial inhibition of food default microorganisms, the use of anti-toxins in agriculture, and the clinical confinement of human safe bacteria. That is, environmental connections between individuals and dynamic farming to increase the frequency of illnesses in certain years may be corresponding to develop the usage of anti-toxins that may potentially choose safe microscopic organisms. It was proven in 1976, that someone may follow *E. coli* who was protected from poultry in the experimental horticulture plot to human ranchers nearby [29]. Recently, it was possible to track links between two ranchers in Denmark, both of whom had MRSA infection. Furthermore, animals were on their 28-mile-distance farmstead. More specifically, a rancher who maintained two horses and two cows was found to have MRSA blood infection. Others have a portion of 10 sheep and ranchers had MRSA-infected wounds [39, 42]; when their case was discovered, they were identified as another MRSA strain that had been accounted for in steers and Danish analysts went out to examine animals on the two homesteads. One cow on one ranch and three sheep on other farms spread new strains. All bacterial samples from the house and the two persons are identical in a few tests and have a similar resistance design; that is, they are defenseless to anti-infection drugs that are not beta lactams (penicillin and cephalosporin). Then, all genomes were sequenced (which was unthinkable in 1976) and compared to how near all instances were. Detaches from ranchers and steers tests are nearly identical (five SNPs), as are disengages from various ranchers and most sheep. There is a difference of 154 SNPs in all instances (single-nucleotide polymorphism—single letter update on 2004 back paper, BP 6.1 antimicrobial opposition 6.1–9 "duplicating mistake" in hereditary code). Because of their relationship, the example created bunches based on two domesticated animals: first, ranchers and cows, and second, ranchers and sheep [43]. Following that, phylogenetic analysis uncovers two distinct gatherings explicitly for horticulture comprising of human cases and their own domesticated animals, while human confines and creatures from a similar farming are distinct with only a few SNP, implying the possibility of zoonotic transmission. Another study recognizes numerous characteristics and changes that are associated with host and harmfulness communications, and that this detach MECC-Mrasa CC130 is occasionally seen in humans. They are said to have been dispatched among animals and mankind [38, 44]. Nonetheless, the examination of this type of proof still has components. This has not been detected before, and the example size is small. It is possible that all hereditary varieties of secludes on specific farming can address the presentation of the two MRSA in the group, rather than a presentation followed by organization. If this happens, the transfer of monster beings can be like zoonosis. "Different hosts" of CCC CC130 MRSA include cows and sheep, as well as ponies, rabbits, felines, canines, deer, canines, mice, and wild avian animals. Examination has clearly supported the notion that sophisticated civilization has increased the possibility of safe microorganisms propagating and thriving in all animals and human surroundings [39, 45]. According to this perspective, as the value of the dollar rises, so will the risk of AMR and, as a result, the necessity to develop new antimicrobial products.

10. Preventive approaches to control *S. aureus*

There is currently no vaccination available to fight carrier diseases. There may also be reasons to investigate illness prevention strategies, particularly in hospitalized patients. Human volunteer hyperimmune whey donors or modest monoclonal antibodies directed at surface-components, such as rules for capsular adherence of proteins or proteins from the surface, can also impede bacterial compliance in Dan, increasing cell phagocytosis. In fact, a vaccine prototype based on *S. aureus* capsular polysaccharide has been developed.

Clinical infections caused by *S. aureus* are expected to remain frequent and severe. Not only have there been waves of growing antibiotic resistance, but the clinical illness spectrum is also changing. We have seen two distinct shifts in the epidemiology of *S. aureus* infections over the last two decades: first, an increase in the number of health care-associated infections, particularly IE and prosthetic device infections, and second, an epidemic of community-associated SSTIs caused by strains with specific virulence factors. There is little question that the landscape of host-pathogen interactions will continue to alter in the next decades [40].

11. Conclusion

S. aureus and many more are very dangerous for human as animals. They caused several diseases in them especially, respiratory problem and others which are described the chapter in brief. Now, some drugs and vaccine should be made to control it as most of the species is untreated and cannot be eradicated. Sulfonamide, penicillin, and streptomycin are used to test antimicrobial time. The assurances of these specialists in terms of feasible control of a broad range of bacterial illnesses are typically filled up with a plethora of antibacterial specialists presently available.

As of today, it is difficult to imagine the fear and stress connected with the recurrence of previous severe illnesses. Is it possible to grasp anti-infection resistance, or are we returning to our inability to cope with harmful microorganisms? There is no legitimate explanation for fear. Although most bacterial illnesses can be easily treated, there are a few of actual difficulties that are not far away.

Acknowledgements

Muhammad Farooq has written the main chapter, Mr. Zia Ullah has helped in design, and Ifra Siddique has made final transcript.

Conflict of interest

"The authors declare no conflict of interest."

Author details

Muhammad Farooq[1*], Ifra Siddique[2] and Zia Ullah[3]

1 Faculty of Veterinary Medicine, University of Teramo, Italy

2 Department of Plant Pathology, University of Agriculture Peshawar, Pakistan

3 Institute of Microbiology, University of Agriculture Faisalabad, Pakistan

*Address all correspondence to: drfarooqnabi@gmail.com

References

[1] Bhakdi S, Tranum-Jensen J. Alpha-toxin of *Staphylococcus aureus*. Microbiological Reviews. 1991;**55**:733

[2] Wilkinson BJ, Easmon CSF, Adlam C. Staphylococci and Staphylococcal Infections. Staphylococci and Staphylococcal Infections: The organism in vivo and in vitro. 1983;**2**:481.

[3] Foster TJ. Potential for vaccination against infections caused by *Staphylococcus aureus*. Vaccine. 1991;**9**:221

[4] Fridkin SK, Hageman JC, Morrison M, Sanza LT, Como-Sabetti K, Jernigan JA, et al. Methicillin-resistant *Staphylococcusaureus* disease in three communities. The New England Journal of Medicine. 2005;**352**:1436-1444. DOI: 10.1056/NEJMoa043252

[5] Schlievert PM. Role of superantigens in human disease. The Journal of Infectious Diseases. 1993;**167**:997

[6] Lyon BR, Skurray R. Antimicrobial resistance in *Staphylococcus aureus*: Genetic basis. Microbiological Reviews. 1987;**51**:88

[7] Rammelkamp CH, Maxon T. Resistance of *Staphylococcus aureus* to the action of penicillin. Experimental Biology and Medicine (Maywood, N.J.). 1942;**51**:386-389. DOI: 10.3181/00379727-51-13986

[8] Kim HK, Falugi F, Missiakas DM, Schneewinda O. Peptidoglycan-linked protein A promotes T cell-dependent antibody expansion during *Staphylococcus aureus* infection. Proceedings of the National Academy of Sciences of the United States of America. 2016;**113**:5718-5723. DOI: 10.1073/pnas.1524267113

[9] Chambers HF. The changing epidemiology of *Staphylococcus aureus*? Emerging Infectious Diseases. 2001;**7**:178-182. DOI: 10.3201/eid0702.700178

[10] Bennett PM. Plasmid encoded antibiotic resistance: Acquisition and transfer of antibiotic resistance genes in bacteria. British Journal of Pharmacology. 2008;**153**(Suppl 1): S347-S357

[11] Wertheim HF, Verveer J, Boelens HA, van Belkum A, Verbrugh HA, Vos MC. Effect of mupirocin treatment on nasal, pharyngeal, and perineal carriage of *Staphylococcus aureus* in healthy adults. Antimicrobial Agents and Chemotherapy. 2005;**49**:1465-1467. DOI: 10.1128/AAC.49.4.1465-1467.2005

[12] Kluytmans J. Nasal carriage of *Staphylococcus aureus*: Epidemiology, underlying mechanisms, and associated risks. Clinical Microbiology Reviews. 1997;**10**:505-520

[13] Kraemer SA, Ramachandran A, Perron GG. Antibiotic pollution in the environment: From microbial ecology to public policy. Microorganisms. 2019;**7**:180

[14] Hayashi S, Mitsuko A, Kimoto M, Furukawa S, Nakazawa T. The DsbA-DsbB disulphide bond formation system of Burkholderia cepacia is involved in the production of protease and alkaline phosphatase, motility, metal resistance, and multi-drug resistance. Microbiology and Immunology. 2000;**44**:41-50

[15] Fuda C, Suvorov M, Vakulenko SB, Mobashery S. The basis for resistance to β-lactam antibiotics by penicillin-binding protein 2a of methicillin-resistant *Staphylococcus aureus*. Journal of Biological Chemistry. 2004;**279**: 40802-40806. DOI: 10.1074/jbc.M403589200

[16] Foster TJ, McDevitt D. Molecular basis of adherence of staphylococci to

biomaterials. In: Bisno AL, Waldvogel FA, editors. Infections Associated with Indwelling Medical Devices. 2nd ed. Washington, D.C.: American Societyfor Microbiology; 1994. p. 31

[17] Licitra G. Etymologia: Staphylococcus. Emerging Infectious Diseases. 2013;**19**:1553. DOI: 10.3201/eid1909.ET1909

[18] Greenwood D, O'Grady F. Scanning electron microscopy of *Staphylococcus aureus* exposed to some common anti-staphylococcal agents. Journal of General Microbiology. 1972;**70**:263-270. DOI: 10.1099/00221287-70-2-263

[19] Foster T. Chapter 12: Staphylococcus. In: Medical Microbiology. 4th ed. Galveston (TX): University of Texas Medical Branch at Galveston, Galveston, Texas; 1996

[20] Touhami A, Jericho MH, Beveridge TJ. Atomic force microscopy of cell growth and divisionin *Staphylococcus aureus*. Journal of Bacteriology. 2004;**186**:3286-3295. DOI: 10.1128/JB.186.11.3286-3295.2004

[21] Tong SYC, Davis JS, Eichenberger E, Holland TL, Fowler VG Jr. *Staphylococcus aureus* infections: Epidemiology, pathophysiology, clinical manifestations, and management. Clinical Microbiology Reviews. 2015;**28**:603-661. DOI: 10.1128/CMR.00134-14

[22] Rupp ME, Archer GL. Coagulase-negative staphylococci: Pathogens associated with medical progress. Clinical Infectious Diseases. 1994;**19**:231

[23] Skinner GRB, Ahmad A. Staphylococcal vaccines—Present status and future prospects. In: Mollby R, Flock JI, Nord CE, Christensson B, editors. Staphylococci and Staphylococcal Infections. Zbl. Bakt. Suppl. 26. Stuttgart: Fischer Verlag; 1994. p. 537

[24] Flores-Tejeida LB, Soto-Zarazua GM, Guevara-Gonzalez R, Escamilla-Garcia A, Gomez-Soto JG. A review of hot and sweet pepper added in animal nutrition: Alternative against the use of antibiotics. XIV International Engineering Congress (CONIIN). 2018;**1**:1-6. DOI: 10.1109/CONIIN.2018.8489822

[25] Baker-Austin C, Wright MS, Stepanauskas R, McArthur JV. Co-selection of antibiotic and metal resistance. Trends in Microbiology. 2006;**14**:176-182

[26] Tenover F, Arbeit R, Archer G, et al. Comparison of traditional and molecular methods of typing isolates of *Staphylococcus aureus*. Journal of Clinical Microbiology. 1994;**32**:407

[27] Vaudaux PE, Lew DP, Waldvogel FA. Host factors predisposing to and influencing therapy of foreign bodyinfections. In: Bisno AL, Waldvogel FA, editors. Infections Associated with Indwelling Medical Devices. 2nd ed. Washington, D.C.: American Society for Microbiology; 1994. p. 1

[28] Archer GL. *Staphylococcus aureus*: A well-armed pathogen. Clinical Infectious Diseases. 1998;**26**:1179-1181

[29] Kluytmans JA, Wertheim HF. Nasal carriage of *Staphylococcus aureus* and prevention of nosocomial infections. Infection. 2005;**33**:3-8. DOI: 10.1007/s15010-005-4012-9

[30] Williams REO. Healthy carriage of *Staphylococcus aureus*: Its prevalence and importance. Bacteriological Review. 1963;**27**:56-71

[31] Kirby WM. Extraction of highly potent penicillin inactivator from penicillin resistant Staphylocooci.

Science. 1942;**99**:452-453. DOI: 10.1126/science.99.2579.452

[32] Bondi JA, Dietz CC. Penicillin resistant Staphylococci. Proceedings of the Society for Experimental Biology and Medicine. 1945;**60**:55-58

[33] Lowy FD. Antimicrobial resistance: The example of *Staphylococcus aureus*. The Journal of Clinical Investigation. 2003;**111**:1265-1273. DOI: 10.1172/JCI18535

[34] Jevons PM. "Celbenin"—Resistant Staphylococci. British Medical Journal. 1961;**1**:124-125

[35] Ito T, Kuwahara-Arai K, Katayama Y, Uehara Y, Han X, Kondo Y, Hiramatsu K. Staphylococcal Cassette Chromosome mec (SCCmec) analysis of MRSA. Methods in Molecular Biology 2014;**1085**:131-148. DOI: 10.1007/978-1-62703-664-1_8

[36] Naimi TS, LeDell KH, Como-Sabetti K, Borchardt SM, Boxrud DJ, Etienne J, et al. Comparison of community- and health care-associated methicillin-resistant *Staphylococcus aureus* infection. JAMA. 2003;**290**:2976-2984. DOI: 10.1001/jama.290.22.2976

[37] Brabban AD, Hite E, Callaway TR. Evolution of foodborne pathogens via temperate bacteriophage-mediated gene transfer. Foodborne Pathogens and Disease. 2005;**2**:287-303

[38] Chee-Sanford JC, Krapac IJ, Yannarell AC, Mackie RI. Environmental impacts of antibiotic use in the animal production industry. Prevention of Infectious Diseases in Livestock and Wildlife (book published in 2012). In: Ecology and Animal. 2012

[39] Rizzo L, Manaia C, Merlin C, Schwartz T, Dagot C, Ploy MC, et al. Urban wastewater treatment plants as hotspots for antibiotic resistant bacteria and genes spread into the environment: A review. Science of the Total Environment. 2013;**447**:345-360

[40] Prevost G, Couppie P, Prevost P, et al. Epidemiological data on *Staphylococcus aureus* strains producingsynergohymenotropic toxins. Journal of Medical Microbiology. 1995;**42**:237

[41] Hall BG, Barlow M. Evolution of the serine β-lactamases: Past, present and future. Drug Resistance Updates. 2004;**7**:111-123

[42] Salyers AA, Amábile-Cuevas CF. Why are antibiotic resistance genes so resistant to elimination? Antimicrobial Agents and Chemotherapy. 1997;**41**:2321-2325

[43] Xiong W, Sun Y, Zhang T. et al. Antibiotics, Antibiotic Resistance Genes, and Bacterial Community Composition in Fresh Water Aquaculture Environment in China. Microb Ecol. 2015;**70**:425-432. https://doi.org/10.1007/s00248-015-0583-x

[44] Anonymous. Antibiotic Fact Sheet: Antibiotic Use in Livestock Production: Ensuring Meat Safety. NW, Washington, D.C.: American Meat Institute; 2010. Available from: http://www.MeatAMI.com

[45] Nielsen KM, Smalla K, van Elsas JD. Natural transformation of Acinetobacter sp. strain BD413 with cell lysates of Acinetobacter sp., Pseudomonas fluorescens, and Burkholderia cepacia in soil microcosms. Applied Environmental Microbiology. 2000;**66**:206-212

Chapter 12

Staphylococcus aureus and the Veterinary Medicine

Muhammad Farhab, Muhammad Tahir Aleem,
Shukseema Shaukat, Ayesha Qadry,
Muhammad Zeeshan Ul Haq, Fateh Ullah,
Muhammad Jawad and Amjad Islam Aqib

Abstract

Staphylococcus aureus has vital importance in veterinary medicine. Within the ruminants, it is one of the major causes of mastitis, the problem that was and is, with no definite solution to date. Along with that, it also affects the health of animals, pets, and poultry in several ways as the tissue tropism for this organism in poultry is the bones and the joints. This review is focused on habitat, species differentiation, differential biochemical tests, pathogenesis, clinical infections, economic importance, public health significance, immune response, the regulation of virulence in the staphylococci, and cytokines response against *S. aureus*.

Keywords: cytokines, superantigens, tissue tropism, virulence, zinc

1. Introduction

Staphylococci are Gram-positive cocci bacteria of 1 pico-meter diameter. They are observed with gram staining under the microscope as a bunch of grapes. The word staphylococcus is originated from the Greek words staphyle and kokkos. Staphyle means the "bunch of grapes", while the word kokkos means "the berry". The normal habitat of staphylococci is skin and mucus membranes. There are approximately 30 species of staphylococcus. They act as commensals but some of them are opportunistic pathogens too. They a famous for their pyogenic infection-causing property. Most staphylococci are facultative anaerobes, non-motile, oxidase-negative, non-spore-forming, and catalase-positive. S. aureus subsp. aureus is the coagulase-positive that has very much importance concerning the disease status of animals. Production of coagulase is directly correlated with the pathogenicity of the staphylococcus i.e. coagulase-negative bacteria are usually non0-pathogenic to animals and humans [1]. They can be grown on non-enriched media. They are facultative anaerobes and non-motile. They are found as commensals on mucous membranes and skin. They are stable in the environment **Figure 1** [99].

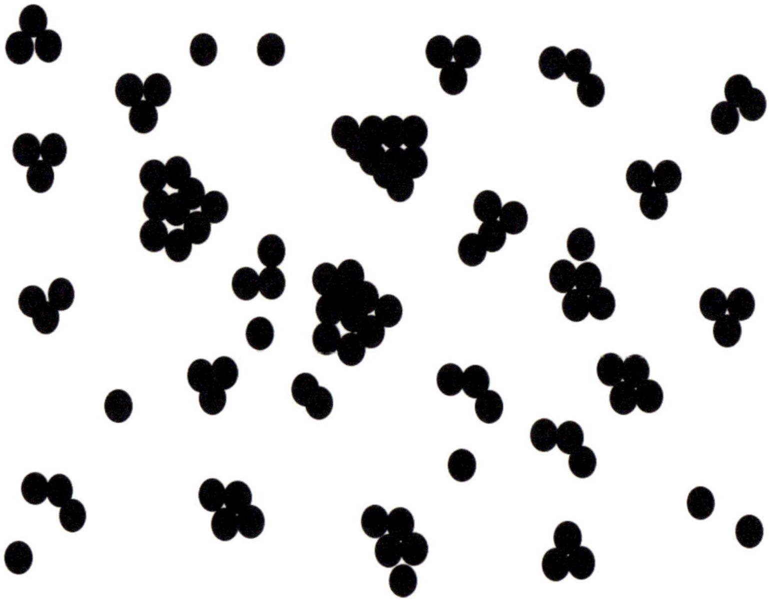

Figure 1.
'Bunches of grapes' appearance of Staphylococci. Modified from [1].

2. Habitat

Staphylococcal species occur on humans and animals on the skin, mucosa of the upper respiratory system, lower urinary, and genital tract, and as transients in the digestive tract. They are stable in the environment, have a selective affinity for particular species. They have limited zoonotic importance [1, 2].

3. Specie differentiation

While confirming a bacterial colony to be a staphylococcus or not, it is necessary to differential differentiate it from closest resembling bacteria named micrococcus

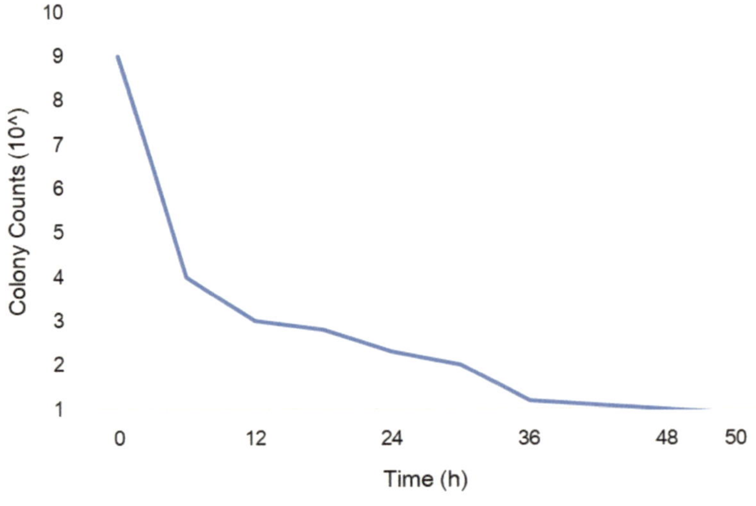

Figure 2.
Growth curve of Staphylococcus aureus within bovine aortic endothelial cells. Modified from [1].

and streptococcus species. The point that differentiates the Staphylococci from staphylococci is that staphylococci are mostly catalase-positive while the streptococci are mostly catalase-negative. Other tests of vital importance within the differentiation of the Staphylococcus species are hemolytic pattern, biochemical profiles, colonial appearance, and rRNA gene restriction patterns [2]. S. aureus and S. intermedius are often confused clinical cases of dogs and cats. Coagulase-negative staphylococci are ordinarily reserved for isolates from pure cultures. Their colonies are white, opaque and up to 4 mm in diameter, some are golden yellow and some have pigmented colonies. Sheep or ox blood agar presents alpha, beta, gamma, and delta hemolysis. Strains of the staphylococcus species are differentiated based on their capability of haemolysin production [1, 2].

The growth curve of *Staphylococcus aureus* within bovine aortic endothelial cells under optimal conditions is presented in **Figure 2**.

4. Biochemical tests for differentiating *Staphylococcus aureus* and Staphylococcus intermedius

A rapid test for the detection of acetoin has been developed [3]. Purple agar, containing bromocresol purple as a pH indicator and 1% maltose, is used to differentiate S. aureus from S. intermedius [4]. Purple is the color of most of the colonies of that bacteria. The energy source used by the *Staphylococcus aureus* in the culture medium is maltose which is utilized by that microbe and the resultant metabolic by-product is acid production. The by-product acid changes the color of the medium and colonies to yellow. Staphylococcus intermedius is a maltose fermenter so it means that it will not affect the color of the medium. There is also the commercial availability of the Biochemical tests which can be used for the confirmation of the staphylococcal species which can further be confirmed by molecular techniques like a polymerase chain reaction and multiplex PCR [5]. There are also studies on the molecular typing of the isolates of different regions of the world. The techniques that are and can be used in near future for the molecular epidemiology of the different isolates of Staphylococcus species can be but not limited to the Multilocus Sequence Typing (MLST) [6–9] and Multilocus variable number of Tandem Repeats (MLV) [10–12].

5. Pathogenesis and pathogenicity

Staphylococci are pyogenic and cause suppurative lesions. Virulent factors for this gram-positive bacterium are capsule, plasmid or phage-mediated, cell wall proteins, teichoic acids, and protein A **Figure 3** [2].

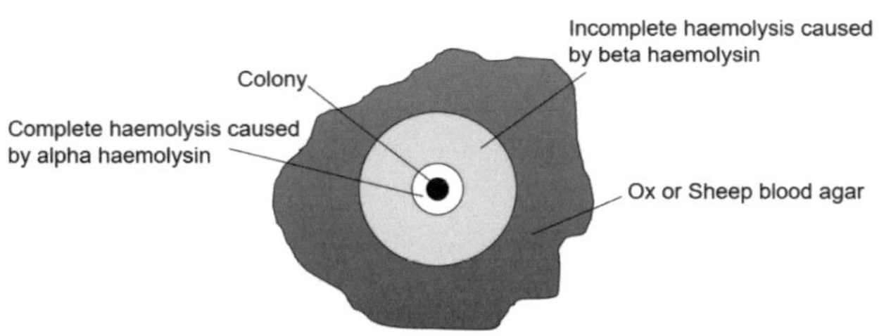

Figure 3.
Sheep or ox blood agar with Double haemolysis of S. aureus. Modified from [1].

6. Clinical infections

Staphylococci infections can be endogenous or exogenous in origin. Many infections are opportunistic and associated with other infections or the immune-compromised state of the host. Coagulase-positive staphylococci are mostly pathogenic. There are no effective vaccines against this malaise to date. Antibiotic sensitivity testing should have to be applied to check the efficacy of the drug against this bacterium. This is because many strains of this bacteria have developed resistance against many antibiotics. Common diseases of veterinary importance the Staphylococci are tick pyaemia, mastitis, botryomycosis, exudative epidermitis, and pyoderma [1].

6.1 Bovine mastitis

Staphylococcal mastitis is a common form of mastitis worldwide. Most infections are subclinical, but they can be acute or chronic, per acute and gangrenous. In gangrenous mastitis, the quarter is cold and blue-black and sloughing by the alpha-toxin causing necrosis of blood vessels and releases lysosomal enzymes [2–4].

6.2 Tick pyaemia

Tick pyaemia of lambs is a disease of hill-grazing regions having the tick Ixodes ricinus. Clinical signs include septicemia and rapid death, localized abscess formation, arthritis, posterior paresis, and ill-thrift. 30% of lambs between half a month old to up to three months of age can be affected. More infections are reported in spring and early summer [4–7].

6.2.1 Diagnosis, treatment and control

In young grazing lambs, clinical signs, microscopy of pus, and isolation and identification are required. Treatment is usually ineffective so control measures should have to be applied as tetracyclines injectables to the susceptible ones. Dipping to avoid tick-control measures should have to be practiced [2–5].

6.3 Exudative epidermitis (greasy-pig disease)

This is the disease pigs that are of up to 3 months old. It is contagious, with excessive sebaceous secretion, and exfoliation of the skin. Clinical signs include anorexia, depression, fever, dermatitis with an exudate. Death may be within 2–4 days with morbidity rate to be 20 to 100%, and mortality rates can be up to 90%. Isolation and identification of this bacteria can be from the vaginal mucosa and skin. Agalactia, weaning, and intercurrent infections are the predisposing factors for this disease [1].

6.3.1 Diagnosis, treatment and control

A high mortality rate in exudative, non-pruritic skin lesions. Along with the isolation and identification of the bacteria is required for confirmatory purposes. Antibiotic therapy with antiseptics is proven to be effective in many cases. Isolation of affected pigs, cleaning, and disinfection of surroundings. Antiseptic application before farrowing is also an effective way of prevention [1–3].

6.4 Botryomycosis

Botryomycosis is chronic, a suppurative granulomatous malaise of horses that is after castration infecting the stump of the scirrhous cord and mammary glands of sows [3–6].

6.5 Staphylococcal infections in dogs and cats

Otitis externa and Pyoderma, endometritis, mastitis, osteomyelitis, and cystitis are reported to be due to the S. aureus in many cases [2–6].

7. Staphylococcosis and poultry

Along with humans and animals, poultry is also susceptible to infections by staphylococcus [13–17]. There are no definitive signs of that bacteria in the poultry and it varies from case to case and the lesions are usually dependent upon the point of entry of the bacteria within the host. Unlike the animals where the staphylococcus mainly targets the skin and mucosa, the skin is less likely to be infected in the poultry and the organs that are more susceptible to the infection of staphylococcus species in poultry are bones, tendons, and joints [14, 16, 18–21]. The infections are characterized by the increased heterophil count and their accumulation into the affected regions [22]. It is also responsible for the acute deaths in layers [23] within the hot climates and is required to be differentially diagnosed with the fowl cholera. Staphylococcal infections in poultry are required to have in-depth studies by future researchers as there is less knowledge about the route of entry, immunity interaction, pathogenesis, and the possible prognosis of that organism. It impedes chronic infections mostly in poultry having poor antibiotic response. Immunization against that pathogen also requires more in-depth studies as the currently available vaccines are not as potent as the poultry business farmers and expecting [23–25].

7.1 Economic importance

Along with the studies that they present acute infection in hot climates, they can infect almost all types of climates and target both poultry and turkey. They have very much economic importance as they decrease the feed conversion ratio, weight gain, egg production, and septicemia. They target the bones resulting in lameness and osteomalacia. Their pathological lesion may lead to the condemnation of the carcass [24, 25]. There is a study correlating the green discoloration of the liver with the staphylococcal infections and it is concluded it these studies that there is a high correlation between the green discoloration of the liver and the staphylococcal infections, and they termed that condition as the "green-liver osteomyelitis complex" [26, 27] of the turkeys. It should have to be remembered that this pathogen is not the only etiological agent for that correlation, other isolates within these studies were Escherichia coli and many others [26–28].

7.2 Public health significance on poultry

Approximately 50% of the *Staphylococcus aureus* strains are responsible for human food poisoning through their enterotoxins [28–32] that are subjected to the condemnation of carcass upon their identification on food processing. Sources of the Staphylococcal infections may be the un-hygienic conditions of the processing plant and the poultry meat handling personals of the processing plant [33–36].

There is also a close associate of the Methicillin-resistant *Staphylococcus aureus* (MRSA) with the poultry meat [37–47]. MRSA has different strains each is resistant to a class of antibiotics as the commonly reported antibiotics against which the MRSA has evolved the disease tolerance includes the semi-synthetic penicillins [48, 49], Methicillin [50], fluoroquinolones [51], Vancomycin [52, 53], Sulphonamides and trimethoprim [54], tetracyclines [55–57], aminoglycosides [58–60], chloramphenicol [61], and clindamycin [62]. MecA gene is reported to be responsible for the methicillin resistance in the *Staphylococcus aureus*. This gene is also attributed to be transmitted from poultry to humans. The most common isolates of MRSA are CC398, ST9 [28–30].

7.3 History and transmission

Firstly reported cases of the isolates have reported the susceptibility of bones with this pathogen and the prominent clinical signs as synovitis and arthritis [63–66]. Navel of the day-old chicks, surgery as trimming, and vaccination in un-hygienic conditions can be the trigger for the infection. Diseases that involve the predilection site to be the immune organs as being directly involved can also the root cause of this infection as the infectious bursal disease [67] and chicken infectious anemia. This is usually fatal as it leads to septicemia. Aged turkeys can have this infection with exposure to the hemorrhagic enteritis virus (HEV) [68]. Genetics of the poultry as the major MHC is also the predisposing factor for the skeletal-related problems of the poultry [69]. The incubation period of 2–3 days is a thumb rule but it is dependent upon several factors as the immune status of the host, the potency, and route of infection of the bacteria as the aerosol and tracheal routes are reported not to be the potent routes of infection [70, 71]. Infections with less than 105 organisms/kg body weight are reported to be defeated by the immune system of a healthy bird [25, 72].

7.4 Clinical signs, morbidity, incubation period, and pathology

Clinical signs of this disease include lameness, depression, pyrexia, and gait abnormalities, and death. Survived animals have arthritis, osteomyelitis [73, 74] unable to stand and sit on the hock and keel [25, 75]. This makes the fragility of the bones, mostly the femur and the tibiotarsus. It also leads to the congestion of the spleen, liver, lungs, and kidneys [23], gangrenous dermatitis, and ultimately the "blue wing disease" that presents the infection to the tip of wings of the birds that are infected with the chicken infectious anemia virus. Other clinical signs include enlarged yolk sac, planter abscess, discolored liver [27, 76]. Usually, the bacteria are not subjected to enough titer that may be the cause of higher mortality rates as compared to another fatal disease as the New Castle disease, etc., under optimal environmental conditions with most of the birds. But this bacterium has also been reported to have very high mortality rates that were primarily due to the immune-compromised state of the birds and the poor management conditions, and this bacteria in these conditions too is not the primary cause of the losses. The common site for the isolation and identification of that agent is the joints [18, 76–78].

7.5 Immune response

There are no convincing reports of the facts the active immunity or passive immunity other than that of the anti-*Staphylococcus aureus* antibodies may have any effect on this bacterium [79, 80]. Immunized hens can have antibodies within their egg yolk that can be used to prevent the bacteria in vitro. Toxoids are ineffective in other species [81, 82], and vaccines have not proven to be a very effective way of controlling the disease [83–86].

7.6 Diagnosis

Isolation and identification of the samples of yolk, joints, and internal organs from the infected bird should have to be practiced. Bacteria are harvested on the blood agar from the sheep or bovine and results are visible within a day of incubation. Selective media for this organism can be used as mannitol salt agar [87–89]. Serology testing includes microtiter plate agglutination assay and indirect immunofluorescent antibody titer assay. It can be differentially diagnosed from the diseases of the joints of the poultry [79, 83].

7.7 Management and control

Sharp objects should not have contact with the birds of the poultry farm, Sanitation and optimal environmental conditions are key to good farming practices that will minimize the chances of infection [22, 67, 90–91]. Nutritionists are also considering the point of adding herbs and plants as Moringa oliefera [92] to boost the immune system, they also claim to have the composition of these herbs that helps the birds to cope up with the pathogens. In ovo inoculation is also advocated to boost the immune system to cope-up with the infectious agents [93]. Passive immunity against this bacterium to the susceptible population is also a rational option to cope up with the disease outbreaks [99].

7.8 Vaccination

Staphylococcal bacterins [81, 94], strain 115 [95], aerosol vaccine S. epidermidis 115 [71, 95–98] and PNSG are available with an aim to prevent the Staphylococcal infections. The capsule of live or dead cells of the Smith diffuse strain of S. aureus is most antigenic and was proved and used as the earliest potent vaccinal candidate, as the antibodies produced against the capsule can deal with the strategy of this bacteria of dodging the phagocytosis [13–19]. The single intraperitoneal injection can protect from the challenge of a lethal dose of 108 CFU [26–27]. Anti-microcapsule vaccines are not proved to be as effective as capsular candidates. Bivalent vaccines are also been approved to be the effective ones. The capsule requires a monophosphoryl lipid A as adjuvant and a booster dose to show an optimal antibody response [98–102].

7.9 Treatment

It is recommended to have antibiotic sensitivity testing before deciding the application of the antibiotic. The commonly used antibiotics against this bacterium are penicillin, tetracycline, streptomycin, novobiocin, sulfonamides, lincomycin, and spectinomycin. Most bacteria to date, are resistant to penicillin and many are resistant to other antibiotics as methicillin too. Vancomycin is considered now to be the most effective antibiotic against this bacterium. It is good to know that the cure rate of Staphylococcal infection with antibiotics does not exceed far beyond thirty percent, so vaccines should be the priority in dairy herd management [99–102].

8. The regulation of virulence in the Staphylococci

Virulence factors are the substances that aid in the pathogenesis of an organism. Pathogenesis of *Staphylococcus aureus* does not depend on a single factor and there are a set of substances that collectively leads to the successful colonization of that bacteria into its host [98–99]. These virulence factors also diversify in their composition of proteins as exoproteins and surface proteins. To date, there are many reports of mutants, which behave differentially concerning the expression of different exoproteins in different environmental conditions [100–102]. Most of the exoproteins are secreted at the post exponential phase. The polysaccharide of the capsule of *Staphylococcus aureus* also acts as the virulent factor. This bacterium can also be classified based on the structure of the capsule into 11 different serotypes [99]. Serotypes 1 and 2 and mucoid, while the serotypes 3 to 11 are microcapsules as which are non-mucoid and have thin capsules [96–101]. Among these 11 serotypes, 5 and 8 are the most prevalent. The capsule is vital to this bacterium as it is responsible for evading the phagocytosis by masking the C3b that is placed on the surface of these bacteria by the host immune cells. The significance of microcapsules in pathogenesis is not well established as there are many controversial studies in this regard. The genes responsible for the formation of microcapsules are cap5H, cap8J, and cap5P. The cap8B and cap5B genes are homologous to each other in several proteins, and cap8B acts as the chain length regulator of the capsule [98–100]. The chemical composition of serotypes 1, 2, 5, and 8 are presented in **Figure 4**.

The agr and sar 16 loci have been extensively studied and believed to have vital importance in the virulence of this bacteria. Alpha toxin is also a virulence factor of Staphyloccocus aureus, which forms the pores to the cells resulting in cytolysis of the surrounding cells of invasion [97–100]. Not all the virulence factors are active throughout the life of the bacteria, but on the as-required basis, to overcome the metabolic burden [96–100]. Currently, the exact mechanism behind these virulence factors is not well elucidated. Staphylococcus is blessed with these virulence factors for its survival in diversified environmental conditions, and the primary purpose of these is not to cause the disease. Passaging the bacteria to nutritive media in vitro leads to the bacteria of less virulency and the passage of bacteria to the live animal or host leads to the bacteria with more virulency [99, 100].

Microbial surface components recognizing adhesive matrix molecules (MSCRAMMS), Sialoprotein, laminin, elastin, etc. are the proteins that are responsible for the adhesion of staphylococcus to its surrounding [98–100].

Type 1: →4)-α-D-GalNAcA*p*(1→4)-α-D-GalNAcA*p*(1→3)-α-D-FucNAc*p*(1→
(A taurine residue is linked by an amide bond to every 4th D-GalNAcA*p* residue.)

Type 2: →4)-ß-D-GlcNAcA*p*(1→4)-ß-D-GlcN(N-acetylalanyl)AcA*p*(1→

Type 5: →4)-3-O-Ac-ß-D-ManNAcA*p*(1→4)-α-L-FucNAc*p*(1→3)-ß-D-FucNAc*p*(1→

Type 8: →3)-4-O-Ac-ß-D-ManNAcA*p*(1→3)-α-L-FucNAc*p*(1→3)-ß-D-FucNAc*p*(1→

(Abbreviations: GalNAcA, N-acetylgalactosaminuronic acid; FucNAc, N-acetyl-fucosamine; GlcNAcA, N-acetyl-glucosaminuronic acid; ManNAcA, N-acetyl-mannosaminuronic acid; O-Ac, O-acetyl)

Figure 4.
The chemical compositions of serotypes 1, 2, 5, and 8. Modified from [99].

To dodge the host immune system is a requirement of the successful colonization of each pathogen. Staphylococcus is also blessed with these factors as protein A for binding the IgG antibodies [99–101].

This bacterium has a system of coordination with environmental conditions as temperature, pH, etc. This system of coordination is named the "two-component systems" having two proteins and a single operon and upon detection of the signal these proteins active certain genes for transcription. A small colony-sized SVC subpopulation is also a potent strategy of this bacteria against the immune system of the host and antibiotic therapy [97, 98].

The bacterial secretions having mitogen properties are also called superantigens. These superantigens are pathogenic and may cause an autoimmune response. They are also responsible to activate macrophages, zinc having a vital role in that, by initiating the IFN-gamma secretion from T cells. Superantigens can initiate an immune response without the increased concentration of IFN-gamma, whereas in mice it is necessary to have the increased concentration of IFN-gamma to initiate the immune response. It is not clear whether the response of MHC I and MHC II are synergistic or not, in the immunologic response against the pathogenesis of Staphylococcus **Figures 5** and **6** [97–101].

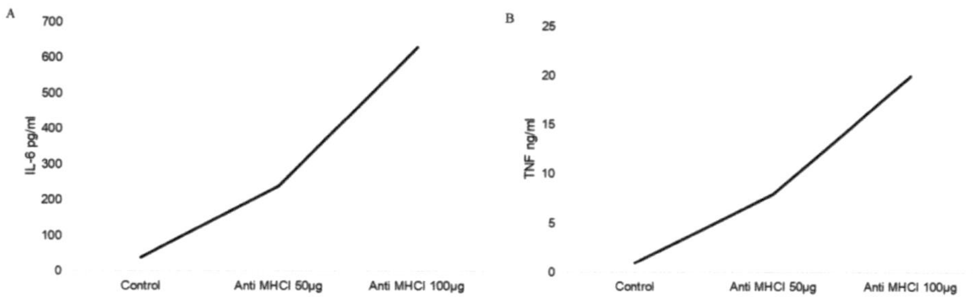

Figure 5.
(A) Response of IL-6 against anti-MHC-I 50 µg and MHC-II 100 µg antibodies incubated with C2D macrophages. (B) Response of TNF against anti-MHC-I 50 µg and MHC-II 100 µg antibodies incubated with C2D macrophages. Modified from [99–102].

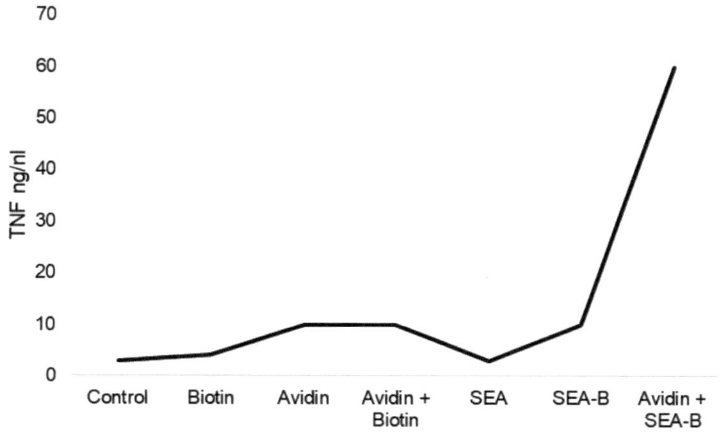

Figure 6.
Response of TNF against various stimuli. (TNF: Tumor Necrosis Factor, SEA: Staphylococcal enterotoxin A, SEA-B: Staphylococcal enterotoxin A). Modified from [99].

9. Endogenous IFN-gamma, TNF, and IL-6 in *Staphylococcus aureus* infection

Endogenous IFN-g plays a detrimental role in S. aureus infection. IFN-g, TNF, and IL-6 levels are elevated within 24 hours of infection even though whether the infection is lethal or non-lethal. In nonlethal cases, Bacteria is not present in the blood but in the kidneys and remains there for up to three weeks of infections. IFN-g peaks again in the spleens and kidneys. Among these three cytokines, the only cytokine that is detected in the serum is IL-6. In lethal infection, IFN-g and IL-6 in the sera and TNF in the kidneys peaked before death [98–102].

10. Conclusion

Staphylococcus aureus has vital importance in the ruminants, as it is one of the major causes of Mastitis. Along with that, it also affects the health of animals, Pets, and Poultry in several ways as the diseases of bones in poultry. The Regulation of Virulence in the Staphylococci mainly are the exoproteins and surface proteins, and capsule, agr, sar 16 loci, and Alpha toxin. Bacteria potentiates cytokines for host resistance [97–101]. IFN-g and TNF play a protective role against Listeria monocytogenes, Mycobacterium species, Salmonella typhimurium, and Francisella tularensis. IFN-g and TNF also mediate gram-negative septic shock and endotoxin shock. Staphylococci induce TNF, interleukin-1, IFN-g, IL-2, and IL-6 in humans and animals [101, 102].

Acknowledgements

I deem it utmost to express my heartiest gratitude to Dr. Shafia Tehseen Gul, Dr. Aisha Khatoon, and Dr. Muhammad Imran Arshad for scholastic guidance, ever encouraging attitude, and valuable suggestions during this project.

Conflict of interest

The authors declare no conflict of interest.

Author details

Muhammad Farhab[1]*, Muhammad Tahir Aleem[2], Shakseema Shaukat[3], Ayesha Qadry[3], Muhammad Zeeshan Ul Haq[4], Fateh Ullah[5], Muhammad Jawad[6] and Amjad Islam Aqib[7]

1 College of Veterinary Medicine, Yangzhou University, Yangzhou, China

2 MOE Joint International Research Laboratory of Animal Health and Food Safety, College of Veterinary Medicine, Nanjing Agricultural University, Nanjing, China

3 Veterinary Research Institute Lahore, Lahore, Pakistan

4 Department of Clinical Medicine and Surgery, University of Agriculture Faisalabad, Faisalabad, Pakistan

5 Department of Clinical Medicine, University of Veterinary and Animal Sciences Lahore, Lahore, Pakistan

6 Islamia College Peshawar, Peshawar, Pakistan

7 Department of Medicine, Faculty of Veterinary Science, Cholistan University of Veterinary and Animal Sciences, Bahawalpur, Pakistan

*Address all correspondence to: farhab.dvm@gamil.com

References

[1] Quinn PJ, Markey BK, Leonard FC, Hartigan P, Fanning S, & Fitzpatrick E. Veterinary microbiology and microbial disease. John Wiley & Sons; 2011.

[2] Thomson-Carter FM, Carter PE, & Pennington TH. Differentiation of staphylococcal species and strains by ribosomal RNA gene restriction patterns. Microbiology. 1989;135:2093-2097.

[3] Davis GHG and Hoyling B. Use of a rapid acetoin test in the identification of staphylococci and micrococci. International Journal of Systematic Bacteriology. 1973;23:281-282.

[4] Quinn PJ, Carter ME, Markey B, Carter GR. Clinical Veterinary Microbiology, Wilfe Publishing, London. 1994. 95-101 p.

[5] Lee YT, Lin DB, Wang WY, Tsao SM, Yu SF, Wei MJ, & Lee MC. First identification of methicillin-resistant *Staphylococcus aureus* MLST types ST5 and ST45 and SCCmec types IV and Vt by multiplex PCR during an outbreak in a respiratory care ward in central Taiwan. Diagnostic microbiology and infectious disease. 2011;70:175-182.

[6] Feil EJ, Cooper JE, Grundmann H, Robinson DA, Enright MC, Berendt T, & Moore CE. How clonal is *Staphylococcus aureus*?. Journal of bacteriology. 2003;185:3307-3316.

[7] Lindsay JA, & Holden MT. Staphylococcus aureus: superbug, super genome?. Trends in microbiology. 2004;12:378-385.

[8] Larsen J, Enright MC, Godoy D, Spratt BG, Larsen AR, & Skov RL. Multilocus sequence typing scheme for *Staphylococcus aureus*: revision of the gmk locus. Journal of clinical microbiology. 2012;50:2538-2539.

[9] Saunders NA, & Holmes A. Multilocus sequence typing (MLST) of *Staphylococcus aureusStaphylococcus aureus*. In Methicillin-Resistant *Staphylococcus Aureus* (MRSA) Protocols. Humana Press. 2007. 71-85 p.

[10] Florentín M, Salinas C, Acuña P, Rodríguez F, & Guillén R. Standardization of automated multi-locus variable number tandem repeats analysis for Methicillin-resistant Staphylococcus aureus *Staphylococcus aureus* typing isolated from invasive infections in paraguayan pediatric population. Revista de salud publica del Paraguay. 2020;10:30-36.

[11] Felix B, Vingadassalon N, Grout J, Hennekine JA, Guillier L, & Auvray F. Staphylococcus aureus strains associated with food poisoning outbreaks in France: comparison of different molecular typing methods, including MLVA. Frontiers in microbiology. 2015;6:882.

[12] Sobral D, Schwarz S, Bergonier D, Brisabois A, Feßler AT, Gilbert FB, & Pourcel C. High throughput multiple locus variable number of tandem repeat analysis (MLVA) of *Staphylococcus aureus* from human, animal and food sources. PLoS One. 2012;7:e33967.

[13] Awan MA, Matsumoto M. Heterogeneity of Staphylococci and other bacteria isolated from six-week-old broiler chickens. Poult Sci. 1998;77:944-949.

[14] Chénier S, and Lallier L. Acantholytic folliculitis and Epidermitis associated with *Staphylococcus hyicus* in a line of White Leghorn laying chickens. Vet Pathol. 2012;49:284-287.

[15] Cheville NF, Tappe J, Ackermann M, and Jensen A. Acute fibrinopurulent blepharitis and conjunctivitis associated with *Staphylococcus hyicus*, *Escherichia*

coli, and Streptococcus sp. in chickens and turkeys. Vet Pathol. 1988;25:369-375.

[16] Scanlan CM, and Hargis BM. A bacteriologic study of scabby-hip lesions from broiler chickens in Texas. J Vet Diagn Invest. 1989;1:170-173.

[17] Tate CR, Mitchell WC, and Miller RG. Staphylococcus hyicus associated with turkey stifle joint osteomyelitis. Avian Dis. 1993;37:905-907.

[18] Frazier MN, Parizek WJ, and Garner E. Gangrenous dermatitis of chickens. Avian Dis. 1964;8:269-273.

[19] Hoffman HA. Vesicular dermatitis in chickens. J Am Vet Med Assoc. 1939;48:329-332.

[20] Rosenberger JK, Klopp S, Eckroade RJ, and Krauss WC. The role of the infectious bursal agent and several avian adenoviruses in the hemorrhagic-aplastic-anemia syndrome and gangrenous dermatitis. Avian Dis. 1975;19:717-729.

[21] Wilder TD, Barbaree JM, Macklin KS, and Norton RA. Differences in the pathogenicity of various bacterial isolates used in an induction model for gangrenous dermatitis in broiler chickens. Avian Dis. 2011;45:659-662.

[22] Andreasen CB, Latimer KS, Harmon BG, Glisson JR, Golden JM, and Brown J. Heterophil function in healthy chickens and in chickens with experimentally induced staphylococcal tenosynovitis. Vet Pathol. 1991;28:419-427.

[23] Bickford AA, and Rosenwald AS. Staphylococcal infections in chickens. Poult Dig. July. 1975:285-287.

[24] McNamee PT, and Smyth JA. Bacterial chondronecrosis with osteomyelitis ('femoral head necrosis') of broiler chickens: a review. Avian Pathol. 2000;29:253-270.

[25] Mutalib A, Riddell C, and Osborne AD. Studies on the pathogenesis of staphylococcal osteomyelitis in chickens. I. Effect of stress on experimentally induced osteomyelitis. Avian Dis. 1983;27:141-156.

[26] McFadden JJ, and Fidler HM. Mycobacteria as possible causes of sarcoidosis and Crohn's disease. Soc Appl Bacteriol Symp Ser. 1996;25:47S–52S.

[27] Clark RS, Barnes HJ, Bickford AA, Chin RP, and Droual R. Relationship of osteomyelitis and associated soft-tissue lesions with green liver discoloration in turkeys. Avian Dis. 1991;35:139-146.

[28] Evans JB, Ananaba RA, Pate CA, and Bergdoll MS. Enterotoxin production by atypical *Staphylococcus aureus* from poultry. J Appl Bacteriol. 1983;54:257-261.

[29] Gibbs PA, Patterson JT, and Thompson. Characterization of poultry isolates of *Staphylococcus aureus* by a new set of poultry phages. J Appl Bacteriol. 1978;44:387-400.

[30] Harvey J, Patterson JT, and Gibbs PA. Enterotoxigenicity of *Staphylococcus aureus* strains isolated from poultry: Raw poultry carcasses as a potential food-poisoning hazard. J Appl Bacteriol. 1982;52:251-258.

[31] Raska K, Matejovska V, Matejovska D, Bergdoll MS, and Petrus P. To the origin of contamination of foodstuffs by enterotoxigenic staphylococci. In: Staphylococci and Staphylococcal Infections. J. Jeljaszewicz, ed. Gustav Fischer Verlag, Stuttgart. 1981;381-385.

[32] Terayama T, Ushioda H, Shingaki M, Inaba M, Kai A, and Sakai S. Coagulase types of *Staphylococcus aureus* from food poisoning outbreaks and types of incriminated foods. Ann Rpt Tokyo Metrop Res Lab Public Health. 1977;28:1-4.

[33] Adams BW, and Mead GC. Incidence and properties of *Staphylococcus aureus* associated with turkeys during processing and further-processing operations. J Hyg. 1983;91:479-490.

[34] Kusch D. Biochemical characteristics and phage-typing of staphylococci isolated from poultry. Zentralbl Bakteriol Parasit Infekt Hyg [IB]. 1977;164:360-367.

[35] Notermans S, Dufrenne J, and van Leeuwen WJ. Contamination of broiler chickens by *Staphylococcus aureus* during processing; incidence and origin. J Appl Bacteriol. 1982;52:275-280.

[36] Thompson JK, and Patterson JT. Staphylococcus aureus from a site of contamination in a broiler processing plant. Rec Agr Res. 1983;31:45-53.

[37] Cuny C, Friedrich A, Kozytska S, Layer F, Nübel U, Ohlsen K, Strommenger B, Walther B, Wieler L, and Witte W. Emergence of methicillin-resistant *Staphylococcus aureus* (MRSA) in different animal species. Int J Med Microbiol. 2010;300:109-117.

[38] Duquette RA, and Nuttall TJ. Methicillin-resistant *Staphylococcus aureus* in dogs and cats: an emerging problem? J Small Anim Pract. 2004;45:591-597.

[39] Fessler AT, Kadlec K, Hassel M, Hauschild T, Eidam C, Ehricht R, Monecke S, and Schwarz S. Characterization of methicillin-resistant *Staphylococcus aureus* isolates from food and food products of poultry origin in Germany. Appl Environ Microbiol. 2011;77:7151-7157.

[40] Kitai S, Shimizu A, Kawano J, Sato E, Nakano C, Uji T, and Kitagawa H. Characterization of methicillin-resistant *Staphylococcus aureus* isolated from retail raw chicken meat in Japan. J Vet Med Sci. 2005;67:107-110.

[41] Lee JH. 2003. Methicillin (Oxacillin)-resistant *Staphylococcus aureus* strains isolated from major food animals and their potential transmission to humans. Appl Environ Microbiol. 2003;69:6489-6494.

[42] Lim SK, Nam HM, Park HJ, Lee HS, Choi MJ, Jung SC, Lee JY, Kim YC, Song SW, and Wee SH. Prevalence and characterization of methicillin-resistant *Staphylococcus aureus* in raw meat in Korea. J Microbiol Biotechnol. 2010;20:775-778.

[43] Mulders MN, Haenen AP, Geenen PL, Vesseur PC, Poldervaart ES, Bosch T, Huijsdens XW, Hengeveld PD, Dam-Deisz WD, Graat EA, Mevius D, Voss A, and Van De Giessen AW. Prevalence of livestock-associated MRSA in broiler flocks and risk factors for slaughterhouse personnel in The Netherlands. Epidemiol Infect. 2010;138:743-755.

[44] Nemati M, Hermans K, Lipinska U, Denis O, Deplano A, Struelens M, Devriese L, Pasmans F, and Haesebrouck F. Antimicrobial resistance of old and recent *Staphylococcus aureus* isolates from poultry: first detection of livestock-associated methicillin-resistant strain ST398. Antimicrob Agents Chemother. 2008;52:3817-3819.

[45] Persoons D, Van Hoorebeke S, Hermans K, Butaye P, de Kruif A, Haesebrouck F, and Dewulf F. Methicillinresistant *Staphylococcus aureus* in poultry. Emerg Infect Dis. 2009;15:452-453.

[46] Weese JS, Archambault M, Willey BM, Hearn P, Kreiswirth BN,

Said-Salim B, McGeer A, Likhoshvay Y, Prescott JF, and Low DE. Methicillin-resistant *Staphylococcus aureus* in horses and horse personnel, 2000-2002. Emerg Infect Dis. 2005;11:430-435.

[47] Weese JS, Avery BP, and Reid-Smith RJ. Detection and quantification of methicillin-resistant *Staphylococcus aureus* (MRSA) clones in retail meat products. Lett Appl Microbiol. 2010;51:338-342.

[48] Chambers HF. The changing epidemiology of *Staphylococcus aureus*? Emerg Infect Dis. 2001;7:178-182. DOI: 10.3201/eid0702.700178

[49] Chambers HF, DeLeo FR. Waves of resistance: *Staphylococcus aureus* in the antibiotic era. Nat Rev Microbiol. 2009;7:629-641. DOI: 10.1038/nrmicro2200

[50] Jevons PM. "Celbenin" – resistant Staphylococci. Br Med J. 1961;1:124-125. PMCID: PMC1952889

[51] Hooper DC. Mechanisms of action and resistance of older and newer fluoroquinolones. Clin Infect Dis. 2000;31:S24–S28. DOI: 10.1086/314056

[52] Sievert DM et al., CDC. Staphylococcus aureus Resistant to vancomycin – United States, MMWR. 2002;51:565-567. PMID: 12139181

[53] Sievert DM, Rudrik JT, Patel JB, McDonald LC, Wilkins MJ, Hageman JC. Vancomycinresistant *Staphylococcus aureus* in the United States, 2002-2006. Clin Infect Dis. 2008;46:668-674. DOI: 10.1086/527392

[54] Then RL, Kohl I, Burdeska A.. Frequency and transferability of trimethoprim and sulfonamide resistance in methicillin-resistant *Staphylococcus aureus* and *Staphylococcus epidermidis*. J Chemother. 1992;4(2):67-71. PMID: 1629749

[55] Trzcinski K, Cooper BS, Hryniewicz W, Dowson CG. Expression of resistance to tetracyclines in strains of methicillin-resistant *Staphylococcus aureus*. J Antimicrob Chemother. 2000;45(6):763-770. PMID: 10837427

[56] Schmitz FJ, Krey A, Sadurski R, Verhoef J, Milatovic D, Fluit AC; European SENTRY Participants. Resistance to tetracycline and distribution of tetracycline resistance genes in European *Staphylococcus aureus* isolates. J Antimicrob Chemother. 2001;47:239-240 DOI: 10.1093/jac/47.2.239

[57] Fluit AC, Florijn A, Verhoef J, Milatovic D. Presence of tetracycline resistance determinants and susceptibility to tigecycline and minocycline. Antimicrob Agents Chemother. 2005;49:1636-1638. DOI: 10.1128/AAC.49.4.1636-1638.2005

[58] Storrs MJ, Courvalin P, Foster TJ. Genetic analysis of gentamicin resistance in methicillin-and gentamicin-resistant strains of *Staphylococcus aureus* isolated in Dublin hospitals. Antimicrob Agents Chemother. 1988;32:1174-1181. PMCID: PMC172372

[59] Freitas FI, Guedes-Stehling E, Siqueira-Júnior JP. Resistance to gentamicin and related aminoglycosides in *Staphylococcus aureus* isolated in Brazil. Lett Appl Microbiol. 1999;29:197-201. PMID: 10530041

[60] Schmitz FJ, Fluit AC, Gondolf M, Beyrau R, Lindenlauf E, Verhoef J, Heinz HP, Jones ME. The prevalence of aminoglycoside resistance and corresponding resistance genes in clinical isolates of staphylococci from 19 European hospitals. J Antimicrob Chemother. 1999;43:253-259. PMID: 11252331

[61] Fayyaz M, Mirza IA, Ahmed Z, Abbasi SA, Hussain A, Ali S. In vitro

susceptibility of chloramphenicol against methicillin-resistant *Staphylococcus aureus*. J Coll Physicians Surg Pak. 2013;23:637-640. DOI: 09.2013/JCPSP.637640

[62] Frank AL, Marcinak JF, Mangat PD, Tjhio JT, Kelkar S, Schreckenberger PC, Quinn JP. Clindamycin treatment of methicillin-resistant *Staphylococcus aureus* infections in children. Pediatr Infect Dis J. 2002;21:530-534. PMID: 12182377

[63] Gwatkin R. An outbreak of staphylococcal infection in barred Plymouth rock males. Can J Comp Med. 1940;4:294-296.

[64] Hole N, and Purchase HS. Arthritis and periostitis in pheasants caused by Staphylococcus pyogenes aureus. J Comp Pathol Ther. 1931;44:252-257.

[65] Jungherr E. Staphylococcal arthritis in turkeys. J Am Vet Med Assoc. 1933;35:243-249.

[66] Lucet A. De l'ostèo-arthrite aigue infectieuse des jeunes oies. Ann Inst Pasteur (Paris). 1892;6:841-850.

[67] Santivatr D, Maheswaran SK, Newman JA, and Pomeroy BS. Effect of infectious bursal disease virus Infection on the phagocytosis of *Staphylococcus aureus* by mononuclear phagocytic cells of susceptible and resistant strains of chickens. Avian Dis. 1981;25:303-311.

[68] Newberry LA, Lindsey DG, Beasley JN, McNew RW, and Skeeles JK. A summary of data collected from turkeys following acute hemorrhagic enteritis virus infection at different ages. In: Proceedings of the 45th NC Avian Dis Conf.; 9-11 October 1994; Des Moines, IA: 1994. p. 63.

[69] Joiner KS, Hoerr FJ, van Santen E, and Ewald S. The avian major histocompatibility complex influences bacterial skeletal disease in broiler breeder chickens. Vet Pathol. 2005;42:275-281.

[70] Cox NA, Bailey JS, Ryser ET, and Marth EH. Incidence and behavior of *Listeria monocytogenes* in poultry and egg products. In: Listeria, Listeriosis and Food Safety, 2nd ed. Ryser, E.T., and E.H. Marth, eds. Marcel Dekker, Inc., New York. 1999;565-600.

[71] Jensen MM, Downs WC, Morrey JD, Nicoll TR, LeFevre SD, and Meyers CM. Staphylococcosis of turkeys. 1. Portal of entry and tissue colonization. Avian Dis. 1987;31:64-69.

[72] McNamee PT, & Smyth JA. Bacterial chondronecrosis with osteomyelitis ('femoral head necrosis') of broiler chickens: a review. Avian Pathology. 2000;29(5), 477-495.

[73] Miner ML, Smart RA, and Olson AE. Pathogenesis of staphylococcal synovitis in turkeys: Pathologic changes. Avian Dis. 1968;12:46-60.

[74] Nairn ME. Bacterial osteomyelitis and synovitis of the turkey. Avian Dis. 1973;17:504-517.

[75] Emslie KR, Ozanne NR, and Nade SML. Acute haemotogenous osteomyelitis: An experimental model. Pathology. 1983;141:157-167.

[76] Bitay Z, Quarini L, Glavits R, and Fischer R. Staphylococcus infection in fowls. Magy Allatorv Lapja. 1984;39:86-91.

[77] Kibenge FSB, Robertson MD, Wilcox GE, and Pass DA. Bacterial and viral agents associated with tenosynovitis in broiler breeders in Western Australia. Avian Pathol. 1982;11:351-359.

[78] Köhler B, Bergmann V, Witte W, Heiss R, and Vogel K. Dermatitis bei broilen durch *Staphylococcus aureus*. Monatsch Veterinaermed. 1978;33:22-28.

[79] Forget A, Meunier L, and Borduas AG. Enhancement activity of homologous anti-staphylococcal sera in experimental staphylococcal synovitis of chicks: A possible role of immune adherence antibodies. Infect Immun. 1974;9:641-644.

[80] Gross WG, Siegel PB, Hall RB, Domermuth CH, and Duboise RT. Production and persistence of antibodies in chickens to sheep erythrocytes. 2. Resistance to infectious diseases. Poult Sci. 1980;59:205-210.

[81] Anderson JC. Staphylococcus. In: Pathogenesis of Bacterial Infections in Animals, 1st ed. C.L. Gyles and C.O. Thoen, eds. Iowa State University Press, Ames, IA, 1986;14-20.

[82] Andreasen JR, Andreasen CB, Anwer M, and Sonn AE. Heterophil chemotaxis in chickens with natural Staphylococcal infections. Avian Dis. 1993;37:284-289.

[83] Andreasen CB, Andreasen JR, Sonn AE, and Oughton JA. Comparison of the effect of different opsonins on the phagocytosis of fluorescein-labeled staphylococcal bacteria by chicken heterophils. Avian Dis. 1996;40:778-782.

[84] Broughan J, Anderson R, and Anderson AS. Strategies for and advances in the development of *Staphylococcus aureus* prophylactic vaccines. Expert Rev Vaccines. 2011;10:695-708.

[85] Schaffer AC, and Lee JC. Vaccination and passive immunisation against *Staphylococcus aureus*. Int J Antimicrob Agents. 2008;32 Suppl 1:S71-78.

[86] Shinefield HR, and Black S. Prevention of *Staphylococcus aureus* infections: advances in vaccine development. Expert Rev Vaccines. 2005;4:669-676.

[87] Kloos WE, and Jorgensen JH. Staphylococci. In: Manual of Clinical Microbiology, 4th ed. E.H. Lenette, A. Balows, W.J. Hausler, Jr., and H.J. Shadomy, eds. American Society of Microbiologists, Washington, DC. 1985;143-153.

[88] Pezzlo M. Identification of commonly isolated aerobic Gram-positive bacteria. In: Clinical Microbiology Procedures Handbook, vol 1. H.D. Isenberg, chief ed. American Society for Microbiology, Washington, DC: 1992. 1.20.1-1.20.12.

[89] Willett HP. Staphylococcus. In: Zinsser Microbiology, 20th ed. W.K. Joklik, H.P. Willett, D.B. Amos, and C.M. Wilfert, eds. Appleton and Lange, Norwalk, CT. 1992;401-416.

[90] Coates SR, Buckner DK, and Jensen MM. The Inhibitory effect of Corynebacterium parvum and *Pasteurella multocida* pretreatment on staphylococcal synovitis in turkeys. Avian Dis. 1977;21:319-322.

[91] Heller ED, Nathan DB, and Perek M. Short heat stress as an immunostimulant in chicks. Avian Pathol. 1979;8:195-203.

[92] Akram M, Saleem I, Farhab M, & Luqman Z. Immunomodulatory Effects of *Moringa Oleifera* Leaf Meal (MOLM) against Newcastle Disease in Broilers. J Nat Appl Sci. 2020;3(2):19-25.

[93] Luqman Z, Masood S, Zaneb H, Majeed KA, Hameed S, Ikram U, & Gulzar S. Effect of in ovo inoculation on Productive Performances and Histo-physiological Traits in Commercial Birds. J sci eng res. 2019;10:1664-1673.

[94] Andreasen JR, Andreasen CB, Anwer M, and Sonn AE. Heterophil chemotaxis in chickens with natural Staphylococcal infections. Avian Dis. 1993;37:284-289.

[95] Meyers CM, and Jensen MM. Staphylococcosis of turkeys. 3. Bacterial interference as a possible means of control. Avian Dis. 1987;31:744-779.

[96] LeFevre SD, and Jensen MM. Staphylococcosis of turkeys. 2. Assay of protein A levels of staphylococci isolated from turkeys. Avian Dis. 1987;31:70-73.

[97] Nicoll TR, and Jensen MM. Preliminary studies on bacterial interference of staphylococcosis of chickens. Avian Dis. 1987;31:140-144.

[98] Wilkinson DM, and Jensen MM. Staphylococcosis of turkeys. 4. Characterization of a bacteriocin produced by an interfering staphylococcus. Avian Dis. 1987;31:80-84.

[99] Honeyman A, Friedman H, and Bendinelli M. Staphylococcus aureus infection and disease. Springer Science & Business Media. 2001. 30 p.

[100] Jenul C, and Horswill AR. Regulation of *Staphylococcus aureus* virulence. Microbiol. spectr. 2019;7(2):7-2.

[101] de Steenhuijsen Piters WA, Sanders EA, and Bogaert D. The role of the local microbial ecosystem in respiratory health and disease. Philos Trans R Soc Lond B Biol Sci. 2015;370(1675):20140294.

[102] Nakane A, Okamoto M, Asano M, Kohanawa M, and Minagawa T. Endogenous gamma interferon, tumor necrosis factor, and interleukin-6 in *Staphylococcus aureus* infection in mice. Infect Immun. 1995;63(4): 1165-1172.